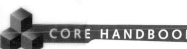

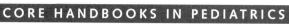
CORE HANDBOOKS IN PEDIATRICS

INHERITED METABOLIC DISEASES

Georg F. Hoffmann, M.D.

Department of Pediatrics
University Children's Hospital
Heidelberg, Germany

William L. Nyhan, M.D., Ph.D.

Department of Pediatrics
University of California San Diego
La Jolla, California

Johannes Zschocke, M.D., Ph.D.

Department of Pediatrics
University Children's Hospital
Heidelberg, Germany

Stephen G. Kahler, M.D.

Victorian Clinical Genetics Services
Murdoch Children's Research Institute
Royal Children's Hospital and the University of Melbourne
Melbourne, Australia

Ertan Mayatepek, M.D.

Department of Pediatrics
University Children's Hospital
Heidelberg, Germany

LIPPINCOTT WILLIAMS & WILKINS
A **Wolters Kluwer** Company

Philadelphia · Baltimore · New York · London
Buenos Aires · Hong Kong · Sydney · Tokyo

Acquisitions Editor: Timothy Y. Hiscock
Developmental Editor: Selina M. Bush
Production Editor: Christiana Sahl
Manufacturing Manager: Tim Reynolds
Cover Designer: Jeane Norton
Compositor: Circle Graphics
Printer: R.R. Donnelley/Crawfordsville

© **2002 by LIPPINCOTT WILLIAMS & WILKINS**
530 Walnut Street
Philadelphia, PA 19106 USA
LWW.com

Printed in the USA

Library of Congress Cataloging-in-Publication Data

Inherited metabolic diseases / Georg F. Hoffmann . . . [et al.].
    p. ; cm. — (Core handbooks in pediatrics)
    Includes bibliographical references and index.
    ISBN 0-7817-2900-9
    1. Metabolic disorders in children—Handbooks, manuals, etc. 2. Metabolism, Inborn errors of—Handbooks, manuals, etc. 3. Metabolism—Disorders—Handbooks, manuals, etc. I. Hoffmann, Georg F. (Georg Friedrich) II. Series.
    [DNLM: 1. Metabolism, Inborn Errors—Child—Handbooks. 2. Metabolism, Inborn Errors—Infant—Handbooks. WD 200.1 I55 2002]
    RJ390 .I54 2002
    618.92′39042—dc

                                                                    2001029920

Care has been taken to confirm the accuracy of the information presented and to describe generally accepted practices. However, the authors and publisher are not responsible for errors or omissions or for any consequences from application of the information in this book and make no warranty, expressed or implied, with respect to the currency, completeness, or accuracy of the contents of the publication. Application of this information in a particular situation remains the professional responsibility of the practitioner.

The authors and publisher have exerted every effort to ensure that drug selection and dosage set forth in this text are in accordance with current recommendations and practice at the time of publication. However, in view of ongoing research, changes in government regulations, and the constant flow of information relating to drug therapy and drug reactions, the reader is urged to check the package insert for each drug for any change in indications and dosage and for added warnings and precautions. This is particularly important when the recommended agent is a new or infrequently employed drug.

Some drugs and medical devices presented in this publication have Food and Drug Administration (FDA) clearance for limited use in restricted research settings. It is the responsibility of the health care provider to ascertain the FDA status of each drug or device planned for use in their clinical practice.

10 9 8 7 6 5 4 3 2 1

To our patients and their families

Contents

V. Selected Groups of Metabolic Diseases

VI. Appendices

♣ Preface

Over the last twenty-five years, the field of inherited metabolic diseases has evolved from a limited group of rare, untreatable, and often fatal disorders to an important cause of acutely life-threatening but, for a substantial number, treatable diseases.

The patient does not come to the physician with the diagnosis; instead, he or she comes with a history, symptoms, and signs. This book starts with these and proceeds logically from questions to answers, often using algorithms. Although metabolic disorders are caused by genetically determined pathobiochemistry, evidence-based guidelines are needed for clinical diagnosis and therapy. We have developed the rational approaches presented in this book for investigations of patients based on our experiences. We have attempted to put special emphasis on acutely presenting disorders and emergency situations.

This system-based and symptom-based approach to inherited metabolic diseases is designed to help colleagues come to the appropriate diagnoses for their patients and to arrange optimal therapy programs. For metabolic and genetic specialists, this book should be particularly helpful as a quick reference for what are, even for the specialist, infrequently encountered presentations.

Georg F. Hoffmann, M.D.
William L. Nyhan, M.D., Ph.D.
Johannes Zschocke, M.D., Ph.D.
Stephen G. Kahler, M.D.
Ertan Mayatepek, M.D.

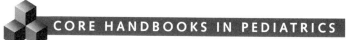

INHERITED
METABOLIC DISEASES

General Introduction

Inherited metabolic diseases are often believed to be disorders that only specialists can understand. Many textbooks leave the uninitiated with complicated biochemical pathways, strange disease names, and the impossible task of reading large lists of single enzyme and protein defects. This handling is unfortunate because metabolic diseases can be understood and remembered in clinically distinct groups that require similar investigations and therapeutic strategies. The aim of this book is to make inborn errors of metabolism accessible to the general clinician and to help with the differential diagnosis in and approach to patients.

Although the individual defects are rare, they represent an important differential diagnosis in many patients who display a wide range of clinical symptoms and signs. The authors feel that a need for a textbook on metabolic disorders that is oriented to the patient rather than to the disease exists. This book discusses treatment strategies in detail only for emergency situations, when the diagnosis may not be known but conditions mandate immediate action. Once a diagnosis is known, well-established, reliable ways exist for obtaining advice from or referral to specialized sources.

This book has six distinct but interdependent parts:

1. Part I provides a comprehensive overview of the major groups of metabolic disorders. Rather than discussing individual defects, it highlights the similarities of the diseases in each group to give simple advice on which investigations are indicated if a particular disease group is suspected. The disease reference table in the appendix provides further information on individual disorders in each group.

2. The second part outlines the general concept of inherited metabolic diseases, placing special emphasis on acutely presenting disorders and emergency situations. It explains the pathophysiology of basic and life-threatening metabolic derangements and gives advice on the most efficient diagnostic and therapeutic strategies.

3. The diagnostic section (Part III) provides an overview and detailed instructions on diagnostic procedures, indications for their implementation, requirements, and problems. This section provides a reference for clinicians planning investigations or tests for a particular patient.

4. The fourth part gives a system-based approach to inherited metabolic diseases. Its aim is to help the clinician understand what symptoms and signs can be caused by which metabolic disorders and to give advice on the most efficient diagnostic strategies.

5. Part V summarizes the characteristics of some especially relevant groups of inherited metabolic diseases. It includes clinical and diagnostic details to facilitate an efficient but complete diagnostic work-up of individual patients.

6. The appendices provides references and background information, including a comprehensive table of diseases that contains

a list of known metabolic disorders under the same headings as the introduction and that provides links to the respective Online Mendelian Inheritance in Man (OMIM) page as well as for enzyme and protein information (Expasy, Swissprot). The internet databases contain a great deal of information for clinicians caring for a patient with an individual disorder.

The authors hope that this book will confirm their belief that the universe of metabolic diseases consists not of many separate single enzyme and protein defects but of a structured interrelationship, which makes this important group of disorders comprehensible to clinicians. This in turn benefits the patients.

I

Inherited Metabolic Diseases: An Overview

1 ❧ Disorders of Intermediary Metabolism

The classical inherited metabolic diseases, or inborn errors of metabolism, are enzyme defects either in the metabolism of amino acids, carbohydrates, and fatty acids or in mitochondrial energy metabolism (Fig. 1.1). These disorders are often dynamic; they fluctuate with changes in the metabolic state of the patient and thus are frequently open to therapeutic intervention. Most of them are readily diagnosed through basic metabolic investigations, which include the following tests: lactate, ammonia, plasma amino acids, urinary organic acids, and an acylcarnitine profile.

DISORDERS OF AMINO ACID METABOLISM

Aminoacidopathies

Typical aminoacidopathies result from abnormalities in the breakdown of amino acids in the cytosol. In addition, the deficiency of several mitochondrial enzymes, such as branched-chain ketoacid dehydrogenase (maple syrup urine disease) or ornithine amino-transferase deficiency (gyrate atrophy of the choroid), are classi-fied as aminoacidopathies as they do not involve CoA-activated metabolites. This distinguishes aminoacidopathies from the organic acidurias, which are considered a separate group of disorders that affect mitochondrial enzymes and CoA-activated metabolites and which have effects on other mitochondrial functions. Clinical symptoms of the aminoacidopathies may be thought of as origi-nating from the accumulation of toxic intermediates, such as phenylalanine, phenylpyruvic, phenyllactic, and phenylacetic acids in phenylketonuria, that cause specific organ damage. Several defects of amino acid metabolism, such as histidinemia, are benign because the metabolites that accumulate are not toxic. The patho-genetic relevance of an inborn error of amino acid metabolism is not always easy to ascertain, as clinical symptoms observed in the child may be coincidental or they may be the reason for performing the analysis in the first place.

Aminoacidopathies are diagnosed through the analysis of plasma (or urinary) concentrations of amino acids and sometimes of urinary organic acids. Most are treatable through the dietary restriction both of protein and of the amino acid involved in the defective pathway, as well as by the avoidance or the prompt treatment of catabolic states that lead to the breakdown of large amounts of protein. Another therapeutic strategy that has been suc-cessful in hepatorenal tyrosinemia is the inhibition of a biochemical step before the actual genetic deficiency, which changes a harm-ful disease into a more benign amino acid accumulation by pre-venting the buildup of more damaging substances downstream.

Organic Acidurias

The classical organic acidurias are deficiencies of enzymes in the mitochondrial metabolism of CoA-activated carboxylic acids, most of which are derived from amino acid breakdown. In this way they are distinguished from disorders of fatty acid oxidation, which also

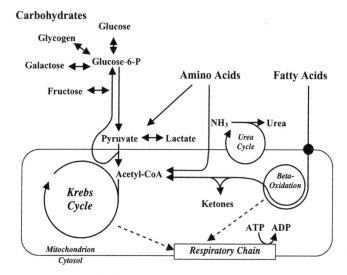

Figure 1.1.   Main pathways of intermediary metabolism.

involve CoA esters but present different diagnostic and therapeutic challenges. The term *organic acidurias* is preferred to the alternative term *organic acidemias* as they are most often detected by analysis of the urine. Biochemically, some of the reactions impaired in the organic acidurias are parallel to the dehydrogenase, hydratase, or ketothiolase reactions of the mitochondrial beta-oxidation cycle. Clinical features frequently include encephalopathy and episodic metabolic acidosis, caused not only by the accumulation of toxic intermediates but also by disturbances of mitochondrial energy metabolism and carnitine homeostasis.

Organic acidurias are diagnosed through the analysis of organic acids in the urine or acylcarnitines in the blood. Treatment is similar to that for the aminoacidopathies and involves the dietary restriction of the relevant amino acid(s) and the avoidance or quick reversal of protein catabolism. However, as the defective enzymes are distant (more downstream) from the respective amino acids, restriction may not lead to a stoichiometric reduction of pathologic metabolites, except for in the case of methylmalonic aciduria. Unexpected fluctuations occur, and complete return to normal intermediary metabolism is usually impossible. Supplementation with carnitine and, in some cases, other substances, such as glycine (to form isovalerylglycine in isovaleric aciduria), is a very useful adjunct to the treatment.

Disorders in the metabolism of biotin, a cofactor of the mitochondrial carboxylases, are included among the organic acidurias. Deficiency of this cofactor of the mitochondrial carboxylases results in multiple carboxylase deficiency, due to insufficient activity of biotinidase or holocarboxylase synthetase. Urinary organic acid analysis usually provides the diagnosis. Programs of neonatal screening now include enzyme analysis of biotinidase in dried blood spots because biotin supplementation provides good treatment for multiple carboxylase deficiency.

Disorders of Ammonia Detoxification

The breakdown of protein produces large amounts of nitrogen in the form of ammonia, a highly neurotoxic substance that is normally converted to urea and excreted in the urine. Defects in enzymes of the urea cycle and other disorders of ammonia detoxification present clinically with encephalopathy and hyperammonemia. Metabolic investigations should include analysis of the amino acids in plasma and urine and of orotic acid in the urine. Treatment involves reducing protein intake, supplementing essential amino acids, avoiding catabolic states, and administering benzoate and/or phenylacetate/-butyrate. These remove nitrogen in the form of alternative conjugates of nonessential amino acids, such as glycine and glutamine.

DISORDERS OF FATTY ACID OXIDATION AND KETOGENESIS

Mitochondrial fatty acid oxidation is required for energy during fasting, either through complete oxidation or through production of ketones in the liver that then serve as an alternative energy source for the brain. Disorders in this pathway typically present as hypoketotic hypoglycemia that leads to coma or convulsions and that is precipitated by fasting. In addition, some disorders cause severe hepatopathy and (cardio-)myopathy, probably as results of the accumulation of toxic metabolites. The diagnosis is best reached in the acute situation through the analysis of free fatty acids, 3-hydroxybutyrate and acetoacetate (ketone bodies), and urinary organic acids, as well as an acylcarnitine profile. The diagnosis is easily missed if samples are obtained in the normal interval between episodes or after the patient has been treated with intravenous glucose and electrolytes and has recovered. Long-term treatment consists of avoidance of fasting. Carnitine supplementation is usually beneficial but must be carefully balanced in some defects, particularly in those that cause cardiomyopathy or hepatopathy.

DISORDERS OF CARBOHYDRATE METABOLISM AND TRANSPORT

The disorders of carbohydrate metabolism and transport display a relatively wide range of clinical features; clinical symptoms may be caused by toxicity, deficiency of energy, hypoglycemia, or storage.

Disorders of Galactose and Fructose Metabolism

Defects in the cytosolic metabolism of galactose and fructose for glycolysis cause disease through accumulation of pathogenic metabolites. Children with galactosemia and fructosemia typically develop evidence of severe damage to the liver and/or kidney after dietary intake of lactose (milk, milk products) or fructose (fruits, sucrose) respectively. Treatment includes the elimination of the intake of galactose or fructose.

Disorders of Glycerol Metabolism

Deficiency of glycerol kinase leads to hypoglycemia, possibly causing neurologic damage. Adrenal insufficiency may also be found because of a contiguous gene deletion syndrome. Some patients with big deletions also have Duchenne muscular dystrophy and ornithine transcarbamylase deficiency.

Disorders of Gluconeogenesis and Glycogen Storage

Typical metabolic features are lactic acidemia and hypoglycemia after relatively short periods of fasting. Variable organ dysfunction, most frequently hepatopathy, may exist. Glycogen storage leads to hepatic enlargement, which in infancy may be massive. In some disorders, such as glycogenosis type III, elevations of the transaminases and creatine phosphate kinase, as well as clinical myopathy, may be seen. Treatments include frequent meals, cornstarch supplementation, and/or continuous overnight tube feeding to avoid hypoglycemia.

Disorders of Carbohydrate Transport

A number of glucose and other carbohydrate carriers exist, so clinical symptoms differ greatly, depending on the tissue localization of the individual defect. Symptoms are frequently gastrointestinal or renal but can also include the central nervous system (deficient glucose transport across the blood/brain barrier, DeVivo syndrome).

MITOCHONDRIAL DISORDERS

Mitochondrial disorders in the strict sense include genetic defects of the pyruvate dehydrogenase complex, the Krebs cycle, and the respiratory electron transport chain, comprising the final pathways of substrate breakdown and the production of ATP. Mitochondrial disorders manifest clinically with signs and symptoms of energy deficiency and a highly variable pattern of organ dysfunctions. In many cases lactic acidemia and progressive neurodegenerative disease are present. Frequently, periods of metabolic stress, such as intercurrent infections, trigger a deterioration of the patient's condition. The diagnostic work-up may be difficult; it should include frequent measurements of blood lactate levels, cerebrospinal fluid (CSF) lactate levels, and plasma amino acids with emphasis on alanine. A search for mutations in mitochondrial DNA should also be conducted. Repeated, careful examinations of organ functions are essential. Treatment options are limited but usually include the intake of various vitamins and cofactors, such as riboflavin, coenzyme Q, or thiamine, as well as dietary management.

VITAMIN-RELATED DISORDERS: COBALAMIN AND FOLATE

Genetically determined or nutritional deficiencies of vitamin cofactors may affect various metabolic pathways and may cause a wide range of clinical symptoms. They can frequently be treated satisfactorily by supplementation of the deficient substance. Of particular importance in intermediary metabolism are cobalamin (vitamin B_{12}) and folate, which are essential for cytosolic methyl group transfer. The cellular methylation reactions require methyl group transfer from serine to S-adenosylmethionine and involve the folate cycle, cobalamin (vitamin B_{12}), and the methionine-homocysteine cycle. A disturbance in this pathway may be caused by methylcobalamin deficiency, a disruption of the folate cycle, or deficient remethylation of homocysteine to methionine. Most disorders of cobalamin metabolism, as well as nutritional deficiency of vitamin B_{12}, cause methylmalonic aciduria. Clinically, disorders of cytosolic methyl group transfer cause an encephalo-neuropathy, often with additional hematologic problems, such as megaloblastic anemia and thromboembolic complications of hyper-homocysteinemia. The diagnosis involves the analysis of urinary organic acids, plasma amino acids (homocysteine), and the levels of folate and cobalamin. Treatment includes supplementation of cobalamin and folate and, in some situations, the addition of betaine and methionine.

DISORDERS OF AMINO ACID TRANSPORT

Deficiencies in the intestinal and/or renal transport of amino acids may be nonsymptomatic, or they may cause symptoms because of deficient absorption of essential amino acids (e.g., tryptophan in Hartnup disease) or because of increased urinary concentration of unsoluble amino acids, causing nephrolithiasis (e.g., cystine in cystinuria). These disorders are diagnosed by the quantitative analysis of amino acids in plasma and urine. Disorders of renal transport are ascertained by calculating the fractional clearances of the respective metabolites.

Treatment depends on the clinical picture. Supplementation with large amounts of these compounds is used to treat deficiency of essential amino acids. The cofactor nicotinic acid, normally made from tryptophan, is used for tryptophan deficiency. In cystinuria, a chelating agent such as penicillamine, which forms a mixed disulfide with cysteine, which is soluble, helps to prevent renal calculi. Calculi that may have formed can be resorbed if they have not incorporated too much calcium.

DISORDERS OF PEPTIDE METABOLISM

The tripeptide glutathione and the gammaglutamyl cycle have multiple functions, ranging from amino acid transport across membranes to detoxification of peroxides, in cellular metabolism.

Deficiencies may cause neurologic and hematologic problems, as well as metabolic malfunctions. Investigations should include the determination of organic acids in the urine and of glutathione in various body fluids. Treatment is largely symptomatic. Certain drugs should be avoided.

Patients with mental retardation or skin problems may have defective breakdown of dipeptides of histidine, such as homocarnosine or carnosine. Those with prolidase deficiency often have ulcers of the skin, particularly of the legs. Investigations should include both amino acid and peptide analysis of the urine. Treatment is symptomatic. Some individuals with dipeptiduria are asymptomatic and do not require treatment.

DISORDERS OF MINERAL METABOLISM

Disorders of Copper Metabolism

Two disorders involve problems with copper metabolism. Wilson disease causes a chronic hepatopathy and symptoms of central nervous dysfunction, whereas patients with Menkes disease suffer from a progressive epileptic encephalopathy in infancy and from abnormalities of hair, connective tissue, and bones. Diagnosis may involve the analysis of copper and ceruloplasmin in serum, the urine, and liver tissue. Treatment in Wilson disease attempts to reduce the copper load, whereas copper should be parenterally administered in Menkes disease.

Disorders of Iron Metabolism

Patients affected with such disorders may present with iron-deficient anemia (e.g., due to insufficient intestinal absorption of iron) or with iron overload and liver dysfunction as in hemochromatosis. Secondary iron overload may be observed in some hemolytic anemias. Treatment is directed at substitution or removal of iron.

Disorders of Zinc Metabolism

Chronic generalized erythrosquamatous skin lesions, alopecia, and central nervous system symptoms characterize acrodermatitis enteropathica. It is diagnosed through the finding of reduced levels of zinc and alkaline phosphatase in the blood and is successfully treated with zinc supplementation.

2 ♣ Disorders of the Biosynthesis and Breakdown of Complex Molecules

Disorders in this group of metabolic conditions frequently show a slow progression of clinical symptoms and thus are less likely to cause acute metabolic crises. They are not usually recognized by basic metabolic analyses; instead, they require specific investigations for their diagnosis.

DISORDERS OF PURINE AND PYRIMIDINE METABOLISM

Deficiencies in enzymes required for the biosynthesis or breakdown of purines and pyrimidines cause neuromuscular abnormalities, nephrolithiasis, gouty arthritis, anemia, or immune dysfunction. They may be recognized through increased or reduced urinary urea relative to creatinine, through urine microscopy, or specifically through the analysis of urinary purines and pyrimidines. Some metabolites of pyrimidine breakdown are recognized only by urinary organic acid analysis.

Treatment for some of these disorders includes allopurinol, which can be used to prevent or to treat nephrolithiasis. A high fluid intake is helpful. Uridine or triacetyluridine can treat some disorders of pyrimidine metabolism, notably orotic aciduria and overactivity of 5'-nucleotidase (nucleotide depletion syndrome). No effective treatment exists for most of the primarily neurologic manifestations of disorders of purine metabolism.

LYSOSOMAL STORAGE DISORDERS

Lysosomes contain a number of hydrolases required for the intracellular breakdown of large lipid and mucopolysaccharide molecules. If one of these enzymes is deficient, its substrate accumulates and causes enlargement and/or functional impairment. Organ systems most obviously involved include the nervous system, the visceral organs, and the connective tissues in different combinations, which are specific according to the individual disorders. Corresponding clinical features include progressive neurologic deterioration, dysmorphic features, and organomegaly. Usually, no metabolic decompensation occurs. Investigations include careful roentgenographic examination of the skeleton for dysostosis multiplex, of leukocytes for vacuoles, and of parenchymatous organs for evidence of storage. The urine may be investigated for abnormal glycosaminoglycans and oligosaccharides. The diagnosis usually requires specific enzyme studies.

For most disorders a specific therapy has not yet been found. Enzyme replacement therapy has been successfully developed for nonneuropathic Gaucher and Pompe diseases. Bone marrow transplantation can be beneficial in the early stages of some disorders, especially mucopolysaccharidosis type I (Hurler disease).

- *Mucopolysaccharidoses* (MPS) typically present with progressive dysmorphic deformities, hepatomegaly, and psychomotor retardation. Analysis of urine for glycosaminoglycans usually provides the diagnosis.

- *Oligosaccharidoses* may resemble the MPS, but many cases show more severe neurologic symptoms, which may be present at birth. Abnormal oligosaccharide patterns in the urine or enzyme analyses provide the diagnosis.
- *Sphingolipidoses and lipid storage disorders* usually present with progressive neurologic deterioration; hepatomegaly is not uncommon. Skeletal deformities and dysmorphic features are rare. The specific diagnosis usually requires enzyme analysis. Electron microscopy followed by molecular analysis generally provides the diagnosis of the neuronal ceroid lipofuscinoses.
- *Mucolipidoses* combine clinical features of the mucopolysaccharidoses and sphingolipidoses; they may reflect the deficiency of several lysosomal enzymes as a consequence of defective enzyme processing that results most commonly from deficiency of N-acetylglucosamine (GlcNAc) phosphotransferase.
- *Lysosomal transport defects* include *cystinosis,* which causes nephropathy and dysfunction of other organs, including the thyroid gland and the eyes (diagnosed on the basis of increased cystine content of leukocytes), and *sialic acid storage disease,* which causes progressive encephaloneuropathy (recognized through elevated free sialic acid in the urine). These disorders result from defective transport of cystine and sialic acid, respectively, out of lysosomes. Oral cysteamine, cysteamine eye drops, and renal transplantation are used to treat cystinosis.

PEROXISOMAL DISORDERS

The biochemical roles of peroxisomes are very diverse. Some functions, such as cholesterol biosynthesis, have only recently been localized to this organelle. Peroxisomal defects usually cause severe, progressive, multisystem disorders.

- *Defects of peroxisome biogenesis* or the activation and beta-oxidation of long-chain fatty acids cause progressive neurologic disease, disturbed organogenesis as in Zellweger syndrome, and abnormalities in hepatic, intestinal, or adrenal function. Usually, analysis of very-long-chain fatty acids in blood or cultured fibroblasts provides the diagnosis. No effective treatment exists.
- *Refsum disease* is a defect in the metabolism of exogenous phytanic acid. It results in slowly progressive neurologic, visual, and auditory abnormalities and often presents in adulthood. It is diagnosed through the quantification of serum phytanic acid. It can be treated by dietary restriction of phytanic acid.
- *Defects of ether phospholipid biosynthesis* cause rhizomelic chondrodysplasia punctata characterized by proximal shortening of the limbs in addition to prominent neurologic and other manifestations. Quantification of plasmalogens in erythrocytes provides the diagnosis for these defects. No effective treatment has been found.

- *Catalase deficiency* is the only known defect of detoxification of oxygen radicals. It causes chronic ulcers in the oral mucosal membranes.
- *Primary hyperoxaluria type I* is the only known defect of glyoxylate metabolism; it causes nephrolithiasis and nephrocalcinosis. It is recognizable by organic acid or high-pressure liquid chromatography (HPLC) analysis for oxalate and glyoxylate. It has been treated by transplantation of the liver and kidney.

DISORDERS OF ISOPRENOID AND STEROL METABOLISM

Many of the reactions in the pathways of isoprenoid and sterol metabolism are localized in the peroxisomes, but some take place in other cellular compartments, such as the endoplasmic reticulum.

- *Mevalonate kinase deficiency* is the only known defect of isoprenoid biosynthesis. It causes dysmorphic features, failure to thrive, mental retardation, and recurrent febrile crises. It has recently been shown to be the cause of the hyperimmunoglobulin D (IgD) syndrome. Treatment is symptomatic.
- *Defects of sterol biosynthesis* cause various structural abnormalities, including the dysmorphic features of the Smith–Lemli–Opitz syndrome and mental retardation. Sterol analysis of plasma, tissues, or fibroblasts provides the diagnosis. Specific treatment by cholesterol supplementation has demonstrated limited success.

DISORDERS OF BILE ACID AND HEME METABOLISM

- *Genetic defects of bile acid biosynthesis* cause symptoms either through bile acid deficiency or through deposition of precursors. The former causes progressive cholestasis and malabsorption, whereas the precursors can lead to progressive neurologic dysfunction and xanthomas. The bile acid biosynthetic pathway is located partly in the peroxisomes and is therefore one of the metabolic processes affected with defects of peroxisome biosynthesis. Diagnosis involves the analysis of urinary bile acids. Treatment with bile acids is effective in the bile acid deficiency states and in down-regulation of bile acid biosynthesis.

  Heme is metabolized to bilirubin and is excreted with bile acids in the bile and urine. *Genetic defects of heme metabolism* may involve specific enzymes or mechanisms of transport into the bile ducts. They cause indirect or direct hyperbilirubinemia. Specific treatment strategies have been developed for some disorders.
- *Porphyrias* are disorders of heme biosynthesis and are usually inherited as autosomal dominant traits. The accumulation of specific intermediary metabolites causes characteristic abdominal, neurologic, and dermatologic symptoms that may be triggered by alcohol, drugs, sunlight, or other factors. The diagnosis involves analysis of porphyrins and porphyrin precursors in urine, feces, and/or erythrocytes. Management may entail the avoidance of precipitating factors.

CONGENITAL DISORDERS OF GLYCOSYLATION (CDG)

Many proteins, including enzymes and transport and membrane proteins, and hormones require glycosylation in the Golgi apparatus or endoplasmic reticulum to render functional glycoproteins. A deficiency of one of the more than 30 different enzymes involved in glycosylation leads to a wide range of structural abnormalities and disturbances of physiologic functions. A disorder from the CDG group should be considered in all patients with unclear multisystem or neurologic dysfunction. Isoelectric focusing of transferrin in serum provides the diagnosis. No effective treatment currently exists for most disorders of this group, except for CDG Ib (mannose phosphate isomerase deficiency), which is quite effectively managed with oral mannose.

DISORDERS OF LIPOPROTEIN METABOLISM

Many disorders of lipoprotein metabolism cause clinical symptoms through the deposition of lipids in tissues and by premature atherosclerosis. Others cause gastrointestinal or peripheral neurologic problems. Quantification of cholesterol and triglycerides and the use lipoprotein electrophoresis can identify them. Many disorders are open to dietary or pharmacologic therapy.

- *Elevated blood cholesterol levels* in hypercholesterolemias and mixed hyperlipidemias cause lipid deposition in the form of xanthomas and xanthelasma. These lead to premature atherosclerosis, especially myocardial infarction and cerebrovascular disease. Therapeutic options include diet, drugs, lipid apharesis, and liver transplantation.
- *Hypertriglyceridemia* may be caused by genetic disorders that affect the utilization of chylomicrons and very-low-density lipoproteins. These disorders may cause failure to thrive, abdominal symptoms, and sometimes severe pancreatitis; they require stringent restriction of dietary fat.
- *Genetic disorders affecting high density lipoprotein (HDL) metabolism* cause a variety of clinical manifestations, including premature atherosclerosis, neuropathy, nephropathy, and corneal clouding. Therapy is symptomatic.
- *Genetic disorders in which low density lipoprotein (LDL) cholesterol and triglycerides are reduced* lead to symptoms of fat malabsorption. Treatment involves restriction of fat and supplementation with fat-soluble vitamins.

3 ♣ Neurotransmitter Defects and Related Disorders

Genetic disorders of neurotransmitter metabolism are beginning to be recognized. These disorders cause severe metabolic encephalopathy, originating either before birth or within the first days of life. The diagnosis usually requires investigation of the cerebrospinal fluid (CSF). This group should be considered in children with neurologic problems whose basic metabolic investigations are normal.

DISORDERS OF GLYCINE AND SERINE METABOLISM

Nonketotic hyperglycinemia is one of the best-known causes of epileptic encephalopathy. Concomitant amino acid analysis of plasma and CSF identifies this condition. Glycine levels in both are elevated, and the CSF-to-plasma ratio specifically is increased. Treatment with dextromethorphan, ketamine, benzoate, or folate has had limited success. Disorders of serine biosynthesis cause neurologic manifestations. Treatment involves serine and glycine supplementation.

DISORDERS OF THE METABOLISM OF PTERINS AND BIOGENIC AMINES

Children affected by disorders of the metabolism of pterins and biogenic amines suffer from progressive developmental retardation, seizures, and encephalopathy. Specific concomitant symptoms of dopamine and/or serotonin deficiency, such as infantile parkinsonism, ptosis, miosis, oculogyric crises, disturbed temperature regulation, or (DOPA-responsive) dystonia, are found. Hyperphenylalaninemia sometimes identifies these diseases, but usually diagnosis is made through the analysis of biogenic amines and pterins in CSF. The deficiency of biogenic amines is treated with L-DOPA in addition to carbidopa and 5-hydroxytryptophan. Additional tetrahydrobiopterin provides treatment for disorders of tetrahydrobiopterin biosynthesis.

- *Disorders of tetrahydrobiopterin biosynthesis and recycling* affect the hydroxylation of phenylalanine and have been called *atypical or malignant phenylketonuria*. The hydroxylations of tyrosine and tryptophan are also disturbed, leading to deficiency of both dopamine and serotonin. Investigations should include the analysis of biogenic amines, pterins, and amino acids in the CSF, as well as that of amino acids in plasma. If the fasting levels of phenylalanine are unremarkable, a pathologic response to oral phenylalanine loading may occur.
- *Disorders of the biosynthesis of biogenic amines* present similarly with progressive extrapyramidal symptoms and encephalopathy. The resultant severe disease is difficult to treat.

DISORDERS OF GAMMA-AMINOBUTYRATE METABOLISM

Disorders of gamma-aminobutyrate (GABA) metabolism cause central nervous dysfunction, including seizures and encephalopathy in many instances. CSF analysis of amino acids and GABA provides the diagnosis. Urinary organic acid analysis may reveal 4-hydroxy-butyric acid indicative of succinic semialdehyde dehydrogenase deficiency. Vitamin B_6–dependent seizures may be associated with high levels of glutamate and low levels of GABA, but they are not caused by glutamate decarboxylase deficiency; their etiology remains unclear. Succinic semialdehyde dehydrogenase deficiency may be treated with vigabatrin.

OTHER NEUROMETABOLIC DISORDERS

An excellent response to treatment with vitamin B_6 or folinic acid provides the diagnosis for *vitamin B_6–dependent* and *folinic acid–dependent seizures* respectively. The diagnosis of the latter can be confirmed by finding a distinct, but as yet unidentified, compound in the analysis of biogenic amines.

Sulfite oxidase deficiency is another cause of infantile seizures and encephalopathy. A sulfite dipstick test of the urine identifies it. Amino acid analysis of plasma and urine may be diagnostic but is less reliable. When it is caused by molybdenum cofactor deficiency, xanthine oxidase deficiency also accompanies it. This second condition may be detected by low uric acid in serum or purine analysis of the urine. No specific treatment exists.

Guanidinoacetate methyltransferase deficiency is a disorder of cytosolic energy metabolism but manifests primarily as a neurometabolic disease with progressive central nervous dysfunction. Decreased plasma and urine concentrations of creatinine and urine analysis for guanidinoacetate provide the diagnosis. A low creatinine concentration is sometimes initially recognized by amino or organic acid analysis in which all the usual components appear elevated because of pathologically decreased creatinine. The disease can be treated with creatine supplementation.

Various cerebral organic acidurias—including Canavan disease, L-2- and D-2-hydroxyglutaric aciduria, 2-ketoglutaric aciduria, fumaric aciduria, and malonic aciduria—present with central nervous dysfunction, which usually is progressive. General metabolic abnormalities are absent, but the specific metabolites are elevated on organic acid analysis of the urine. The molecular basis of Canavan disease has been established, but the bases of other defects are unknown. No specific treatment currently exists.

II

Approach to the Patient with Metabolic Disease

4 ❖ When to Suspect Metabolic Disease

HISTORY

Family History

A careful family history may reveal important clues that point toward the diagnosis of an inborn error of metabolism. Most metabolic disorders are inherited as autosomal recessive traits, which may be suspected if the parents are consanguineous or if the family has a confined ethnic or geographic background. Carriers for particular disorders and, as a consequence, affected children may be more frequent in remote villages, close-knit communities (e.g., the Amish in Pennsylvania), certain ethnic groups (e.g., Ashkenazi Jews), or countries that have seen little immigration over many centuries (e.g., Finland).

Quite often specialist investigations begin only after a second child is affected. Older siblings may be found to suffer from a disorder similar to that of the index patient or to have died from an acute unexplained disease classified as "sepsis with unidentified pathogen," "encephalopathy," or "sudden infant death syndrome" (SIDS). The last is a frequent determination in disorders of intermediary metabolism that have acute lethal presentations, such as disorders of ammonia detoxification, organic acidurias, or fatty acid oxidation disorders.

The written clinical descriptions of complex conditions can be inconsistent or even misleading when assessing the medical records of previously affected, undiagnosed family members. Depending on the presumptive diagnosis at that time, important clinical clues may be missing. Sometimes, parents are more reliable sources of information. On the other hand, the clinical expression of the same inborn error of metabolism may vary, even within families. A wide range of different mutations with different degrees of disease severity is found in some more common Mendelian disorders. Disease manifestations are especially variable in females with X-linked traits because of differences in the lyonization of the X chromosome in carrier females (e.g., ornithine transcarbamylase deficiency). Similarly, dominant disorders with variable penetrance may cause erratic clinical problems in different members and generations even of one family, as in Segawa syndrome due to guanosine 5'-triphosphate (GTP) cyclohydrolase deficiency.

As a result of the successful treatment of disorders of intermediary metabolism in which toxic small molecules accumulate, more relatively healthy, affected women are reaching the reproductive age. If they become pregnant, their fetuses may be harmed by pathologic amounts of toxic metabolites from the mother, although the children themselves are heterozygous and thus are not affected. Maternal phenylketonuria (PKU) is especially important, as it is likely to become a major health problem. Some women at risk may not even know they are affected by PKU if they have discontinued dietary treatment and medical follow-up in late childhood. However, they will remember that they had followed a special diet, and the physician should ask about such diets in the patient's past. Mothers, in some cases, have been diagnosed with mild PKU only after classic maternal PKU syndrome has been diagnosed in their child. Other maternal conditions may cause postnatal "metabolic" disease in the neonate or infant (e.g., methylmalonic aciduria and hyperhomocysteinemia in fully breastfed children of mothers ingesting a vegan diet, which causes nutritional vitamin B_{12} deficiency).

Prenatal Development and Complications of Pregnancy

Toxic small molecules that accumulate in many disorders of intermediary metabolism do not harm the fetus because they are removed via the placenta and are metabolized by the mother. Children affected by such disorders usually have a completely normal intrauterine development and normal birth measurements at term. In contrast, disorders that interfere with cellular energy metabolism (e.g., mitochondrial disorders) may impair fetal organ development and prenatal growth, causing structural (particularly cerebral) abnormalities, dysmorphic features, and dystrophy. Structural abnormalities and dysmorphic features may be even more pronounced in disorders of the biosynthesis of complex molecules necessary for developmental pathways and networks. Notable examples are the defects of sterol biosynthesis that interfere with cholesterol-dependent signaling pathways of development (e.g., the Smith–Lemli–Opitz syndrome).

Disorders affecting the breakdown of complex molecules, such as lysosomal storage disorders, cause specific dysmorphic characteristics, as in Hurler disease, and when severe, may present at birth. Mothers carrying a fetus affected by long-chain hydroxyacyl-CoA dehydrogenase (LCHAD) deficiency or carnitine palmitoyl-transferase II deficiency, and defects of fatty acid beta-oxidation, have an increased risk of developing acute fatty liver of pregnancy, preeclampsia, or hemolysis, elevated liver enzymes, and low platelets (the HELLP syndrome). Systematic studies showed that fetal LCHAD deficiency is found in a significant number of women with acute fatty liver of pregnancy but in only a very small percentage of those with the far more common HELLP syndrome in which acute fatty liver is absent. Acylcarnitine analysis in a dried blood spot provides the means of screening the neonates of such mothers for fatty acid oxidation disorders.

Age of Presentation and Precipitating Factors

Figure 4.1 depicts the typical age of manifestation for different groups of metabolic disorders in the first year of life. Usually, disorders of intermediary metabolism that cause symptoms through the accumulation of toxic molecules ("intoxication") display no symptoms in the first hours of life. They present after exposure to the respective substrate derived from catabolism or diet. Postnatal protein breakdown requires amino acid catabolism and nitrogen detoxification. Patients with acute aminoacidopathies (e.g., maple syrup urine disease), classic organic acidurias, or urea cycle defects most frequently develop progressive symptoms between day 2 and day 5 of life. Subsequent risk periods include the second half of

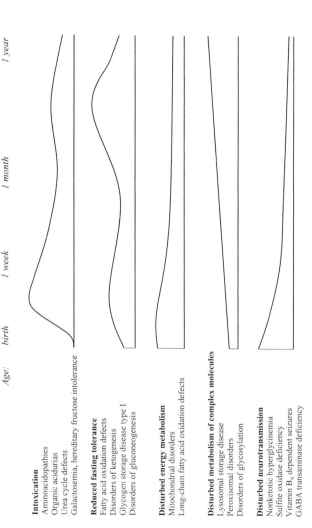

Intoxication
Aminoacidopathies
Organic acidurias
Urea cycle defects
Galactosemia, hereditary fructose intolerance

Reduced fasting tolerance
Fatty acid oxidation defects
Disorders of ketogenesis
Glycogen storage disease type I
Disorders of gluconeogenesis

Disturbed energy metabolism
Mitochondrial disorders
Long-chain fatty acid oxidation defects

Disturbed metabolism of complex molecules
Lysosomal storage disease
Peroxisomal disorders
Disorders of glycosylation

Disturbed neurotransmission
Nonketotic hyperglycinemia
Sulfite oxidase deficiency
Vitamin B$_6$ dependent seizures
GABA transaminase deficiency

Figure 4.1. Typical age of manifestation of metabolic disorders in the first year of life. Abbreviation: GABA, gamma-aminobutyrate.

the first year of life (particularly 6 to 8 months of age), when children begin solid meals with higher protein content and an overnight fast, and late puberty and puerperium, when hormonal changes and a reduced growth rate change the metabolic state. Catabolic states resulting from infections, fever, vaccinations, high-dose steroid therapy, surgery, accidents, and prolonged fasting can trigger the disorder throughout life.

Of the disorders of carbohydrate metabolism, galactosemia often presents after the introduction of milk (which contains the galactose–glucose disaccharide lactose) in the first week of life. Children with hereditary fructose intolerance develop symptoms after the introduction of fruits, vegetables, and particularly table sugar (the fructose–glucose disaccharide sucrose) to their diet, often between 4 and 8 months of age.

Disorders with a reduced fasting tolerance include genetic defects of fatty acid oxidation and ketogenesis, as well as deficiencies in producing and releasing glucose. They typically present during periods of reduced food intake and/or increased energy requirement, such as prolonged fasting or metabolic stress, and the age of presentation thus overlaps with that of the "intoxication" disorders. However, disorders with reduced fasting tolerance occur less frequently or have less severe symptoms in the postnatal period. They present more frequently in the second half of infancy and occur in association with infections.

Disorders of energy metabolism frequently are symptomatic at birth but may present at any time of life, depending on the severity of the genetic defect and on the organs involved. Major alterations in carbohydrate intake or in the ingestion of large amounts of rapidly absorbed carbohydrates may trigger acute decompensation in mitochondrial disorders. Long-chain fatty acids that interfere with energy metabolism in some beta-oxidation defects cause the clinical features of a mitochondrial disorder during fasting periods. Mitochondrial disorders also display a marked and frequently irreversible deterioration of the clinical condition with intercurrent illnesses.

Disorders in the metabolism of complex molecules rarely show acute metabolic crises but do present with variable and often progressive organ dysfunction throughout childhood. Usually, no precipitating factors are found. The clinical presentation of neurotransmitter defects and related disorders depends on the ontogenetic expression of neurotransmitter systems and receptors. Affected children often show symptoms immediately after birth; symptoms of intrauterine epilepsy may even provide evidence of prenatal disease. In general, no precipitating factors exist.

PHYSICAL EXAMINATION

Every child suspected of suffering from an inborn error of metabolism requires a thorough physical examination and a careful evaluation of organ functions, aided by routine laboratory and imaging investigations. In addition, hearing and vision should be examined at specialist appointments. Depending on the presenting symptoms and the clinical course, the physician should reevaluate the patient every 6 months with a detailed physical examination. Even if the patient does not complain about additional manifestations, detecting them is of great importance, particularly if the final diagnosis is unknown.

The involvement of multiple organ systems provides one of the strongest arguments in favor of an inherited metabolic disease. This is especially valid for defects of organelle metabolism, such as mitochondrial or peroxisomal disorders, or for the quickly enlarging group of glycosylation defects or congenital disorders of glycosylation (CDG) syndromes. Structural abnormalities, such as dysmorphic features or malformations, may result from disorders in the metabolism of complex molecules, as well as from disorders affecting mitochondrial energy metabolism; however, other disorders of intermediary metabolism do not typically display them. Generalized organomegaly often suggests a lysosomal storage disorder, whereas isolated hepatomegaly occurs in a great variety of enzyme defects. Urine color and body odor can provide diagnostic clues, as will be discussed later. The appendices lists differential diagnoses of characteristic symptoms and signs.

UNUSUAL ODOR

Unaccustomed odors can alert the physician to a number of metabolic diseases (Table 4.1). The most commonly encountered is the sweet smell of acetone found in the acute ketoacidosis of diabetes mellitus and the organic acidemias. Other characteristic odors are that of maple syrup urine disease (MSUD), the acrid smells of isovaleric acidemia and glutaric aciduria type II, and the odor of phenylacetic acid in PKU. The phenylacetic acid odor is much more

Table 4.1.   **Diagnostic utility of unusual odors**

Odor	Substance	Disorder
Animal-like	Phenylacetate	Phenylketonuria
Maple syrup	Sotolone	Maple syrup urine disease
Acrid, short-chain acid	Isovaleric acid	Isovaleric acid, glutaric acid type II
Cabbage	2-OH-butyric acid	Tyrosinemia type I, methionine malabsorption
Rancid butter	2-Keto-4-methiolbutyric acid	Tyrosinemia type I
Rotten fish	Trimethylamine, dimethylglycine	Trimethlaminuria, dimethylglycinuria

prominent in patients with urea cycle defects and can be treated with sodium phenylacetate or phenylbutyrate. Trimethylaminuria and dimethylglycinuria have very prominent unpleasant odors. Such odors can be very useful in suggesting a diagnosis or an appropriate test, but their absence does not mean the physician should discard a potential diagnosis as certain people cannot detect some odors. Many physicians, for example, cannot detect the ketotic patient by smell. In other conditions the acute metabolic crisis leads to a cessation of oral intake and vigorous parenteral fluid therapy, causing the odor to disappear long before the patient reaches the referral hospital.

The odor of maple syrup led to the recognition and original description of MSUD before it was recognized as a disorder in the metabolism of the branched-chain amino acids. A keen sense of smell can still be useful in detecting this disease, but the seriousness of the presentation of metabolic imbalance and the readiness of clinicians to analyze amino acids in plasma are such that most patients diagnosed today do not trigger the smell test. They are thus diagnosed and treated before the smell is evident. This is also true of acute exacerbation in established patients. Testing for urinary ketones with dinitrophenyl hydrazine (DNPH) and organic acid analysis of the urine are also useful for diagnosing this disease.

The odor of the patient with isovaleric acidemia has been described as like that of sweaty feet, but it does not smell anything like a locker room. The smell is penetrating and pervasive and is readily recognized. It is the odor of a short-chain volatile acid. The same smell may be appreciated in patients with multiple acyl-CoA dehydrogenase deficiency (glutaric aciduria type II) during times of acute illness.

Now that developed countries all screen newborns for PKU, patients with this disease are rarely diagnosed because of the characteristic odor, but some clinicians have diagnosed patients this way before the development of screening. The odor has been described as musty, barny, animal-like, or wolflike. It is actually the odor of phenylacetic acid. Because physicians now treat patients who have defects in the urea cycle with phenylacetic acid or its precursor phenylbutyric acid, specialists in inherited metabolic disease have become accustomed to this odor.

Patients with hepatorenal tyrosinemia and other nonmetabolic patients with hepatic cirrhosis may have a very unpleasant odor resulting from the accumulation of methionine.

The classic unpleasant odor is that of patients with trimethylaminuria. Trimethylamine smells like spoiled fish. The compound is a major end product of nitrogen metabolism of teleost fish, which convert it to the oxide and employ the resulting compound to balance their osmotic pressure with surrounding seawater. In man, trimethylamine is formed from dietary trimethylamine oxide in fish and from choline absorbed in the intestine and is transported to the liver, which, for detoxification, produces the trimethylamine oxide that is ultimately excreted in the urine. Patients with trimethylaminuria have an inborn error in the metabolism of the oxide, caused by defective activity of hepatic trimethylamine

N-oxide synthetase. The metabolic abnormality does not appear to produce a disease as we usually understand it. Nevertheless its consequences are terrible for it produces an strong, unpleasant odor that can lead to social ostracism, poor performance in school, depression, loss of employment, and even suicide, at times. Diagnosis is important because a diet low in fish, liver, and egg yolks usually eliminates the odor. Gas chromatography, gas chromatography–mass spectroscopy (GC-MS), fast-atom bombardment–mass spectroscopy (FAB-MS), or nuclear magnetic resonance (NMR) spectroscopy is used to identify the compound, enabling diagnosis. Loading with choline to increase excretion may be necessary for diagnosis of patients who have found dietary ways of minimizing their odor. Using a morning specimen of urine for reference, a 5-g oral supply of choline bitartrate (three doses over a 24-hour period) was found to increase trimethylamine excretion by a factor of 44, to 1.098 μmol/mg creatinine. (Normal individuals excrete 0.0042 to 0.405 μmol/mg creatinine.) Biopsies of the liver have provided measurement of the activity of the enzyme, a flavin-containing monooxidase designated FMO3.

Researchers have identified several mutations in the FMO3 gene on chromosome 1q23–25. For instance, some patients with severe trimethylaminuria and no enzyme activity *in vitro* carry the P153L mutation. Other patients with a mild phenotype and a mild or intermittent odor of trimethylamine carried an allele with two common polymorphisms—E158K, in which a 472G→A mutation coded for a lysine instead of a glutamate, and E308G, in which a 923A→G mutation coded for glycine instead of glutamate. Patients generally are heterozygous for this allele and a disease-producing mutation, but one was homozygous for the variant allele. The variant allele is common in Caucasian populations. In Germans, for example, allele frequency is 20%.

Dimethylglycinuria is a newly recognized inherited error of metabolism that also causes a fishy odor. The defective enzyme is the dimethylglycine dehydrogenase, which catalyzes the conversion of dimethylglycine to sarcosine. A missense mutation in the gene was identified in an affected patient. Trimethylamine is absent from the patient's urine. A complaint of muscle fatigue, as well as elevated levels of creatine kinase in the serum, was present. ^{1}H-NMR spectroscopy readily detected dimethylglycine, and ^{13}C-NMR spectroscopy and GC-MS of nonextracted urine confirmed its presence. However, detecting the compound by GC-MS after the usual ethylacetate extraction was impossible.

COLOR OF THE URINE OR DIAPER

Since at least the time of Hippocrates, physicians have understood that the color of the urine may provide the clue to the diagnosis. Garrod's recognition of the significance of the dark urine of patients and families with alkaptonuria led to the conceptualization of the inborn errors of metabolism.

Alkaptonuria surprisingly is infrequently recognized in this way; many patients reach adulthood and clinical arthritis before diagnosis. This results from many factors, including the fact that the black pigment forms with time and oxygen and that flushing eliminates it. When attempting to make a visual diagnosis, alkalinizing and shaking the urine and looking for the fine black precipitate in excellent light conditions works best. In the past, when infants wore cloth diapers that were laundered with strong alkaline soap, the conditions were perfect, making reaching a diagnosis based on black pigment in the diaper possible. Now, children often wear plastic disposable diapers, which generally turn pink on contact with alkaptonuric urine. Therefore, clinicians can still make an early diagnosis by examining the diaper.

Alkaptonuric urine also gives a positive test for reducing substance and is glucose-negative, which may be a signal for the diagnosis. Homogentisic acid also reduces the silver in photographic emulsion, and alkaptonuric urine has been used to develop a photograph, an interesting qualitative test for the diagnosis. Quantitative analysis of homogentisic acid in the urine confirms the diagnosis (Table 4.2).

Examination of the Urine for the Significance of Color

Various nonmetabolic conditions may affect the color of urine; thus, examination of the significance of urine color can permit the diagnosis of a variety of conditions in addition to inherited metabolic diseases. Normally, urine has an amber color from the pigment urochrome. Pale, dilute, or watery urine results from a plentiful fluid intake or from diuresis, as in diabetes mellitus, diabetes insipidus, or the recovery phase of a tubular necrosis. Very dark urine or concentrated urine results from dehydration. A pale urine with a high specific gravity suggests diabetes mellitus. A dark urine with a low specific gravity suggests the presence of urobilin or bilirubin, which is best checked for by analysis of the blood. Very bright yellow urine may be seen in infants who ingest large amounts of carotene, but the skin of such infants is usually carotenemic. Urine may be red because of hematuria, but microscopic analysis readily reveals this; such a specimen is not the subject of differential diagnosis by color. Free hemoglobin in the urine appears brown or black when methemoglobin is formed. The most famous example of this is the black water fever of malaria.

Dark Brown or Black Urines

In addition to alkaptonuria, hemoglobinuria and myoglobinuria both produce a brown or dark urine. The dipstick for hemoglobin or the benzidine test detects both. Hematuria often accompanies hemoglobin in the urine. Hemoglobinuria in the absence of red cells in the urine is often accompanied by evidence of hemolysis, such as anemia, reticulocytosis, or hyperbilirubinemia, whereas myoglobinuria is often associated with muscle pain or cramps and with the elevation of creatine phosphokinase and uric acid. An attack of myoglobinuria should signal a work-up for a disorder of fatty acid oxidation (see Chapter 1). It also appears as a result of enzyme defects localized to muscle tissue, such as myophosphorylase deficiency (McArdle disease) and myoadenylate deaminase deficiency. Melaninuria, which also produces brown or black urine, occurs in disseminated melanotic sarcoma.

Table 4.2. Syndromes of abnormally colored urine or diapers

Color	Conditions	Confirmation
Dark brown or black urine or diapers		
Alkaptonuria (pampers become red)	Standing, alkaline	Homogentisic aciduria Clinitest positive
Melaninuria		Disseminated melanotic sarcoma
Red urine or diapers		
Hematuria		Microscopic
Hemoglobinuria, myoglobinuria		Microscopic, guaiac, benzidine
Beets (anthrocyanins)		History
Red dyes (Monday morning disorder, rhodamine B)		History
Red diaper syndrome (*Serratia marcescens*)	24–36 hours of oxidation after passage	Culture, neomycin treatment
Phenolphthalein		History, pH sensitive
Green-blue urine		
Blue diaper syndrome (indigotin)		Tryptophan malabsorption, indicanuria, indoleacetic aciduria
Biliverdin (obstructive jaundice)		Serum bilirubin
Methylene blue (ingestion, treatment)		History
Orange sand		
Urate overproduction (urates may stain diaper red in neonatal period)		Chemical assay for uric acid, blood, and urine; HPRT

Abbreviation: HPRT, hypoxanthine-guanine phosphoriboryl transferase.

Red Urine

Porphyrias are the major metabolic cause of red urine. Congenital erythropoietic porphyria is an autosomal recessive disease caused by mutations in the gene for uroporphyrinogen synthase. Uroporphyrin and coproporphyrin are found in the urine. Porphyria manifests a variable phenotype that ranges from nonimmune hydrops fetalis to a mild adult-onset form with only photosensitive cutaneous lesions. A pink, red, or brown stain in the diapers often is the first sign of the disease. These patients also develop erythrodontia, in which ultraviolet illumination reveals a red fluorescence of the teeth.

Red urine may also occur with the ingestion of large quantities of colored foods. The anthrocyaninuria of beet ingestion is quite common. Blackberries may also cause red urine. Red food colorings, such as rhodamine B, have led to red urine in so many children after weekend parties that the condition was termed the *Monday morning disorder of children*. Phenolphthalein in laxatives may also cause red urine.

In the neonatal period distinct red spots appear in the diaper where crystals of ammonium urate have dried out. In the past, when cloth diapers were used and accumulated for a while before laundering, a red diaper syndrome was recognized in which the color developed after 24 hours of incubation from the growth (in the diaper) of the chromobacterium *Serratia marcescens*, which produces pigment after aerobic growth at 25° to 30°C, not in the infant's intestine.

Green or Blue Urine

Blue pigment found in urine containing urochrome usually produces a green color. The blue diaper syndrome produces a blue-colored urine, caused by a disorder of the intestinal absorption of tryptophan. This disorder was first described in two siblings who also had hypercalcemia and nephrocalcinosis. In this condition, tryptophan is not efficiently absorbed, so intestinal bacteria convert it to indole metabolites that are absorbed and excreted in the urine. The blue color comes from the oxidative conjugation of two molecules of indican to the substance indigotin, or indigo blue, a water-insoluble dye. Giving the patient oral tryptophan load increases the excretion of indole products. The condition is rare as additional patients have not been reported since the initial report in 1964.

Indoles, including indican, are also found in the urine of patients with Hartnup disease, in which defective renal tubular reabsorption exists, as well as in the intestinal absorption of a number of amino acids, including tryptophan. However, blue diapers or urine have not been reported.

Biliverdin, the oxidation product of bilirubin, is excreted in the urine; therefore, jaundiced patients, particularly those with chronic obstructive jaundice, may have green urine.

Benign pigments, such as those in methylene blue, found in some tablets, or indigo–carmine, found in foods, can also color the urine.

ROUTINE LABORATORY INVESTIGATIONS

Unexpected findings in a "routine" laboratory specimen require critical evaluation. Particularly in patients with unusual and unexplained symptoms, they may indicate an inborn error of metabolism and can help direct specific diagnostic investigations. Table 4.3

Table 4.3. **Routine laboratory investigations**

Finding	Indicative of
Anemia (macrocytic)	Disturbances in cobalamin or folic acid metabolism
Reticulocytosis	Glycolysis defects, disorders of the γ-glutamyl cycle
Vacuolized lymphocytes	Lysosomal storage disorders
↑ Alkaline phosphatase	Bile acid synthesis defects
↓ Cholesterol	Sterol synthesis defects, lipoprotein disorders
↑ Triglyceride	Glycogen storage disorders, lipoprotein disorders
↑ CK	Mitochondrial disorders, fatty acid oxidation defects, glycogen storage disease types II and III, glycolysis defects, muscle-AMP-deaminase deficiency, dystrophinopathies
↑ α-Fetoprotein	Ataxia telangiectasia, hepatorenal tyrosinemia
↓ Glucose in cerebrospinal fluid	Mitochondrial disorders, glucose transport protein deficiency
↑ Uric acid	Glycogen storage disorders, disorders of purine metabolism, fatty acid oxidation defects, mitochondrial disorders
↓ Uric acid	Disorders of purine metabolism, molybdenum cofactor deficiency
↓ Creatinine	Creatinine synthesis defect
↑ Iron, transferrin	Hemochromatosis, peroxisomal disorders
↑ Copper (in urine and liver)	Wilson disease, peroxisomal disorders
↓ Ceruloplasmin	Wilson disease, Menkes disease, aceruloplasminemia
Hypothyroidism, hypoparathyroidism	Mitochondrial disorders, CDG syndromes

Abbreviations: AMP, adenosine monophosphate; CDG, congenital disorders of glycosylation; CK, creatine kinase.

gives a collection of such unexpected laboratory abnormalities that may suggest certain metabolic disorders.

WHEN NOT TO SUSPECT A METABOLIC DISEASE

Inborn errors of metabolism may be a factor in the differential diagnosis of a great variety of clinical problems. Sometimes, deciding that specialized metabolic investigations are unwarranted is difficult. The decision about whether to undertake such investigations obviously depends on secondary factors such as local or national availability, costs of the test, likelihood of litigation, and the personal experience of the clinician. Excluding disorders for which effective treatments are available is imperative, whereas in cases of slowly progressive, and by experience often incurable, disorders, diagnostic procedures should be stepwise and should depend on the results of the first investigations and on the appearance and development of signs and symptoms with time.

The diagnosis of some metabolic disorders involves procedures that are stressful, such as sedation or lumbar puncture, or that are potentially dangerous for the child (e.g., fasting or loading studies). These procedures can often be stressful for the parents also. Therefore, psychosocial factors should be part of any diagnostic work-up as families need to be guided and supported. In the worst cases, a specific diagnosis with an unfavorable prognosis that shatters the expectations of the parents can even damage the parent–child relationship. However, for most families, a specific diagnosis, no matter how negative, will be one of the most important supports for coping. A timely genetic diagnosis, followed by appropriate counseling, is especially critical for young families.

Children with moderate developmental delay, isolated delay in speech development in early childhood, moderate failure to thrive, and frequent infections or occasional seizures (e.g., during fever) do not usually mandate specialized metabolic investigations. An inborn error of metabolism is also unlikely in the healthy sibling of an infant who died of SIDS, provided that that child had been previously asymptomatic. Key factors in evaluating symptoms are their isolated appearance versus the presence of additional pathology, however subtle (i.e., the lack or presence of additional neurologic and/or systemic abnormalities), and a static versus progressive clinical course. Multisystem progressive disorders are much more likely to result from inborn errors of metabolism.

ADDITIONAL READINGS

Moolenaar SH, Poggi-Bach J, Engelke UFH, et al. Defect in dimethylglycine dehydrogenase, a new inborn error of metabolism: NMR spectroscopy study. *Clin Chem* 1999;45:459–464.

Saudubray JM, Charpentier C. Clinical phenotypes: diagnosis/algorithms. In: Scriver CR, Beaudet AL, Sly WL, et al., eds. *The metabolic and molecular bases of inherited disease,* Vol. 1. New York: McGraw-Hill; 1995:327–400.

Zschocke J, Kohlmueller D, Quak E, et al. Mild trimethylaminuria caused by common variants in FMO3 gene. *Lancet* 1999;354:834–835.

5 ♣ Patient Care and Treatment

Care and treatment of patients with an inherited metabolic disease require both a detailed knowledge of the natural history of the disease and a comprehensive understanding of the molecular basis and the pathophysiologic consequences of gene defects. Continuous sympathetic support and guidance of patients and their families are essential for optimal outcome. Inherited metabolic diseases are chronic conditions that involve various organ systems and that often show progressive pathology. In addition, several genetic aspects, such as passing on a disease to one's children, the implications of consanguinity, the possibility of carrier detection, and prenatal or preimplantation diagnosis, create a severe psychosocial burden for individuals and families. Thus, an equally diverse multidisciplinary approach to care and treatment is needed.

Primary correction of the genetic defect (i.e., gene or molecular therapy) has not yet been established for any inherited metabolic disease. Treatment usually attempts to circumvent or to neutralize the genetic block (e.g., through reducing dietary phenylalanine in phenylketonuria). In addition, symptomatic treatment of the disease (e.g., medication for seizures or a portable electric wheel chair) is essential for health and/or improved quality of life. The overall goal is to help the patient achieve optimal development during childhood and maximal independence, social integration, and self-esteem as an adolescent and adult. These goals can only be achieved by a multidisciplinary approach. Care and treatment of the patient and the family should involve different medical specialties, as well as associated professions, such as dietitians, nurses, psychologists, physiotherapists, social workers, speech therapists, and teachers. Families may gain valuable emotional support and much practical advice from meeting other similarly affected families. Ideally, a specialist in inherited metabolic diseases coordinates all aspects of care and treatment of the patient in close collaboration with the local family doctor or pediatrician.

A detailed coverage of the diverse issues of the long-term care and treatment of inherited metabolic diseases is beyond the scope of this book. Treatment is discussed in detail only where it is practically relevant for physicians who are faced with an acute presentation of a metabolic disorder or its complications in a patient. The book describes the principles of rational therapy for individual disorders. For detailed information on the treatment of individual metabolic disorders and of specific manifestations, the authors refer the reader to the respective parts of the major textbooks.

6 ♣ Metabolic Emergencies

GENERAL CONSIDERATIONS

Patients presenting with episodes of acute, life-threatening illness constitute the most demanding problems for rapid diagnosis and treatment in the field of genetic disease. This is the mode of presentation of a considerable number of inherited metabolic diseases (Table 6.1). It is particularly characteristic of the organic acidurias, the disorders of the urea cycle, maple syrup urine disease (MSUD), nonketotic hyperglycinemia, and the disorders of fatty acid oxidation. The lactic acidemias may present in this way, but generally their presentation is more indolent. Disorders that present with potentially lethal metabolic emergencies usually do so first in the neonatal period or early infancy. In fact, before expanded neonatal screening, many such infants probably died without diagnosis.

Acute infection and its attendant catabolism often precipitate episodes of acute illness and metabolic decompensation. Surgery or injury may also induce catabolism. The duress of birth may be sufficiently catabolic to induce an early neonatal attack. The diseases in which the fundamental defect is in an enzyme involved in the catabolism of a component of food, such as protein, often involve a buildup of body stores of toxic intermediates until the levels are great enough to produce metabolic imbalance. Such patients may have cycles of acute illness that result in admission to the hospital, cessation of feedings, and administration of parenteral fluids and electrolytes, which result in recovery and discharge; this is then repeated with readmission to the hospital until physicians finally reach a diagnosis and initiate the appropriate therapy. In the disorders of fatty acid oxidation, fasting brings on episodes of metabolic emergency. These can occur when the infant begins to sleep longer, or more commonly, when intercurrent infection leads to vomiting or failure to feed.

The classic presentation of the diseases that produce metabolic emergencies is for an initial acute occurrence in infancy, often in the neonatal period, followed by recurrent episodes of metabolic decompensation, usually with infection. Nevertheless, some patients with these diseases, usually those with variant enzymes in which some residual activity occurs, may first present in childhood or even in adulthood. The diseases of fatty acid oxidation typically require fasting for 16 to 24 hours before metabolic imbalance ensues. Some people reach adulthood without ever fasting that long. Nevertheless, the first episode may be lethal, regardless of age.

The initial clinical manifestations of metabolic emergency are often vomiting and anorexia or failure to take feedings. Rapid deep breathing in the acidotic infant may follow, and a characteristic ketotic odor may occur. The patient may rapidly progress through lethargy to coma, or convulsions may develop. Hypothermia can be the only manifestation besides failure to feed and lethargy. He or she may further advance to apnea and, in the absence of intubation and assisted ventilation, death.

The initial laboratory evaluation (Table 6.2) involves tests, particularly clinical chemistry, that are readily available in most hos-

Table 6.1.   Metabolic diseases presenting as acute overwhelming disease

Disorder	Detect	Definitive diagnosis
Maple syrup urine disease	Urinary 2,4-DNP	Branched-chain amino acidemia Branched-chain ketoacid decarboxylase
Organic acidurias, Isovaleric aciduria	Smell	Isovaleric acid in blood, isovaleryl-glycinuria
Methylmalonic aciduria	Methylmalonic acid in urine	Methylmalonic acid in blood and urine, methylmalonyl-CoA mutase, complementation assay
Propionic aciduria	Hyperglycinemia, urinary organic acid pattern	Propionic acidemia, propionyl-CoA carboxylase
Multiple carboxylase deficiency	Urinary organic acid pattern	Biotinidase, holo-carboxylase synthetase
D-2-Hydroxyglu-taric aciduria	Urinary organic acid pattern	Isomer differentiation of 2-hydroxyglutaric acid
Urea cycle defects	Blood NH$_3$, plasma amino acids, urinary orotic acid	Ornithine transcarba-mylase, carbamyl phosphate synthetase, N-acetyl-glutamate synthetase, argininosuccinate synthetase, argini-nosuccinate lyase, HHH syndrome
Disorders of fatty acid oxidation	Hypoketotic hypoglycemia	Acylcarnitine profile, enzyme assay, MCAD DNA
Lactic acidemias	Lactate, alanine	Enzyme assay, mitochondrial DNA
Hyperglycinemia, nonketotic	Glycinemia, CSF glycine	Glycine cleavage enzyme in liver
Methylenetetra-hydrofolate reductase deficiency	Homocysteinemia, hypomethio-ninemia	Enzyme assay

continued

Table 6.1.   *Continued.*

Disorder	Detect	Definitive diagnosis
Sulfite oxidase deficiency	Sulfite test, amino acid pattern	Sulfite oxidase
Adenylosuccinate lyase deficiency	Succinyladenosine, SAICAriboside	Enzyme assay
Lysosomal acid phosphatase deficiency		Lysosomal acid phosphatase
Adrenogenital syndrome	17-Ketosteroids	Pregnanetriol, testosterone
Fructose intolerance	Fructosuria	Hepatic fructose-1-P-aldolase
Galactosemia	Urinary reducing substance	Galactose-1-phosphate-uridyl transferase

Abbreviations: CSF, cerebrospinal fluid; DNP, 2, 4-dinitrophenol; HHH, hyperammonemia, hyperorninthinemia, homocitrullinuria; MCAD, medium-chain acyl-CoA dehydrogenase; SAICA, succinylaminoimadazole carboxamide.

Table 6.2.   **Initial laboratory investigations**

Blood:	Electrolytes—bicarbonate, anion gap
	Blood gases—pH, pCO_2, HCO_3, pO_2
	Ammonia
	Glucose
	Lactate, pyruvate
	Calcium
	3-Hydroxybutyrate
	Uric acid
	Creatine phosphokinase
	Complete blood count
Urine:	Ketones
	Reducing substance
	Dinitrophenylhydrazine (DNPH)
	Sulfites (sulfite test)
	Benzidine, guaiac
Store at $-20°C$: ($-4°F$)	Urine
	Heparinized plasma
	Cerebrospinal fluid
Store at $4°C$: ($39°F$)	Heparinized whole blood

pital laboratories. The most important for early discrimination are the electrolytes and the ammonia. Blood gases often give the first data for a very sick infant. They provide some of the same information as do electrolytes on the presence or absence of metabolic acidosis. In general, doing every test on the list when an admitted patient is suspected of having a metabolic emergency is advised. Acidosis and hyperammonemia indicate an organic acidemia. Hyper- ammonemia and alkalosis characterize urea cycle defects. Hypoglycemia with elevation of uric acid and creatine phosphokinase (CPK) occurs in disorders of fatty acid oxidation. If ketones are absent from the urine, this is almost certainly the diagnostic category. Their presence does not rule it out; the blood level of 3-hydroxybutyrate is a better indicator of the adequacy of ketogenesis. Hypocalcemia may be a nonspecific harbinger of metabolic disease.

Elevated levels of lactate are significant in the absence of cardiac disease, shock, or hypoxemia. Such levels occur in organic acidemias and even hyperammonemias, as well as in the lactic acidemias of mitochondrial disease (see page 47). A normal pH in the blood does not rule out lactic acidemia; the pH usually remains neutral until lactic acid concentrations reach 5 mM. The blood count helps to indicate the presence or absence of infection. More important, neutropenia with or without thrombocytopenia or even with pancytopenia characterizes organic acidemia, whereas patients with mitochondrial disease sometimes develop thrombocytosis.

The dinitrophenylhydrazine (DNPH) test is positive in any disorder in which large amounts of ketones are found in the urine. It is particularly useful as a spot indicator for the presence of MSUD. A positive urine-reducing substance may be the first indicator of galactosemia. Today in most developed countries, this disorder is generally discovered through routine neonatal screening for the defective enzyme. Chemical testing for blood in the urine is also useful for detecting hemoglobinuria and myoglobinuria, with the latter indicating a crisis in a disorder of fatty acid oxidation. The test for sulfite indicates the presence of sulfite oxidase deficiency, either as an isolated condition or as a result of molybdenum cofactor deficiency, which may present with intractable seizures shortly after birth.

In a seriously ill infant saving some blood and urine (Table 6.2) while this initial testing is proceeding is advised. Then, if the initial indicators point to an area of metabolic disease, these samples can be processed appropriately, obviating such problems as a later lack of availability of urine in an infant in whom dehydration and shock lead to renal tubular necrosis. Further testing requires a biochemical genetics laboratory expert for the execution of these procedures. Programs of proficiency testing indicate that not all laboratories that undertake these specialized procedures perform them properly.

With acidosis that suggests organic aciduria, the assay of choice is organic acid analysis of the urine. A positive DNPH in the absence of acidosis or with mild acidosis indicates the need for amino acid analysis of the plasma for MSUD. Hyperammonemia without acidosis, indicating a urea cycle defect, should be followed by amino acid analysis of the plasma and analysis of the urine for orotic acid. This can be done either by organic acid analysis or better by a specific assay for orotic acid. In an infant with an elevated plasma concentration of glycine, the clinician should obtain cerebrospinal fluid (CSF) simultaneously and analyze it for glycine to permit a definitive diagnosis of nonketotic hyperglycinemia. Following initial testing that indicates a disorder of fatty acid oxidation, definitive testing is comprised of organic acid analysis of the urine, an acylcarnitine pattern of the blood, and a medium-chain acyl-CoA dehydrogenase (MCAD) assay of the DNA. In most of these patients quantification of concentrations of carnitine in blood and urine is useful.

Precise molecular diagnosis is made by enzyme assay, usually of lymphocytes or cultured fibroblasts, or by determination of the mutation in the DNA. DNA analysis is particularly useful in those situations in which a common mutation occurs, such as the A985G mutation in the MCAD gene in Caucasians.

Neonates

The classic presentation of the metabolic disorders that lead to medical emergencies involves life-threatening illness in the newborn period. These infants are usually healthy when born, and in classic presentations a period of apparent well-being before the onset of symptoms follows. This free period can be as short as 12 hours or less. It is usually at least 48 hours and can be as long as 6 to 8 months. Nevertheless, within 24 hours of the appearance of the initial symptom, the infant is commonly in the intensive care unit with artificial ventilation.

The most important key to the diagnosis of a metabolic disease in such an infant is a high index of suspicion. Some alerting signals occur (Table 6.3). The picture of overwhelming illness in a neonate most often suggests a diagnosis of sepsis. Once the blood

**Table 6.3. Clinical features suggesting
the presence of metabolic disease in an infant**

Overwhelming illness in the neonatal period
Vomiting, pyloric stenosis
Acute acidosis, anion gap
Massive ketosis
Hypoglycemia
Coagulopathy
Deep coma
Seizures, especially myoclonic
Chronic hiccups
Unusual odor
Extensive dermatosis, especially monilial
Family history of siblings dying early

culture is negative, some alert physicians initiate a metabolic work-up in such an infant. This approach of checking for sepsis and then initiating a metabolic work-up may provide an earlier diagnosis than, unfortunately, is usual in the diagnosis of most neonates with metabolic disease. Nonetheless, one should keep in mind that some patients with metabolic disease may actually present in the newborn period with septicemia. Before the advent of newborn screening for galactosemia, physicians who recognized that these patients present with neonatal *Escherichia coli* sepsis often made the earliest diagnoses of this disease. The authors have also encountered positive blood cultures and clinical sepsis in citrullinemia, propionic aciduria, and other disorders. Cerebral hemorrhage and pulmonary hemorrhage may complicate the initial episode of metabolic imbalance. Coagulopathy may be the first sign of the presence of hepatorenal tyrosinemia.

Many metabolic diseases, particularly the organic acidurias and the hyperammonemias, present first with vomiting. This has led frequently to a diagnosis of pyloric stenosis or duodenal obstruction, resulting in a number of pyloromyotomies or other explorations. This should not cause the alert physician to miss organic acidurias because in all such patients, results of electrolyte analysis are available. Pyloric stenosis causes alkalosis, so a patient who appears to have pyloric stenosis and has acidosis is suffering from an organic aciduria even if someone can feel an olive. Electrolyte analysis is also useful in suggesting a diagnosis of adrenal insufficiency or adrenogenital syndrome, especially in males in which the physical sign of ambiguous genitalia is missing. Patients with adrenal disease have hyponatremia and hyperkalemia, and some present with poor sucking or a complete inability to feed. An odd smell may help in the diagnosis of metabolic disease, especially in that of isovaleric aciduria and MSUD (see Table 4.1).

The critically ill infant is often first seen in a coma in an intensive care unit. Figure 6.1 shows an algorithmic approach to the infant in coma. Initial evaluation of NH_3, pH, and electrolytes permits early separation, for instance, into those with elevated ammonia and no acidosis, most of whom have urea cycle defects (see "Work-up of the Patient with Hyperammonemia," page 69), and those whose ammonia is elevated or normal but who have metabolic acidosis and usually massive ketosis, who often have an organic aciduria. Patients with lactic acidemia and pyroglutamic aciduria may present with neonatal acidosis but not usually with coma. The patient with MSUD may be convulsant or opisthotonic, as well as comatose; but usually little or no acidosis is present, and the DNPH test is positive.

Comatose patients without hyperammonemia or acidosis and a negative DNPH most commonly have nonketotic hyperglycinemia. The identical presentation can be seen in babies suffering from sulfite oxidase deficiency, adenylosuccinate lyase deficiency, methylenetetrahydrofolate reductase deficiency, or leukotriene C_4-synthesis deficiency. A urinary sulfite test must therefore be

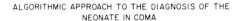

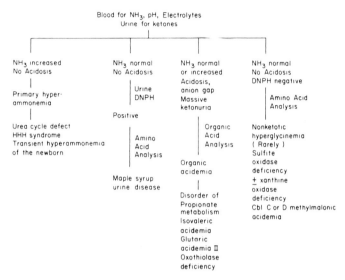

ALGORITHMIC APPROACH TO THE DIAGNOSIS OF THE
NEONATE IN COMA

Blood for NH₃, pH, Electrolytes
Urine for ketones

Figure 6.1.   The metabolic diagnosis of a newborn infant in a coma. Abbreviations: DNPH, dinitrophenylhydrazine; HHH, hyperammonemia, hyperornithinemia, homocitrullinuria.

done on every child presenting with catastrophic encephalopathy, and specific tests for homocysteine in blood, as well as urinary purine analysis, should be ordered. Leukotrienes are best analyzed in CSF, which must be stored at −70°C or on dry ice or liquid nitrogen, as an intermediate measure. If intractable seizures dominate the clinical picture, folinic acid–responsive seizures should be considered, as should pyridoxine-responsive (B₆-responsive) seizures. If a therapeutic trial with 100 mg pyridoxine intravenously is negative, it should be followed by the administration of three doses of folinic acid, 5 mg/kg/day, either intravenously or orally. Severe neonatal/infantile epileptic encephalopathy is one indication for specialized CSF testing of metabolic pathways of brain metabolism, especially of neurotransmission (see Chapter 8, "Specialized CSF and Urine Analyses for Neurometabolic Disorders"). Defects in the metabolism of biogenic monoamines are diagnosed in this manner, as is gamma-aminobutyrate (GABA) transaminase deficiency. A patient in a coma may also have hypoglycemia.

Ketosis and acidosis in the neonatal period are almost certain indicators of metabolic disease. Ketosis is rare in newborns. Even the neonatal diabetic is not ketotic, so urine is often not tested at this time. However, this is a mistake because infants with organic aciduria have massive ketosis. A reasonable position for a clinician might be that any infant admitted to a neonatal intensive care unit with a life-threatening nonsurgical illness should be tested for blood pH, NH_3, electrolytes, glucose, and ketonuria. One could also argue that valuable time could be saved by testing at the outset for lactate and amino acids in the blood, organic acids in the urine, and acylcarnitines in blood spots.

Infancy

The infant with a metabolic emergency that presents after the neonatal period may experience a period of some months of failure to thrive. Such an infant may feed poorly and may vomit frequently, but he or she generally avoids the metabolic crisis until the advent of an intercurrent infection or until a switch from human to cow's milk. Such an infant may then promptly develop the picture of life-threatening illness just like that of the newborn. The etiologies are often the same—organic acidurias, hyperammonemias, hepato-renal tyrosinosis, and fructose intolerance.

The disorders of fatty acid oxidation (see "Approach to the Child Suspected of Having a Disorder of Fatty Acid Oxidation," pg. 65) classically present at 7 to 12 months of age, consistent with the age when infants begin to sleep longer or the timing of the first intercurrent infection that leads to prolonged fasting because of anorexia or vomiting. One must remember, however, that they can present first at any age in which these conditions are met. The infantile presentation of these diseases is with hypoketotic hypoglycemia. Clinically, convulsions or coma may exist. Cardiac arrhythmias are common. Assessing the level of glucose in the blood and the adequacy of ketogenesis is important. Urine that is negative for ketones in the presence of hypoglycemia is very helpful, but if ketones are found in the urine, evaluate for ketogenesis by testing the blood for the concentrations of free fatty acids and 3-hydroxybutyrate. Roentgenographic examination of the chest, electrocardiography, and echocardiography should be carried out.

Muscle tone is affected in a variety of infants with metabolic diseases. These include the organic acidurias and the disorders of fatty acid oxidation, which are classically complicated by metabolic emergencies. Thus, inclusion of a work-up for metabolic disease in the hypotonic or floppy infant may provide data important for treatment before the first episode of metabolic decompensation occurs, which often leads to death or mental retardation.

Neutropenia, thrombocytopenia, and even pancytopenia occur concomitantly to a number of metabolic diseases, notably the organic acidurias and the cobalamin-related disorders. Recognition of this association in infancy may lead to an early diagnosis and can forestall what is usually the most life-threatening crisis—the first one.

The infant thought to have Reye syndrome is an excellent candidate for a diagnosis of an inborn error of metabolism. Single-episode Reye syndrome was once relatively common but is not any longer, presumably because of the sparing use of salicylates in acute viral illness. Today most infants with the typical Reye presentation of hypoglycemia, hyperammonemia, and elevated transaminases have an inherited metabolic disease. Most of them have medium-chain acyl-CoA dehydrogenase (MCAD) deficiency or ornithine transcarbamylase (OTC) deficiency, but any disorder of fatty acid oxidation or of the urea cycle may produce this picture (see "Work-up of the Patient with Hypoglycemia," page 55 and "Work-up of the Patient with Hyperammonemia," page 69). The authors have diagnosed the hyperammonemia, hyperornithinemia, homocitrullinuria (HHH) syndrome in an infant thought to have Reye syndrome. The liver biopsy in this infant had the typical Reye picture of microvesicular steatosis, as have infants with the other metabolic diseases. Therefore, a positive liver biopsy can not constitute the diagnosis. A metabolic work-up is required.

The differential diagnosis of primary metabolic coma in infancy overlaps with the experiences in the neonatal period as shown in Fig. 6.1 and described earlier. In later infancy patients with defective B_{12} metabolism—including cobalamin C disease and transcobalamin II deficiency, as well as breast-fed infants of either mothers on a vegan diet or mothers suffering from unrecognized pernicious anemia—may also present in this way. A patient in coma may also have hypoglycemia (see "Work-up of the Patient with Hypoglycemia," pg. 55). If hypoglucorrachia is found, a very specific cause can be defective glucose transporter 1 (GLUT1) protein, the facilitative glucose transporter of the brain. This diagnosis, also termed De Vivo syndrome, can be anticipated from a pathologically decreased CSF/blood glucose ratio, < 0.35 (normal mean, 0.8 ± 0.1) in the absence of pleocytosis or elevated CSF lactate. Care must be taken to perform the lumbar puncture and determinations of blood sugar at least four hours postprandially.

Older Children and Adults

Any of the disorders that present in early infancy may develop repeated attacks of metabolic emergency at any age, despite generally successful therapy. Late-onset forms of many of the diseases that present classically in infancy also occur, although this is generally rare. They are more common for the urea cycle defects; therefore, ammonia should be determined in every patient with unexplained coma. The lateness of onset is usually a function of the fact that the variant enzyme resulting from the mutation has greater residual activity than does that of the patient with the early neonatal presentation. Nevertheless, the dangerous nature of these diseases is clearly indicated by the fact that episodes of metabolic imbalance occurring in childhood, adulthood, or even old age may be quickly fatal. This is particularly true of urea cycle defects; OTC deficiency also is notoriously unpredictable. A series of readily manageable hyperammonemic episodes may be followed by one that leads promptly to cerebral edema, herniation, and death. The authors have also observed carbamylphosphate synthetase deficiency that led to edema in a first episode in adults up to the age of 50. Branched-chain ketoaciduria has been reported in a small number of late-presentation patients. As in the case of urea cycle defects, a late-onset patient is still in danger of dying from the first or a subsequent episode of metabolic imbalance.

The defects in fatty acid oxidation may present late simply because the patient has never fasted long enough, prior to the occurrence, to exhaust liver glycogen and to call upon oxidation of fats. Thus an MCAD deficiency can first present in an adult as a fatal episode of hypoketotic hypoglycemia. Other diseases of fatty acid oxidation present later with acute rhabdomyolysis and cardiac arrhythmias. These patients usually have elevated levels of CPK and uric acid at the time of the crisis. Others may present with acute cardiac failure, a consequence of accumulated cardiomyopathy year after year and of the depletion of body stores of carnitine.

Mitochondrial diseases (see "Mitochondrial Disease" under "Work-up of the Patient with Lactic Acidemia") may present at any age; commonly they present first in childhood and adulthood. The first episode could include coma with lactic acidosis and ketoacidosis. More commonly, particularly in the mitochondrial encephalomyelopathy, lactic acidemia, and strokelike episodes (MELAS) disease (see "Mitochondrial Disease" under "Work-up of the Patient with Lactic Acidemia," page 47), a stroke or strokelike episode occurs. Such episodes have also been seen in propionic aciduria, methylmalonic aciduria, OTC deficiency, and congenital disorders of glycosylation (CDG syndromes). Patients with mitochondrial disease often have abnormal neuroimaging studies. In addition to evidence of stroke obtained by computed tomography (CT) or magnetic resonance imaging (MRI), areas of increased signal appear in the basal ganglia and elsewhere. Many have the radiologic appearance of Leigh syndrome. The authors have diagnosed the neurodegeneration, ataxia, and retinitis pigmentosa (NARP) mutation in a patient who carried a radiologic diagnosis of acute demyelinating encephalomyelitis (ADEM).

Recurrent exaggerations of neurologic and psychiatric symptoms often leading to metabolic coma are a major presenting feature of several late-onset inborn errors of metabolism in older children and adults. Clinical and laboratory presentations are especially variable and require a high index of suspicion on the part of the physician. The "Work-up of the Patient with Acute or Recurrent Neurologic or Psychiatric Features" (see page 74) section discusses these constellations and the most important diagnostic approaches.

WORK-UP OF THE PATIENT WITH METABOLIC ACIDOSIS AND MASSIVE KETOSIS

A number of metabolic diseases present with acidosis (Table 6.4), most of them for the first time in the neonatal period. The metabolic acidosis may be caused by the accumulation of the carboxylic acid itself, as in the case of lactic acidemia, pyroglutamic aciduria, or hawkinsinuria in infancy. However, in many of the most severe acidoses, the acidosis is caused by a massive ketoacidosis in which acetoacetic acid and 3-hydroxybutyric acid accumulate in the blood and the urine tests strongly for ketones. These constitute

Table 6.4. Metabolic diseases that may present with acute metabolic acidosis

Disorder	Detect or suspect	Definitive diagnosis
Propionic aciduria, ketotic hyperglycinemia	Massive ketosis	Methylcitraturia, propionic acidemia, propionyl-CoA carboxylase
Methylmalonic aciduria	Propionic acidemia, hyperglycinemia Massive ketosis, methylmalonic acid in urine	Methylmalonic acid in blood and urine, methylmalonyl-CoA mutase, complementation analysis
Isovaleric aciduria	Acrid smell	Isovalerylglycinuria, isovaleric acid in blood, hydroxyisovaleric aciduria
Multiple carboxylase deficiency	Hydroxyisovaleric aciduria, 3-methylcrotonylglycinuria, methylcitrate	Biotinidase, holocarboxylase synthetase
Oxothiolase deficiency	Massive ketosis, tiglylglycinuria	3-Oxothiolase
Methylcrotonyl-CoA carboxylase deficiency	3-Methylcrotonylglycinuria	3-Methylcrotonyl-CoA carboxylase
Maple syrup urine disease	Urinary 2,4-DNP	Branched-chain amino acidemia, branched-chain keto acid dehydrogenase

Lactic acidemia	Growth retardation, ataxia, stroke, hyperalaninemia, lactic acid in blood and CSF	Defective fructose-1,6-diphosphatase or pyruvate dehydrogenase, mitochondrial DNA, electron transport chain enzymes
Lysosomal acid phosphatase deficiency		Lysosomal acid phosphatase
Pyroglutamic aciduria		Pyroglutamic acid in blood or urine
Hawkinsinuria	Iodoplatinate	Cysteinyl-dihydrocyclohexyl acetic acid
Ketolysis defects	Ketosis	Cytosolic or mitochondrial acetoacetyl-CoA thiolase, succinyl-CoA, 3-oxoacid-CoA transferase
SCHAD deficiency	Hypoglycemia	SCHAD

Abbreviations: CSF, cerebrospinal fluid; 2,4-DNP, 2,4-dinitrophenol; SCHAD, short-chain hydroxyacyl-CoA dehydrogenase.

classic metabolic emergencies where making the diagnosis as soon as possible and beginning therapy, even before the precise diagnosis is known (see "Emergency Treatment of Inherited Metabolic Diseases"), is critical. Incorporating testing of the urine for ketones into the work-up of a severely ill infant is important. Until the recognition of the organic acidurias, medical thinking was that ketonuria did not occur in the neonatal period; therefore, testing for ketones early in life is often neglected. Their presence can signify an underlying metabolic diagnosis.

Ketosis can be readily quantified by measuring the concentration of 3-hydroxybutyrate in the blood. Normally, this is less than 1.0 mmol in the nonfasting state; it usually is less than 0.1 mmol in children and adults. Levels of 2 to 3.5 mmol are achieved after a 24-hour fast. Infants and children with ketoacidosis may have levels of more than 7 mmol.

Massive ketosis and metabolic acidosis are the hallmarks of the organic acidurias. Those most frequently encountered are propionic aciduria, methylmalonic aciduria, multiple carboxylase deficiency, isovaleric aciduria, and 3-oxothiolase deficiency (Table 6.4). 3-Hydroxyisobutyric aciduria causes episodic ketoacidosis and may otherwise mimic lactic acidemia. 3-Hydroxyisobutyryl-CoA deacylase deficiency, or methacrylic aciduria, may also present with ketoacidosis and 3-hydroxyisobutyric aciduria.

The initial episode may begin with vomiting, anorexia, and lethargy but progresses rapidly to life-threatening acidosis, dehydration, coma, and apnea. In the absence of intubation and assisted ventilation, the infant or child dies.

A clinical clue to the diagnosis is acidosis with vomiting. Some infants with organic aciduria have been thought to have pyloric stenosis and some have been treated surgically; however, pyloric stenosis and its attendant vomiting lead to alkalosis. A patient who seems to have pyloric stenosis but has paradoxical acidosis is suffering from an organic aciduria.

These infants also are often thought to have sepsis, and some even have positive blood cultures. Certainly septic infants can be acidotic, but they are not ketotic, at least in the neonatal period. Therefore, an infant with real or apparent sepsis and massive ketonuria should be investigated and treated for an organic aciduria.

Patients with these disorders go on to have recurrent episodes of acidosis, which are always heralded by ketonuria. These occur in response to the intake of the usual amounts of protein before a specific diagnosis and the introduction of dietary therapies and, in patients with an established diagnosis and an appropriate therapeutic regimen, they result from infection.

The results from the clinical chemistry laboratory indicate severe acidosis. The arterial pH may be from 6.9 to 7.2. The serum concentration of bicarbonate is low, possibly 5 mEq/L or less. The anion gap is increased, and the pH of the urine is less than 5.5. An acidosis with a high urinary pH signifies a renal tubular acidosis, but these disorders are usually chronic problems, not acute metabolic emergencies. In the acute crisis of the organic acidurias, levels of lactic acid in the blood are also elevated, possibly contributing to the acidosis.

Hypoglycemia, hypocalcemia, and, at least in the neonatal period, hyperammonemia may also be found, and each may be symptomatic. Hyperammonemia leads to respiratory alkalosis. Elevated ammonia in a patient with acidosis indicates that the diagnosis is an organic aciduria. Routine clinical hematology may also indicate the presence of an organic aciduria, especially in a very young infant. These disorders lead regularly to neutropenia, often to thrombocytopenia, and sometimes to anemia. Pancytopenia and acidosis occur in infants with sepsis; they also appear in infants with organic aciduria. If large amounts of ketones also occur in the urine, the patient has an organic aciduria. Chronic moniliasis may also indicate the presence of an organic aciduria. In a patient with a known diagnosis, abnormal hematologic findings and moniliasis indicate a lack of metabolic control.

The definitive diagnosis of an organic aciduria is made by gas chromatography mass spectrometry (GC-MS). Using this, the presence of isovalerylglycine indicates the diagnosis is isovaleric aciduria; methylmalonate, methylmalonic aciduria; methylcitrate, 3-hydroxypropionate; methylcitrate and tiglylglycine, propionic aciduria; tiglylglycine and 2-methyl-3-hydroxybutyrate, 3-oxothiolase deficiency; and 3-hydroxyisovalerate, 3-methylcrotonylglycine, 3-hydroxypropionate, and methylcitrate, multiple carboxylase deficiency.

Among the organic acidurias, 3-oxothiolase deficiency is the most likely to present in a cryptic fashion. For reasons that are unclear, the key metabolites may not be found in the urine at the time of the acute crisis, as they are somehow masked by the massive quantities of acetoacetate and 3-hydroxybutyrate. On the other hand, when the patient is well, the tiglylglycine and 2-methyl-3-hydroxybutyrate may be missing from the urine. In such a situation, an isoleucine loading test will reveal the characteristic presence of these organic acid products of isoleucine.

Quantification may also be important in diagnosis. For instance, the presence of 3-hydroxyisovalerate, 3-hydroxypropionate, and methylcitrate may suggest a diagnosis of multiple carboxylase deficiency; but these compounds are also found in propionic aciduria because 3-hydroxyisovalerate increases in any patient with ketosis. The two are readily distinguished by quantification. In multiple carboxylase deficiency, the amounts of 3-hydroxyisovalerate are large and those of the other compounds are small, whereas in propionic aciduria, the reverse is found. The distinction is important because to send a patient home with biotin and no restriction of protein intake under the assumption that the diagnosis is multiple carboxylase deficiency could be lethal in propionic aciduria.

Propionic aciduria may also be recognized by nuclear magnetic resonance (NMR) spectroscopy, and most of the organic acidurias may be detected by tandem mass spectrometry analysis of the blood or urine for acylcarnitines (see "Tandem Mass Spectrometry" in Chapter 9).

Once this biochemical genetic diagnosis is made, definitive molecular diagnosis may be undertaken at the level of the enzyme or gene. Enzyme analysis is often made by analyzing freshly isolated leukocytes, but for precision in diagnosis, especially at a distant laboratory, establishing a fibroblast culture, sending a confluent culture, and ensuring enzymatic analysis of viable cells is usually preferable.

Most of the other disorders listed in Table 6.4 do not usually present as a metabolic emergency, although they do cause acidosis. Pyroglutamic aciduria may present, on rare occasions, with severe acidosis without ketonuria; but more commonly, the acidosis is mild or absent. MSUD, on the other hand, presents as a metabolic emergency, but the acidosis is usually absent or minor. In MSUD the DNPH test is very useful for detecting large quantities of the keto acid derivatives of the branched-chain amino acids. GC-MS analysis of the organic acids of the urine will identify these keto acids and their hydroxy acids. The specific pattern is diagnostic of MSUD, as is the analysis of the amino acids of the plasma.

Ketoacidosis occurs in diabetes mellitus, a diagnosis that is readily made clinically. A diabetic infant or child is unlikely to be missed if routine clinical chemistry is employed. At times, however, physicians mistake organic aciduria for diabetes when an isolated elevation of glucose occurs at the time of presentation in ketoacidosis. Such patients with organic aciduria may show elevated ammonia or lactic acid in the blood, which provide the keys to the diagnosis. The hyperglycemia also is transient and responds extremely quickly to a small amount of insulin. Disorders of carbohydrate metabolism—sometimes von Gierke glucose-6-phosphatase deficiency, but also fructose-1,6-diphosphatase deficiency and glycogen synthase deficiency—can have impressive levels of ketones in the blood. However, these disorders seldom present with an acute metabolic acidotic emergency. Instead they occur with hypoglycemia (see "Work-up of the Patient with Hypoglycemia," page 55). Ketosis is seldom considered in the lactic acidoses (see "Work-up of the Patient with Lactic Acidemia," pg. 47). However, the authors have repeatedly observed crises of ketoacidosis in patients with episodic illness in electron transport abnormalities, such as the NARP mutation. These episodes respond to the administration of parenteral glucose and water (see "Emergency Treatment of Inherited Metabolic Diseases," pg. 80).

The disorders of ketolysis may present with a more or less pure ketoacidosis in which no hypoglycemia, hyperglycemia, organic aciduria, lactic acidemia, or hyperammonemia occur. Patients with these diseases are believed to have defective peripheral utilization of acetoacetate and 3-hydroxybutyrate. The prototype condition is cytosolic acetoacetyl-CoA thiolase deficiency. At least one patient with this disorder has been reported to suffer from moderate hypoglycemia; others had elevated concentrations of both lactate and pyruvate and a normal lactate-to-pyruvate ratio. Other ketolytic defects include the mitochondrial acetoacetyl-CoA thiolase deficiency and succinyl-CoA:3-oxoacid-CoA transferase deficiency. The latter catalyzes the conversion of acetoacetate to acetyl-CoA. Patients with this disorder are ketotic despite eating.

WORK-UP OF THE PATIENT WITH LACTIC ACIDEMIA

The lactic acidemias represent a family of disorders of pyruvate metabolism. Under these disorders large elevations of pyruvate concentration might be expected but are seldom seen. Accumulating pyruvate leads not to large elevations of pyruvate concentration but to conversion to its two sinks, lactate and alanine (Fig. 6.2).

Genetically determined causes of lactic acidemia fall into two categories, defects in gluconeogenesis and defects in oxidation. In the work-up distinguishing clearly into which of the two categories each patient falls is important. The distinction is useful in determining optimal therapy, even in those patients in whom a molecular diagnosis remains elusive. Definitive diagnosis documents deficiencies in the activity of a growing group of enzymes and mutations in DNA, especially in mitochondrial DNA.

The first step in investigating a patient with lactic acidemia is to document that the level of lactic acid in the blood or CSF is truly elevated. The most common situation in which the concentration of lactic acid in blood is elevated is factitious, the result of improper technique, the use of a tourniquet, or difficulty in drawing the blood. That levels vary is true; even in patients with known mitochondrial disease, the concentration of lactic acid is not always increased. Lactic and pyruvic acids are located distant from many of the enzymatic steps that are defective, especially those of the electron transport chain.

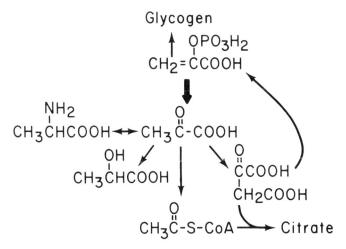

Figure 6.2. Pathway of pyruvate metabolism with pyruvate in the center and the lactate and alanine sinks to the left.

For the evaluation of energy metabolism, lactate should be determined repeatedly throughout the day (especially before and after meals). Determining levels of pyruvic acid and alanine in the blood, as well as of lactic acid, is also useful. Alanine is not falsely raised by problems of technique. One must, in obtaining samples for lactic acid evaluation be sure to use blood that is flowing freely (i.e., without a tourniquet). The concentrations of lactate and alanine in the CSF should also be determined, particularly in those who appear to have mitochondrial disease with neurologic symptoms despite normal levels of lactate in the blood. Many have elevated concentrations of lactate in the CSF while the plasma level is normal, slightly, or intermittently elevated. Lactate-to-creatinine ratios in urine are less sensitive. Raised urinary lactate does, however, support the significance of questionable increased lactate levels in blood. If consistent elevation of urinary lactate is found more often than that of blood lactate, predominant or even isolated disease of the kidney should be considered. Also, in a phenomenon seemingly unrelated to the underlying mitochondrial disorder, patients sometimes show a constant thrombocytosis.

Before embarking on a specific investigation for lactic acidemia, excluding conditions that cause secondary lactic acidemia is important. Patients with hypoxemia, hypoventilation, shock, or hypoperfusion are, in general, readily recognizable as patients with sepsis, cardiac, or pulmonary disease. Anaerobic exercise also produces lactic acidemia, but this is seldom clinically relevant except in the convulsing patient. A variety of inherited metabolic diseases produce secondary lactic acidemia, including propionic, methylmalonic, isovaleric, 3-hydroxy-3-methylglutaric, and pyroglutamic acidurias. Each of these conditions can be excluded by organic acid analysis.

An uncommon cause of lactic acidosis is D-lactic acidemia, resulting from absorption of D-lactic acid produced by intestinal bacteria (see Chapter 17). Most such patients have obvious malabsorption or short-gut syndromes, metabolic acidosis, and massive lactic aciduria, found by colorimetric test or by urinary organic acid analysis. Testing for lactate is now usually done in an enzymatic assay that is specific for L-lactate so that this situation is often not even recognized. The discrepancy between urine and blood lactate levels, plus the history, is the key to diagnosis. A short course of treatment with oral neomycin or metronidazole will cause a dramatic fall in D-lactate production, and the lactic acidemia will disappear.

Specific Work-up

Once investigators have determined that a patient has lactic acidemia, the redox status and the response to a carbohydrate load should be evaluated first (see Chapter 11, "Pre- and Postprandial Investigations" and "Glucose Challenge"). Lactate should be determined both preprandially and postprandially, together with pyruvate, 3-hydroxybutyrate, and acetoacetate, preferably from the same samples collected into tubes prefilled with perchloric acid. In addition plasma glucose must be determined. Elevated ratios of the cytosolic (lactate to pyruvate > 20), as well as of the mitochondrial redox status (3-hydroxybutyrate to acetoacetate > 3), point to a disturbance of oxidative phosphorylation. An elevated ratio of lactate:pyruvate without elevation of the 3-hydroxybutyrate:acetoacetate ratio indicates severe pyruvate carboxylase deficiency (see Table 11.4). These patients can also have elevated levels of the amino acids citrulline and lysine, as well as hyperammonemia.

A postprandial rise of lactate (> 20%) occurs in pyruvate dehydrogenase deficiency and in glycogen storage diseases types 0, III, and VI. In primary defects of the respiratory chain, the redox state may become more abnormal, and a rise of total ketone bodies (paradoxical ketonemia) may occur. A postprandial fall of lactate occurs in glycogen storage disease type I and in defects of gluconeogenesis.

The differentiation between problems in gluconeogenesis or oxidation (Fig. 6.3) can be best achieved by evaluating the response to a prolonged fast (Table 6.5 and Chapter 11). An intravenous catheter should be inserted to facilitate drawing samples. Before the initiation of fasting, blood should be obtained to test for glucose, lactate, pyruvate, and alanine. In this method of fasting, 0.5 mg of glucagon is given intramuscularly after 6 hours to deplete the liver of glycogen made from glucose; the glucose response is then determined at 15, 30, 45, 60, and 90 minutes. The response to glucagon should be a sizable increase in glucose (> 20%), except in glycogenosis type I (see Chapter 11, "Glucagon Stimulation"). As the fast is continued for 18 to 24 hours or until the development of hypoglycemia, the body depends on gluconeogenesis to maintain normal levels of glucose in the blood. Hypoglycemia (blood glucose < 40 mg/dL = 2.3 mM) at any time signals the conclusion of the fast. If the patient is asymptomatic, glucagon is given again. If the glucose does not rise at this time, the defect is in gluconeogenesis. Glucose is given intravenously to restore normoglycemia without waiting for the usual interval of a glucagon test; in the presence of any symptoms, it should be given immediately without testing glucagon responsiveness. Concentrations of lactic and pyruvic acids, alanine, acylcarnitines, free fatty acids, and ketone bodies are determined at the end of the fast. In a hypoglycemic patient, concentrations of insulin, growth hormone, and glucagon are also evaluated at the time the fast is terminated.

Fed and fasted responses to glucagon can provide a discrimination between glycogenosis type I and glycogenosis type III. In suspected glycogen storage diseases, testing the response to glucagon in the fed, as well as the fasted, state is often helpful. After a fast of 24 hours or fasting to mild hypoglycemia, administration of glucagon yields a flat response in glycogen storage diseases types I and III. On the other hand, when glucagon is given 2, 3, or 6 hours after a meal, the blood glucose rises in type III glycogen storage disease, reflecting the release of glucose molecules on the outer branches by phosphorylase. In type I glycogen storage disease,

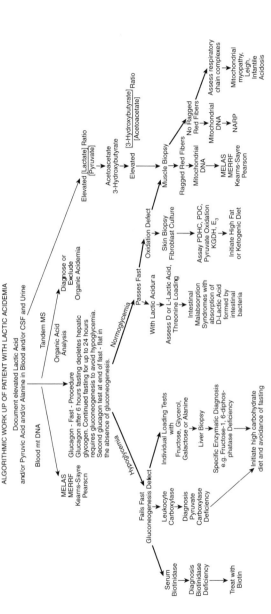

Figure 6.3. An approach to the stepwise evaluation of a patient with lactic acidemia. Abbreviations: E_3, estriol, MELAS, mitochondrial encephalomyelopathy, lactic acidemia, and strokelike episodes; MERRF, myoclonic epilepsy with ragged red fibers; MS, mass spectroscopy; mt, mitochondrial; NARP, neurodegeneration, ataxia, and retinitis pigmentosa; PDHC, pyruvate dehydrogenase complex.

Table 6.5.   Twenty-four-hour fast for lactic acidemia

Protocol and specimens

Begin fast at time $T = 0$ at 4 P.M. The first 16 hours are the least hazardous, so they should happen overnight.

T(ime) = 0 (4 P.M.): End of last meal with documented intake

$T = 1$ (5 P.M.): Serum glucose, electrolytes, phosphate, transaminases, uric acid. Lactate, pyruvate, 3-hydroxybutyrate, acetoacetate from perchloric acid tube. Plasma alanine. Plasma for acylcarnitines. Can be spotted on Guthrie card. Blood sample should be collected as back-up.

$T = 6$ (10 P.M.): Blood glucose

$T = 6$ (10 P.M.): 1 mg glucagon is given by IM or IV after flushing the line with 5 mL 5% albumin.

$T = 6{,}15'$: Blood glucose

$T = 6{,}30'$: Blood glucose

$T = 6{,}45'$: Blood glucose

$T = 7{,}30'$: Blood glucose

$T = 9$ (1 A.M.): Blood glucose

If any glucose level from the 9 and after blood draws is

   > 85 mg/dL (4.7 mM), collect glucose levels q 3 hours.

   > 65 but < 85 mg/dL (3.6–4.7 mM), collect glucose levels q 2 hours.

   > 50 but < 65 mg/dL (2.8–3.6 mM), collect glucose levels q 1 hour.

   > 40 but < 50 mg/dL (2.2–2.8 mM), collect glucose levels q ½ hour.

$T = 15$ (7 A.M.): Serum glucose, electrolytes, phosphate, uric acid. Lactate, pyruvate, 3-hydroxybutyrate. Plasma alanine.

$T = 24$ (4 P.M.) or at the time of development of hypoglycemia: Serum glucose, electrolytes, phosphate, uric acid, transaminases, creatine kinase. Blood gases. Lactate, pyruvate, 3-hydroxybutyrate, acetoacetate collected in perchloric acid tube. Plasma alanine, free fatty acids. Plasma acylcarnitines. Collect urine for quantitative analysis of organic acids.

If blood sugar is < 40 mg/dL (2.3 mM) draw samples as above and in addition for insulin, growth hormone, and glucagon. Give 1 mg glucagon by IM or IV and collect blood glucose at 15 min. If glucose rises, collect at 30 and 45 min, followed by 3–5 mL 10% glucose per kg of body weight per hour. In the presence of any symptoms or if glucose does not rise, give 2 mL of 20% or 4 mL of 10% glucose per kg of body weight intravenously as a bolus, followed by 3–5 mL 10% glucose per kg of body weight per hour until normoglycemia is restored and the patient can resume adequate oral intake.

Abbreviations: IM, intramuscularly; IV, intravenously.

minimal production of glucose occurs in response to glucagon whether fed or fasted, whereas lactate increases markedly.

In the further work-up of a patient with a defect in gluconeogenesis who fails the fasting test, an assay of biotinidase in serum or blood spot and of carboxylase activity in leukocytes or fibroblasts is convenient. In this way a definitive diagnosis of multiple carboxylase deficiency (due to holocarboxylase synthetase or biotinidase deficiency) or of pyruvate carboxylase deficiency can be made. Patients with disorders of gluconeogenesis in whom these are not the diagnoses, such as those with fructose-1,6-diphosphatase deficiency, require liver biopsy for definitive enzyme assay; but the diagnosis will be indicated and effective treatment can be instituted on the basis of fasting and loading data. Information about the area of the defect may be obtained by loading tests, with fructose (see Chapter 11), alanine, or glycerol. Each compound is given orally as a 20% solution 6 to 12 hours postprandially in a dose of 1 g/kg.

Most patients who pass the fasting test have defects in the oxidation of pyruvate, reflecting mitochondrial dysfunction. The elucidation of oxidation defects is initiated by obtaining a skin biopsy for fibroblast culture. The physician can order a diet high in fats and low in carbohydrates with vitamin supplementation while waiting for sufficient quantities of cells for analysis. Fibroblasts may be assayed for defects in the pyruvate dehydrogenase complex (PDHC). Mutational analysis can also test for defects in the first enzyme of the complex, pyruvate decarboxylase or E1α. Measuring respiratory chain complex activities and identifying the cause of the dysfunction may require lengthy laboratory investigations. A more immediate answer may be obtained by analyzing blood for abnormalities in mitochondrial DNA (see Chapter 10).

Mitochondrial DNA and Oxidative Phosphorylation

Mitochondrial dysfunction is an important aspect of many disorders of intermediary metabolism. Mitochondrial functions can be thought of in two categories: metabolic processes that take place in the mitochondria but that are more or less under the direct control of the nuclear DNA (e.g., propionic aciduria due to propionyl-CoA carboxylase deficiency, OTC deficiency in the urea cycle) and disorders that involve oxidative phosphorylation and the electron transfer chain, which are disorders of mitochondrial number, regulation, posttranslational modification, signaling, import, quality control, folding, and assembly of the oxidative phosphorylation apparatus as a whole.

At conception two copies of the nuclear DNA, one from each parent, are found. This leads to the familiar dominant, recessive, and X-linked inheritance. The fertilized oocyte has several thousand mitochondria, essentially all of which are from the mother. The result of maternal inheritance of mitochondria is that familial mitochondrial disorders typically affect all the children of affected women but none of the children of affected men. The mitochondria in the oocyte may have identical DNA (called *homoplasmy*) or may vary (called *heteroplasmy*). The mitochondrial DNA is a circular structure of 16,569 base pairs (bp), which codes for the two ribosomal RNAs and 22 tRNAs needed for protein synthesis within the mitochondria, and 13 other peptides for components of the respiratory chain. All the other proteins within the mitochondria, perhaps 1,000 in all (including roughly 70 components of the respiratory chain), must be imported after synthesis from instructions encoded in nuclear DNA. Many copies of the mitochondrial DNA exist within each mitochondrion, and many thousands of mitochondria can be found in each cell, except for erythrocytes, which lose them as they mature.

Mutations in mitochondria may be inherited in heteroplasmic or homoplasmic form from the mother. Only the mildest mutations can be tolerated in the homoplasmic mode. Heteroplasmic mutations may be quite devastating to the function of an individual mitochondrion, but if they are present in only a small percentage of mitochondria, or cells, they can be tolerated. The threshold proportion for symptoms varies for different mutations and tissues.

After fertilization and the beginnings of cell division in early embryogenesis, the mitochondria also replicate and populate the developing embryo. Variations in the assortment of normal and mutant mitochondria can lead to great variation in tissue distribution and in the consequent expression of mitochondrial dysfunction. In addition, mitochondria proliferate throughout life, so that within the various tissues an opportunity for the proportion of normal and mutant to change occurs, often with an increase in abnormal forms and a worsening of symptoms.

Mutations in mitochondria may arise at any time from conception onward and can lead to dysfunction of one or many organs. In such a situation, the family history is negative and heteroplasmy exists. This transpires for a large deletion that arises spontaneously, deleting about a third of the mitochondrial DNA and resulting in the Kearns-Sayre syndrome of ophthalmoplegia, ataxia, and heart block, as well as in the Pearson marrow–pancreas syndrome.

Some have said that the greater the number of organ systems involved is, the greater the likelihood that the patient has a mitochondrial disorder. Mitochondrial disorders can involve any tissue (so they are sometimes generically called *mitochondrial cytopathies*) and can present at any age with any degree of severity. Table 6.6 lists symptom clusters that are associated with mitochondrial dysfunction. An otherwise unexplained combination of symptoms in different organ systems constitutes the strongest indicator of a mitochondrial disease.

The consideration of mitochondrial disease proceeds along three axes—clinical symptoms, functional assays, and molecular analysis. Molecular defects can be in the mitochondrially encoded tRNAs, mitochondrial and nuclear-encoded subunits of the oxidative phosphorylation complexes, and many other proteins. As many areas of overlap—different syndromes from the same mutation, different functional impairments with the same syndrome, and so on—occur, investigations are necessarily wide-ranging. Functional

**Table 6.6. Some common aspects
of mitochondrial dysfunction**

Organ or tissue	Types of dysfunction
Brain—cerebral hemispheres	Seizures, dementia, infarcts, strokelike episodes, myoclonus, parkinsonism, migraine, leukoencephalopathy
Cerebellum	Ataxia
Optic nerve, retina	Optic atrophy, pigmentary degeneration
Extraocular muscles	Ophthalmoplegia
Ear	Deafness
Skeletal muscle	Myopathy
Bone marrow	Pancytopenia or failure of specific cell lines
Heart	Cardiomyopathy, conduction defects
Liver	Hepatic dysfunction, bile stasis, liver failure, cirrhosis
Intestine	Obstipation, pseudoobstruction
Testis, ovary	Gonadal failure
Kidney	Tubulopathy, Fanconi syndrome
Pancreas	Diabetes, exocrine failure, pancreatitis
Endocrine organs (thyroid, parathyroid, adrenal, etc.)	Failure of hormone secretion
Growth	Failure to thrive, wasting
Blood, cerebrospinal fluid, urine	Increased lactate

deficiencies of a single complex may be due to a mutation of one of the proteins; mutations at a deeper level (e.g., tRNA Leu) may result in disturbed function of several complexes.

More than 100 pathogenic point mutations and 200 deletions, insertions, and rearrangements have been identified since the first mitochondrial DNA mutations were described in 1988 (www.gen. emory.edu/mitomap.html). Most laboratories in this field can look for the common mutations associated with disorders such as MELAS, myoclonic epilepsy and ragged red fibers (MERFF), or NARP and can do Southern blot analyses, searching for deletions such as those seen in the Pearson marrow–pancreas syndrome and Kearns–Sayre syndrome.

The nuclear-encoded oxidative phosphorylation disorders and other mitochondrial syndromes have been difficult to elucidate. The techniques of molecular biology are starting to reveal the basis of these problems (e.g., SURF1 mutations in cytochrome oxidase [COX] deficiency and thymidine phosphorylase deficiency in myoneurogastrointestinal disorder and encephalopathy [MNGIE]). At present, extended biochemical analyses in fresh muscle remain the gold standard for diagnosing many defects of the respiratory chain. These analyses help to determine defects of regulation, posttranslational modification, signaling, import, quality control, folding, and assembly of the oxidative phosphorylation apparatus as a whole. Table 6.7 lists some of the common mitochondrial syndromes and their causes. Chapter 19 provide further discussion of mitochondrial disorders.

WORK-UP OF THE PATIENT WITH HYPOGLYCEMIA

Hypoglycemia must be recognized promptly and treated effectively to prevent permanent damage to the brain. Treatment means bringing the blood glucose to a normal concentration and maintaining that concentration. Rational treatment demands a specific diagnosis of the disease causing the hypoglycemia. Determination of the blood concentrations of insulin, growth hormone, and cortisol at the time of hypoglycemia leads to the definition of the classic forms of hypoglycemia. Liver disease must be excluded as a cause. The metabolic causes of hypoglycemia may be elucidated by the response to fasting and determination of the levels of free fatty acids, acetoacetate, and 3-hydroxybutyrate in the blood. These permit the distinction of ketotic hypoglycemia, which includes the disorders of carbohydrate metabolism and the transient disorder called *ketotic hypoglycemia*, from hypoketotic hypoglycemia, which, in the absence of hyperinsulinemia, includes most of the disorders of fatty acid oxidation.

Acute hypoglycemia is a manifestation of a variety of different disorders. Its prompt recognition and reversal are critical because this absence of substrate for cerebral metabolism can lead to permanent damage of brain just as surely as lack of oxygen. The acute episode can also be fatal. Its management requires providing the patient with enough glucose to bring its blood concentration to normal and then to keep it there. Hypoglycemia is defined as a serum concentration of glucose of less than 50 mg/dL or as a concentration in whole blood of less than 45 mg/dL. Low concentrations of glucose are so common in the neonatal period that neonatologists often define hypoglycemia as a concentration of less than 30 to 35 mg/dL and in preterm infants, as less than 25 mg/dL. However, little evidence exists to show that the brain of the very young is more tolerant of hypoglycemia than that of adults, and therefore, the authors prefer to maintain concentrations of glucose of more than 40 mg/dL in every age group.

The classic symptoms of hypoglycemia are sweating, pallor, irritability, and tremulousness, but considerable variability may occur even in the same individual; convulsions or coma may be the initial manifestation, particularly in the neonate. Vomiting may be present, but this may be the result of an intercurrent illness that induces the acute hypoglycemic episode. Headache, lethargy,

(*text continues on page 60*)

Table 6.7. Mitochondrial syndromes

Syndrome	Common mutations	Genome/inheritance	Ataxia	Myoclonic epilepsy	Generalized seizures	Lactic acidosis	Stroke or strokelike episodes	Retinopathy
MELAS	Mito—tRNA Leu 3243; tRNA Ser; Complex III, subunit III; ND subunits	M/He				++	++	
MERFF	Mito—RNA Lys (A8344G), tRNA Leu, tRNA Ser	M/He	+	++	++	+		+
Kearns-Sayre syndrome (KSS)	Large deletions (most common 4977bp) of mtDNA	M; sporadic	++				+	++
CPEO (several forms)	Mito—tRNA Leu; Nucl—ANT1	M/He; N/AD				+		
Mitochondrial myopathy	Mito—COX def; tRNA Leu; Complex III (cytochrome b); Complex I							
NARP	ATPase 6 (Complex V) (nt 8993)	M/Het	++		++			++
Infantile myopathy		N/AR				+		

Ophthalmoplegia	Myopathy	Cardiomyopathy	Heart block, conduction disturbance, etc.	Hearing loss	Hepatic dysfunction	Pancreatic insufficiency	Intestinal dysmotility	Bone marrow failure	Endocrine failure, including diabetes	Comments
	++					+				
	++			+						Slow growth
++, ptosis	++ RRF		++	++		+			+	Dementia, sudden death
++, ptosis	+ RRF									Cataracts, depression, bulbar weakness
	++ RRF									Myoglobinuria
	+									Neuropathy, dementia
	++									Renal involvement

continued

Table 6.7. *Continued.*

Syndrome	Common mutations	Genome/inheritance	Ataxia	Generalized seizures	Lactic acidosis	Stroke or strokelike episodes
Leigh disease	Nuclear— SURF1 (COX), PDH, PC. Mito– ATPase 6 (complex V)–T8993G; tRNA Lys A8344G; Complex I (ND5, ND6)	M/He; N/AR; XL	++	++	++	+
LHON	Complex I–ND4, others	M/Ho or He				
MNGIE	Thymidine phosphory- lase	N/AR				
Depletion of mitochondrial DNA		N/AR				
Pearson marrow– pancreas syndrome	Deletions (identical to CPEO, KSS)	M, spo- radic				
Sideroblastic anemia and ataxia			++			

Legend: ++ = prominent; + = often present.
Abbreviations
Syndromes: CPEO, chronic progressive external ophthalmoplegia; LHON, Leber hereditary optic neuropathy; MELAS, mitochondrial encephalomyelopathy with lactic acidosis and strokelike episodes; MERRF, myoclonic epilepsy with ragged red fibers; MNGIE, myoneurogastrointestinal disorder and encephalopathy; NARP, neurodegeneration ataxia and retinitis pigmentosa; RRF, ragged-red fibers.

Ophthalmoplegia	Myopathy	Cardiomyopathy	Heart block, conduction disturbance, etc.	Hearing loss	Hepatic dysfunction	Pancreatic insufficiency	Intestinal dysmotility	Bone marrow failure	Endocrine failure, including diabetes	Comments
++	+	+								Apnea/ hyperpnea, regression, spongiform lesions in basal ganglia and brainstem
			+							Male predominance, some recovery of vision
++	RRF		+				++			Wasting, peripheral neuropathy, leukoencephalopathy
	++				++					Renal tubulopathy; encephalopathy
						++			++	2-Oxoadipic and 2-aminoadipic aciduria, may progress to KSS, episodes of acidosis, coma
									++	

Mutations: ANT1, adenine nucleotide transporter I; COX, cytochrome c oxidase (complex IV); ND, NADH ubiquinone oxidoreductase (Complex I); nt, nucleotide; PC, pyruvate carboxylase; PDH, pyruvate dehydrogenase; SURF1, gene.
Genome Inheritance: AD, autosomal dominant; AR, autosomal recessive; He, heteroplasmic; Ho, homoplasmic; M, mitochondrial; N, nuclear; XL, X-linked.

altered behavior, or psychosis may occur in older children and adults; apnea, tachypnea, cyanosis, or hypothermia may occur in the newborn. Some individuals for whom very low levels of glucose are a chronic occurrence, such as patients with von Gierke disease or glycogen synthase deficiency, tolerate surprisingly low levels without symptoms. In addition, sudden drops in glucose levels are more apt to induce symptoms than those achieved slowly.

Algorithmic Approach to Diagnosis

Definitive diagnosis elucidates the cause of the hypoglycemia. This is an essential feature of the design of therapy. Diagnosis also permits prognostication of the hypoglycemia as of either a transitory or a potentially recurrent nature (Fig. 6.4).

The diagnostic work-up is best initiated when an acute attack of hypoglycemia occurs. At this time blood can be obtained to test for insulin, growth hormone, and cortisol to discover the common endocrine causes of hypoglycemia. This blood also permits tests of hepatic function to reveal disease of the liver (a very common cause of hypoglycemia), along with specialized tests, such as the blood concentrations of free fatty acids, acetoacetate, 3-hydroxybutyrate, and plasma alanine, which determine whether the hypoglycemia is ketotic or hypoketotic (Fig. 6.4). More often, clinicians must evaluate the patient after treating the acute attack when euglycemia has been restored. In this situation a controlled monitored fast is required to reproduce the hypoglycemic state and to initiate the work-up (see Chapter 11) (Fig. 6.5).

The clinical history may guide the differential diagnosis. The age of the patient may help as certain types of hypoglycemia are commonly encountered at different ages. Transient neonatal hypoglycemia is a condition found in the first days of life, and it occurs particularly in preterm and small-for-gestational-age (SGA) babies. Ketotic hypoglycemia commonly is a transient disease with onset usually between 1 and 2 years of age; it disappears by 6 to 8 years of age. Endocrine and metabolic causes may present first at any age, including the stressful first days of life, but the usual age of occurrence is after 7 months, when infants sleep longer and are more likely to acquire infectious illnesses that lead to anorexia or vomiting and hence to fasting.

Patients with disorders of carbohydrate metabolism become hypoglycemic after short periods of fasting. Six to 8 hours of fasting leads to hypoglycemia in a patient with glycogenosis type I or glycogen synthase deficiency. Conversely, even an infant may have to fast for 16 to 24 hours before exhausting stores of glycogen so that fatty acid oxidation must be carried out to avoid hypoglycemia. Hypoglycemia resulting from the ingestion of a toxin, such as salicylate or ethanol, is usually evident from the history. However, covert administration of insulin in the Munchausen by proxy syndrome is more difficult to suspect. Hyperinsulinemia with a normal C-peptide reveals this situation.

The physical examination is useful in leading to the diagnosis of specific syndromes in which hypoglycemia is common. Macro-

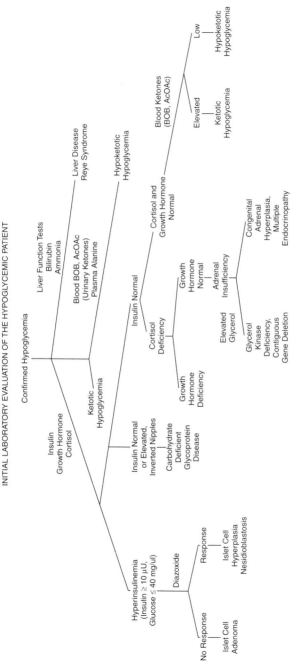

Figure 6.4. An algorithmic approach to the definitive diagnosis of the cause of hypoglycemia. Abbreviations: AcOAc, acetoacetic acid; BOB, 3-hydroxybutyric acid.

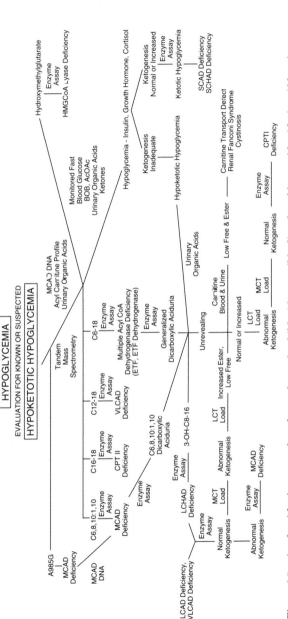

Figure 6.5. An algorithmic approach to the work-up of a child with a possible disorder of fatty acid oxidation. Abbreviations: AcOAc, acetoacetic acid; BOB, 3-hydroxybutyric acid; CPT, carnitine palmitoyltransferase; DNA, deoxynucleic acid; ETF, electron transfer flavoprotein; HMG, 3-hydroxy-3-methylglutaric acid; LCAD, long-chain acyl-CoA dehydrogenase; LCHAD, long-chain hydroxyacyl-CoA dehydrogenase; LCT, long-chain triglycerides; MCAD, medium-chain acyl-CoA dehydrogenase; MCT, medium-chain triglycerides; SCAD, short-chain acyl-CoA dehydrogenase; SCHAD, short-chain hydroxyacyl-CoA dehydrogenase; VLCAD, very long-chain acyl-CoA dehydrogenase.

somia in an infant with full rounded cheeks and a plethoric, edematous appearance alerts the practitioner to the danger of hypoglycemia in the infant of the diabetic mother. These children also have a behavioral phenotype of drowsiness, hypotonia, a long latency for response, and only brief periods of alertness. Macrosomia and hypoglycemia also occur in the Beckwith–Wiedemann syndrome, accompanied by macroglossia, omphalocele, and hepatomegaly. In both syndromes hypoglycemia is transitory, lasting 1 to 3 days. A micropenis may be the only external clue to the presence of panhypopituitarism. Some such infants have midline defects, such as clefts of the lip and palate. Hepatomegaly is characteristic of even very young infants with glycogen storage disease. In the older child, this cause of hepatomegaly can sometimes be differentiated from that originating in acute liver disease by its lack of tenderness.

The initial laboratory evaluation of the hypoglycemic patient (Fig. 6.4) rests on tests readily available in the clinical laboratory. Hyperinsulinemia is present when the insulin value is 10 U/mL or more in the presence of a plasma glucose concentration of 40 mg/dL or less. Many of the infants labeled as having idiopathic hypoglycemia, the infants of diabetic mothers, and those with leucine-sensitive hypoglycemia have hyperinsulinism. Persistent or recurrent hyperinsulinemic hypoglycemia results from hyperplasia of the beta cells of the pancreatic islets, referred to as nesidioblastosis or, less commonly in older children, as *islet cell adenoma*. In both conditions a relative absence of ketosis and a substantial risk of damage to the brain are found. Some patients without adenomas respond to diazoxide with a lessening of hypoglycemia. Most of the patients from either group who have persistent hyperinsulinemia require surgical removal of most of the pancreas. Hypoglycemia also occurs in patients with a variety of tumors that secrete insulinlike material. An interesting, newly elucidated cause of hyperinsulinemic hypoglycemia, known as the hyperinsulinism–hyperammonemia syndrome, results from mutations in the gene for glutamate dehydrogenase. Concentrations of ammonia in these patients, although clearly elevated, are not very high, and patients do not demonstrate symptoms attributable to hyperammonemia. Changes in protein intake do not change the hyperammonemia. Persistent hyperinsulinemic hypoglycemia of infants also results from mutation in the pancreatic beta cell sulfonylurea receptor gene (SUR 1) and in the inward rectifier potassium channels gene (KIR 6.2), as well as in the glucokinase gene.

Patients with hypoglycemia and normal levels of insulin may have deficiency of cortisol with or without growth hormone deficiency and may be diagnosed as having one of the classic endocrine disorders (Fig. 6.4).

Patients in whom endocrine evaluations are normal may have ketotic or hypoketotic hypoglycemia (see Figs. 6.4 and 6.5). This distinction can sometimes be made on the basis of the presence or absence of ketonuria at the time of hypoglycemia. However, the presence of ketones in the urine may be misleading. Many patients with later documented disorders of fatty acid oxidation have been initially missed because of positive tests for ketones in the urine. Quantitative assays of acetoacetate and 3-hydroxybutyrate in the blood along with the levels of free fatty acids clearly show that such a patient is hypoketotic at the time of hypoglycemia.

Ketotic Hypoglycemia

Ketotic hypoglycemia is the name of a very common disorder of late infancy and childhood that seldom begins before 18 months and that disappears by 4 to 9 years of age. In actuality, a number of disorders exist in which abundant amounts of ketones accompany hypoglycemia. Massive ketosis is the hallmark of the organic acidurias (see "Work-up of Patients with Metabolic Acidosis and Massive Retosis," page 41), in which hypoglycemia sometimes accompanies the acute attack of ketoacidosis. The other molecularly defined conditions in which ketosis accompanies hypoglycemia are disorders of carbohydrate metabolism, notably glycogenoses types 0 and III.

The syndrome known as ketotic hypoglycemia presents classically with symptomatic hypoglycemia in the morning after a long fast. Often, an intercurrent illness that causes the child to miss dinner precipitates it. At the time of the hypoglycemia, tests of the urine for ketones are positive; and concentrations of acetoacetate and 3-hydroxybutyrate in the blood are elevated. Analysis of amino acids indicates that the concentration of alanine is low. This is often a hallmark of a problem with gluconeogenesis.

Physical examination is often unremarkable, but the patient may be short and may have diminished subcutaneous fat; the history may include low birth weight. Glucagon administered at the time of hypoglycemia is followed by little or no increase in glucose concentration.

In patients seen after recovery from hypoglycemia, the syndrome may be reproduced by fasting (see Chapter 11, "Monitored Prolonged Fast"); but in some patients this test may be negative. In these patients a test of a ketogenic diet containing 67% of the calories as fat initiated after an overnight fast may reproduce the syndrome; as before, no response to glucagon is found.

Disorders of Carbohydrate Metabolism

Patients with glycogenosis type III, a consequence of deficiency of the debrancher enzyme, also have low blood concentrations of alanine consistent with their very active gluconeogenesis. They are distinguished on examination from those with ketotic hypoglycemia because they have quite large livers. They do not respond to glucagon after fasting, but they do respond to the fed glucagon test (Chapter 11, "Glucagon Stimulation").

Patients with glycogenosis type I or von Gierke disease, by contrast, have very high concentrations of alanine. Hypoglycemia occurs early in life and recurs. Concentrations of lactate are high, and ketonuria is frequent. Hypercholesterolemia and hypertriglyceridemia lead ultimately to cutaneous xanthomata. Hyperuricemia may lead to gouty arthritis or renal disease. The liver is quite large, stature is short, and the face may appear cherubic. In these patients the glucagon test is flat under all conditions. The enzyme deficiency is in glucose-6-phosphatase. Patients with disorders of gluconeogenesis, such as glycerol kinase deficiency, pyruvate carboxylase deficiency, pyruvate carboxykinase deficiency, or fructose 1,6-diphosphatase deficiency, often have high concentrations of alanine and lactate in the blood as well. Definitive diagnosis is by enzyme assay in leukocytes or fibroblasts or, in the case of fructose-1,6-diphosphatase deficiency, by biopsy of the liver. Hypoglycemia during a monitored fast (see "Work-up of the Patient with Lactic Acidemia," page 47) may reveal these disorders, especially if glucagon is given after 6 hours to deplete glycogen in the liver. The glycemic response to glucogen is normal at 6 hours. Loading tests with fructose (see Chapter 11, "Fructose Challenge"), glycerol, or alanine may clarify what enzyme to assay. Patients with glycerol kinase deficiency may have adrenal insufficiency as part of an X-chromosomal contiguous gene deletion syndrome. Some may also have OTC deficiency and Duchenne muscular dystrophy.

Glycogen Synthase Deficiency

Deficiency of glycogen synthase is a rare, unique cause of hypoglycemia in which a distinctive pattern of biochemical abnormality is found. Patients have fasting hypoglycemia, usually without acidosis but with high concentrations of acetoacetate and 3-hydroxybutyrate along with ketonuria. Thus, this is a ketotic hypoglycemia. Concentrations of alanine and lactate are low at times of hypoglycemia, but feeding the patient or a glucose tolerance test (see Chapter 11, "Glucose Challenge") leads to hyperglycemia and elevated concentrations of lactate in the blood. Glucagon during fasting has no effect on blood concentrations of glucose, lactate, or alanine, whereas the fed glucagon test yields a glycemic response. Diagnosis by enzyme assay requires a biopsy of the liver, but mutational analysis can define the defect in the gene.

APPROACH TO THE CHILD SUSPECTED OF HAVING A DISORDER OF FATTY ACID OXIDATION

Disorders of fatty acid oxidation usually present initially with hypoketotic hypoglycemia. Hyperammonemia may suggest Reye syndrome. Sudden infant death syndrome (SIDS) is another acute presentation. Some patients present more chronically with myopathy or cardiomyopathy. Medium-chain acyl-CoA dehydrogenase (MCAD) deficiency is the only common disorder, and most patients have the same mutation. Therefore, modern work-up begins with assay of the DNA for the A985G mutation. Mutations not revealed in this way are now assayed by tandem mass spectrometry for the acylcarnitine profile; this may indicate the diagnosis and the appropriate enzymatic assay. Organic acid analysis should reveal the diagnosis in those with 3-hydroxy-3-methylglutaryl-CoA lyase deficiency. Patients for whom these measures do not provide a diagnosis undergo an algo-rithmic investigation, central to which is a prolonged monitored fast (see Chapter 11). These measures are followed with loading tests with specific lipids.

Most patients with disorders of fatty acid oxidation present with hypoglycemia. The classic initial presentation is with hypoketotic hypoglycemia, usually at 6 to 12 months of age fol-lowing a period of fasting of more than 12 hours and induced by the vomiting or anorexia of an intercurrent respiratory or gas-trointestinal infection. The hypoglycemia may manifest itself as lethargy, or a seizure may be the first signal. It may progress rapidly to coma. Hyperammonemia may be present, which has led to a diagnosis of Reye syndrome. Liver biopsy in such a patient may reveal microvesicular fat, which may seem to confirm the diagno-sis of Reye syndrome. Most patients that are diagnosed with Reye syndrome today actually have a disorder of fatty acid oxidation. A few have a urea cycle defect. Orotic aciduria, a hallmark of OTC deficiency, has been seen as an acute presentation in disordered fatty acid oxidation.

The other major presentation is myopathic. This may be acute, with muscle pains and rhabdomyolysis, with or without hypo-glycemia. It may be chronic, with weakness and hypotonia. Also common is presentation with cardiomyopathy. The first manifes-tations in some patients are those of congestive heart failure. Arrhythmias are also common, especially in the acute episode of metabolic imbalance.

A third presentation is with SIDS. One prevalent scenario has been diagnosis of a disorder of fatty acid oxidation, most commonly MCAD deficiency, in an infant and the subsequent discovery that a previous sibling died of SIDS. The authors have obtained blood samples representing the previous infant that were saved from neonatal screening programs and have diagnosed MCAD deficiency by DNA analysis. This type of posthumous diagnosis has also been made by assay for octanoylcarnitine. Furthermore, disorders of fatty acid oxidation have been detected in studies of sudden infant death by assay of postmortem liver for deficiency of carnitine and by GC-MS for the presence of key organic acids.

In the patient presenting with hypoglycemia, a negative test for ketones in the urine helps to suggest the diagnosis. In this situa-tion hypoglycemia is clearly hypoketotic. However, these patients may be treated with parenteral glucose in the emergency room and the first urine analysis may be done hours or days after the hypoglycemia has resolved, making this clue to the diagnosis unavailable. More commonly, the diagnosis may be missed because ketones appear in the urine at the time of acute illness. These pa-tients can readily be shown to be hypoketotic by analyzing the blood, but this does not exclude the possibility that the urine test for ketones may be positive. Documenting that hypoglycemia is hypoketotic is best accomplished by quantifying the concentra-tions of free fatty acids, acetoacetate, and 3-hydroxybutyrate in the blood, as is most commonly done in the context of a controlled or monitored fast (see Chapter 11). This approach is mandated because the stability of acetoacetate requires planning ahead for its analysis and because it is seldom considered at the time of the initial acute episode. Nevertheless, a good idea of the presence of hypoketosis can be obtained simply by assaying 3-hydroxybutyrate and free fatty acids in the blood at the time of the acute hypoglycemic illness.

Clues from the routine clinical chemistry laboratory that suggest the presence of a disorder of fatty acid oxidation include elevated levels of uric acid and CPK. Uric acid determinations are not regularly included in metabolic panels for pediatric patients, so they may have to be ordered separately, as may tests for CPK; but levels of more than 1,000 U/L commonly occur on presentation. Transaminase levels also may be elevated. Analysis of organic acids in the urine may reveal dicarboxylic aciduria, and its pattern may provide direction as to the site of the enzymatic defect. During intervals between episodes of illness, these patients usually appear completely well. Abnormalities, such as the dicarboxylic aciduria and elevations of uric acid and CPK, usually disappear completely. The patient is often first seen in consultation after the initial hypoglycemia has been treated; none of the abnormalities that occur in the acute situation are present. Therefore, a systematic algorithmic approach to the work-up is important (Fig. 6.5). In a patient suspected of having a disorder of fatty acid oxidation, the algorithm starts with an assay of the blood for DNA, for the common mutation in MCAD deficiency, for an acylcarnitine profile, and for the organic acids of the urine.

MCAD deficiency is the only common disorder of fatty acid oxidation. Its frequency has been estimated at one in 6,000 to 10,000 Caucasians. Most patients have the same mutation, an A985G change that makes a protein containing glutamic acid in which a lysine occurs in the normal enzyme. So this single DNA-diagnostic approach can be expected to yield a rapid diagnosis in many patients with this group of disorders. The acylcarnitine profile resulting from assay by tandem mass spectrometry can also detect MCAD deficiency. In this instance octanoylcarnitine is the key compound; hexanoylcarnitine may be present as well. In a patient negative for the A985G mutation and positive in the acylcarnitine assay, enzyme analysis documents MCAD deficiency. In that case, testing for the 4-bp deletion, which with A985G accounts for 93% of the MCAD mutations, may be useful; a rapid test exists for this as for A985G. Acylcarnitine assay may also point to enzyme assay for carnitine palmitoyltransferase (CPT) deficiency, very-long-chain acyl-CoA dehydrogenase (VLCAD) deficiency, or multiple acyl-CoA dehydrogenase (MAD) deficiency. Acylcarnitine profiles are usually obtained by tandem mass spectrometry and can be done on as little as a drop of dry blood. These profiles are usually not quantified. Stable isotope dilution GC-MS has provided quantitative profiling of acylcarnitine in plasma.

Organic acid analysis can be expected to reveal 3-hydroxy-3-methylglutarate (HMG) in the presence of HMG-CoA lyase deficiency. This compound is abundant in the urine of affected patients even after recovery from the acute hypoglycemic episode. In most of the other disorders, organic acid analysis is more often normal than abnormal in intervals between episodes of acute illness.

In many patients (essentially all who would not be detected by the tests mentioned in the previous three paragraphs), a controlled, prolonged fast (see Chapter 11) is necessary to document that the hypoglycemia really is hypoketotic and to determine the nature of the defect. In response to this long fast the body's first step is lipolysis, which releases free fatty acids. In patients with disorders of fatty acid oxidation, concentrations of free fatty acids are higher than are those of 3-hydroxybutyrate in the blood when hypoglycemia develops. In addition, fatty acids that accumulate in the presence of defective oxidation undergo omega-oxidation to dicarboxylic acids, giving an elevated ratio of dicarboxylic acids to 3-hydroxybutyrate in the analysis of organic acids of the urine. The nature of the dicarboxylic aciduria at the time the hypoglycemia develops may indicate the site of the defect. Thus C8 to C10 dicarboxylic aciduria appears in MCAD deficiency, and 3-hydroxy long-chain acids occur in LCHAD deficiency.

Patients during the long fast must be monitored closely to avoid symptomatic hypoglycemia. Testing should be done where the staff is experienced in the protocol. An intravenous line should be placed to ensure access for therapeutic glucose. Blood concentrations of glucose are monitored regularly at the bedside. In abnormalities of fatty acid oxidation, fasting must last long enough to exhaust stores of glycogen and to require the mobilization of fat and its oxidation.

Analysis of the concentrations of carnitine in the plasma and the urine, and its esterification may suggest the answer, particularly if free carnitine in the blood is low and if large amounts of esters are being excreted in the urine. Transport of long-chain fatty acids into the mitochondria, where beta-oxidation takes place, requires carnitine; the entry of carnitine into cells such as muscle requires a specific transporter that may be deficient as a cause of hypoketotic hypoglycemia. Assays of carnitine in the blood and urine reveal very low levels of free and esterified carnitine in these patients.

In patients with normal or increased blood and urine carnitine levels, a long-chain triglycerides (LCT) load may reveal abnormal ketogenesis, and a medium-chain trygglyceride (MCT) load may indicate normal ketogenesis. In such patients MCT administration may even reverse fasting-induced hypoglycemia; enzyme assay reveals the deficiency of carnitine palmitoyl transferase (CPT I). Esterification of carnitine with fatty acids acyl-CoA ester is catalyzed by acyltransferases, such as CPT I. The transport of acyl-carnitines across the mitochondrial membrane is catalyzed by carnitine translocase. Hydrolysis, which releases free carnitine and the fatty acid acyl-CoA, is catalyzed by a second acyltransferase, CPT II. Each of these three enzymatic steps has documented, known inborn errors of metabolism.

When the carnitine ester level of the urine is high and the free carnitine level of the blood is low, the metabolic block causes the accumulation of acyl-CoA compounds that are esterified with carnitine and then are excreted in the urine, particularly in disorders of beta-oxidation.

In beta-oxidation two carbons shorten the fatty acid successively, releasing acetyl-CoA. Specific dehydrogenases with overlapping specificities for chain length include short-chain acyl-CoA dehydrogenase (SCAD), medium-chain acyl-CoA dehydrogenase (MCAD), long-chain acyl-CoA dehydrogenase (LCAD), and very-long-chain acyl-CoA dehydrogenase (VLCAD). In addition, a tri-functional enzyme catalyzes 3-hydroxyacyl-CoA dehydrogenation (LCHAD), 2-enoyl-CoA hydration, and 3-oxoacyl-CoA thiolysis. Diseases involving defects in each of these steps have been defined. All patients with these diseases would be expected to have abnormal ketogenesis following an LCT load. When they are tested with MCT, MCAD patients display abnormal ketogenesis, whereas those with LCAD, LCHAD, and VLCAD deficiency have normal ketogenesis. This testing is followed up via assay for the specific enzyme or enzymes, as suggested in Fig. 6.5.

The enzyme assays for specific disorders are technically demanding and are generally not available. A reasonable step following the fast, if a disease is not identified, is to pursue a more general study of metabolism in cultured cells in which the oxidation of fatty acids of varying chain length is studied *in vitro* or in which carnitine esters are separated and identified after oxidation with ^{14}C- or ^{13}C-labeled long-chain fatty acids, such as hexadecanoate. Impaired oxidation of long-chain fatty acids, such as palmitate *in vitro*, may also be seen in patients with mitochondrial disorders (see "Work-up of the Patient With Lactic Acidemia, page 47"). These patients may also have hypoketotic hypoglycemia with increased levels of 3-hydroxydicarboxylic acids because of a failure to oxidize the nicotinamide adinine dinucleotide (NADH) produced in the 3-hydroxyacyl-CoA dehydrogenase step via the electron transport chain. They usually display lactic acidemia.

WORK-UP OF THE PATIENT WITH HYPERAMMONEMIA

Elevated concentrations of ammonia occur episodically in a variety of inherited diseases of metabolism. These include not only the disorders of the urea cycle but also organic acidurias and disorders of fatty acid oxidation. Effective management is predicated on a precise diagnosis and understanding of the nature of the patho-physiology. A systematic progression from routine clinical chemistry to more specific analyses of amino acids, organic acids, and acylcarnitines leads to the diagnosis. Liver biopsy is required for enzymatic diagnosis of carbamyl phosphate synthetase deficiency and OTC deficiency, as well as of N-acetylglutamate synthetase deficiency.

Deficiencies of enzymes of the urea cycle and some other disorders, such as the organic acidemias and the disorders of fatty acid oxidation, present with hyperammonemia. Normally, values of NH_3 are below 110 µmol/L (190 µg/dL) in newborns and below 80 µmol/L (140 µg/dL) in older infants to adults. In the newborn period a diagnostic work-up for hyperammonemia is warranted with values of > 150 µmol/L (260 µg/dL) and in older infants to adults, at values > 100 µmol/L (175 µg/dL). The classic onset of urea cycle defects is with a sudden, potentially lethal neonatal coma. The male with OTC deficiency (E.C.2.1.33) exemplifies the classic presentation, but distinct disorders result from deficient activity with each of the enzymes of urea cycle (Fig. 6.6).

Figure 6.7 shows the work-up of an infant in hyperammonemic coma. The differential diagnosis is very important because different disorders require different treatments. The work-up must proceed with dispatch to make the correct diagnosis and to institute appropriate therapy in time to prevent death or permanent damage to the brain. The initial steps in the algorithm are available in the routine clinical chemistry laboratory. Definitive diagnosis requires the services of a biochemical genetics laboratory.

The first step in evaluating a patient, especially an infant in a coma, is to measure the concentration of ammonia in the blood. The following step is to quantify serum concentrations of bicarbonate, sodium, chloride, and the anion gap and to test the urine for ketones. Acidosis and/or an anion gap suggest that the disorder does not involve the urea cycle. (Such disorders usually present with respiratory alkalosis.) The acidotic patient with massive ketosis has an organic aciduria, such as propionic aciduria, methylmalonic aciduria, isovaleric aciduria, or multiple carboxylase deficiency. The specific diagnosis is made by quantitative analysis of the organic acids of the urine or of the acylcarnitines from dried blood spots. The disorders of fatty acid oxidation, which may present with hyperammonemia, are characteristically hypoketotic. However, testing the urine for ketones may be misleading. The authors have observed highly positive urinary ketostick tests in patients with disorders of fatty acid oxidation. Quantification of concentrations of free fatty acids together with acetoacetic and 3-hydroxybutyric acid in the blood of those patients reliably indicates defective ketogenesis. The acute crises in these patients often display hypoglycemia; consequently, clinicians have sometimes diagnosed Reye syndrome. The authors have reported an acute hyperammonemic episode in a teenage girl with medium-chain acyl-CoA dehydrogenase deficiency that met all the criteria for a diagnosis of OTC deficiency, including orotic aciduria. However, when the biopsied liver was tested for OTC activity, it was normal. A patient with hyperammonemic coma resulting from a urea cycle defect may develop hypoxia leading to lactic acidosis. Adequate oxygenation and perfusion should be assured before excluding a diagnosis of urea cycle defect and pursuing one of organic acidemia.

The definitive diagnosis of a urea cycle abnormality is initiated by the quantitative assay of the concentrations of amino acids in blood and urine. The plasma concentrations of amino acids provide the diagnosis in patients with argininemia and citrullinemia. Study of the urine is required in argininosuccinic aciduria.

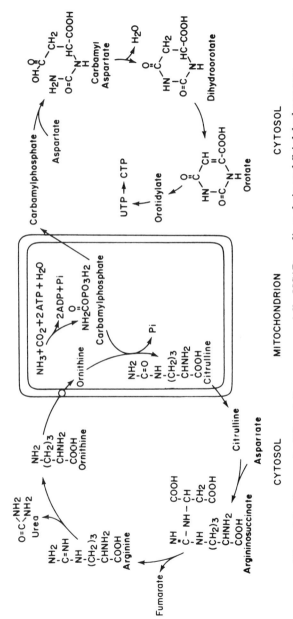

Figure 6.6. Urea cycle. Abbreviations: esp., especially; MCAD, medium-chain acyl-C.A dehydrogenase.

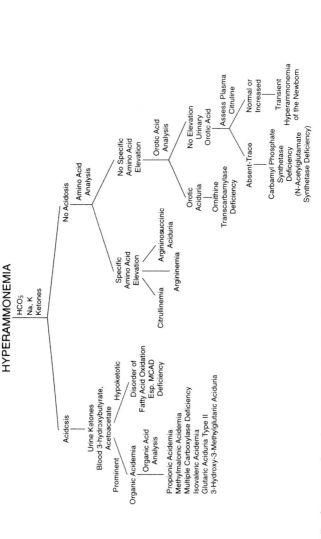

Figure 6.7.   An approach to the stepwise evaluation of a patient with hyperammonemia. Abbreviations: esp., especially; MCAD, medium-chain acyl-CoA dehydrogenase.

In hyperammonemic patients that have been found not to have a diagnostic abnormality in the concentration of an amino acid, the urine should be tested for orotic acid. This can be a part of organic acid analysis by GC-MS, or a specific assay can be performed for the compound. Orotic aciduria is found in patients with OTC deficiency. It also occurs in citrullinemia and in argininemia. In a patient without an elevation of a specific amino acid and without orotic aciduria, the usual diagnosis is carbamylphosphate synthetase (CPS) deficiency. N-acetylglutamate synthetase deficiency presents with an undistinguishable clinical and biochemical constellation but is much rarer. Transient hyperammonemia of the newborn may also present this way, but for reasons that are unclear, encounters with this disorder are much less likely to occur than they were 20 years ago. Failure of immediate closure of the ductus aranchii after birth is thought to result in transient hyperammonemia of the newborn because portal blood bypasses the liver.

The definitive diagnoses of CPS, OTC, and N-acetylglutamate synthetase deficiencies are made by assaying enzyme activity in biopsied liver. If a transient hyperammonemia of the newborn is suspected, waiting to perform the liver biopsy is suggested because the elevated ammonia in this disorder could resolve within 5 days. In addition, the waiting period gives the clinician time to bring the patient's blood concentration of ammonia under control. The level of citrulline in the blood may also help in distinguishing CPS deficiency from transient hyperammonemia of the newborn in which citrulline is usually normal or elevated. In neonatal CPS, OTC, or N-acetylglutamate synthetase deficiencies, citrulline is barely detectable. In citrullinemia, concentrations of citrulline in plasma usually exceed 1,000 µmol/L. They are elevated to levels of 150 to 250 µmol/L in argininosuccinic aciduria and to 54 ± 22 µmol/L in transient hyperammonemia in the newborn. The normal range is 6 to 20 µmol/L. Persistent hypocitrullinemia can, in general, be viewed as a marker for disorders of mitochondrial urea cycle enzymes (N-acetylglutamate synthetase, carbamylphosphate synthetase I, and ornithine carbamoyltransferase), as well as for deficient pyrroline-5-carboxylate synthetase. Citrulline synthesis is directly coupled to ATP concentration. Consequently, hypocitrullinemia can also be observed in patients with respiratory chain disorders, especially those caused by NARP mutation.

Amino acid analysis also reveals regularly elevated concentrations of glutamine in patients with hyperammonemia. Concentrations of alanine are also usually elevated, as are those of aspartic acid in some patients. These are nonspecific findings. They are not helpful in differentiating among the different causes of hyperammonemia. They are potentially helpful in diagnosis, as sometimes an elevated level of glutamine occurs in a patient that has not been expected to have hyperammonemia. Although concentrations of ammonia may vary from hour to hour, the elevated concentration of glutamine signifies a state in which chronic over-abundance of ammonia has occurred. The transamination of pyruvic acid to alanine and oxaloacetic acid to aspartic acid, as well as of 2-oxoglutaric acid to glutamic acid and its subsequent amidation to glutamine, are detoxification responses to the presence of excessive quantities of ammonia.

Amino acid analysis may also reveal elevations of tyrosine, phenylalanine, and the branched-chain amino acids. If these are substantial, the possibility of a primary liver disease should be carefully investigated.

Some patients with defects of the urea cycle and residual enzyme activity, especially many females with OTC deficiency, display completely unremarkable values of NH_3, amino acids, and orotate in between crises. Therefore, investigating the cause of an unexplained symptomatic episode of hyperammonemia in detail even after the patient recovers is essential, even in adults or aged adults. In those instances in which the amino acids are normal, the allopurinol loading test may reveal the diagnostic direction (see Chapter 11).

The differential diagnosis of hyperammonemia also includes the HHH syndrome, which results from deficiency of the ornithine transporter in the mitochondrial membrane, and lysinuric protein intolerance. HHH signifies hyperammonemia, hyperornithinemia, and homocitrullinuria. Suspicion is usually first aroused by identifying large amounts of homocitrulline in the urine. Very low levels of lysine in the blood indicate lysinuric protein intolerance. Patients with this condition are characterized by failure to thrive; and when body stores of lysine are very depleted, the characteristic amino aciduria may not be present. It returns when the diagnosis is made and blood amino acid concentrations are brought to normal. The metabolic abnormalities become more obvious by calculating the fractional clearances of lysine and other dibasic amino acids. The concentration of citrulline in the blood may be high. Finally, symptomatic hyperammonemia may also result from a urinary tract infection in which the infecting proteus mirabilis has urease activity, which produces ammonia from urea.

WORK-UP OF THE PATIENT WITH ACUTE OR RECURRENT NEUROLOGIC OR PSYCHIATRIC FEATURES

Acute or recurrent attacks of neurologic or psychiatric symptoms, such as coma, ataxia, or abnormal behavior, are a major presenting feature of several late-onset inborn errors of metabolism. The initial diagnostic approach to these disorders is based on a few metabolic screening tests. Therefore, the biologic fluids must be collected at the same time during the acute attack. Having specimens from both before and after treatment can also be useful. Some of the most significant metabolic manifestations, such as acidosis and ketosis, may be moderate or transient, depending on symptomatic treatment. On the other hand, at an advanced state of organ dysfunction, many laboratory abnormalities (e.g., metabolic acidosis, lactic acidemia, hyperammonemia, and signs of liver failure) may be secondary consequences of hemodynamic shock. Figures 6.8, 6.9, and 6.10 present flow charts for the differential diagnosis and diagnostic approach to acute neurologic manifestations, such as ataxia and psychiatric aberrations.

Neurologic disease is the most common and important consequence of inherited metabolic diseases. The brain appears to possess restricted capabilities for repair so that even slow but continuous or repeated insults can result in lasting or progressive neurologic disease. Mental capacities are being requested at an ever-increasing level in modern human society, and even marginal insufficiencies can have a profoundly negative effect on the status and well-being of the individual.

Acute attacks of neurologic or psychiatric manifestations, such as coma, intractable seizures, ataxia, or abnormal behavior resulting from inherited metabolic diseases, require prompt and appropriate diagnostic and therapeutic measures. In an occurrence of acute metabolic cerebral edema, quick recognition and treatment is essential. Too often, physicians pursue only a diagnosis of encephalitis. Cerebral edema is observed particularly in acute hyperammonemias (most frequently OTC deficiency) or MSUD. In contrast to respiratory chain defects or organic acidurias that involve the mitochondrial metabolism of CoA-activated compounds, the metabolic block in urea cycle defects and MSUD does not directly interfere with mitochondrial energy production, and the typical signs of acute mitochondrial decompensation, such as lactic acidosis, may be lacking. They may develop later as the patient's condition deteriorates. Acute hemiplegia may be a presenting symptom; it has also been reported in patients with organic acidurias, particularly with propionic aciduria and methylmalonic aciduria, as well as in phosphoglycerate kinase deficiency.

An acute onset of extrapyramidal signs during the course of a nonspecific intercurrent illness, minor surgery, accident, or even immunizations may initially be misinterpreted as encephalitis; however, this onset is a conspicuous feature of several metabolic disorders. In glutaric aciduria type I (GA1), a dystonic dyskinetic movement disorder results from the acute destruction of the basal ganglia, specifically the striatum. The acute encephalopathic crisis in GA1 typically occurs between the ages of 6 and 18 months. Affected children may have had mild neurologic abnormalities before the acute episode; frequently they are macrocephalic. Almost half of the patients with Wilson disease present with neurologic symptoms, usually after the age of 6 years. Dysarthria, incoordination of voluntary movements, and tremor are the most common signs. Involuntary choreiform movements may also occur, and gait may be affected.

Acute strokelike episodes occur in several metabolic disorders. They are the hallmark feature of the MELAS syndrome, a disorder caused by mutations in the tRNA$^{Leu(UUR)}$ gene in the mitochondrial DNA. Eighty percent of patients carry the mutation

(*text continues on page 79*)

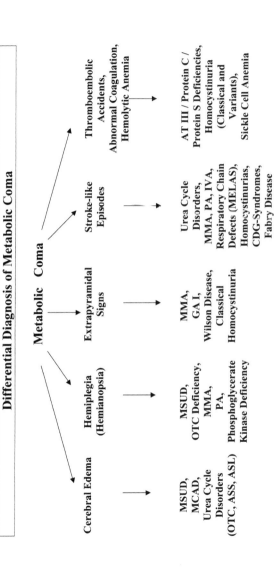

Figure 6.8.   Differential diagnosis of metabolic coma. Abbreviations: ASS, argininosuccinate synthase deficiency; ASL, argininosuccinate lyase deficiency; AT, antithrombin; CDG, carbohydrate deficient-glycoprotein; GA I, glutaric aciduria type I; IVA, isovaleric aciduria; MCAD, medium-chain acyl-CoA dehydrogenase deficiency; MELAS, mitochondrial encephalopathy, lactic acidemia, and strokelike episodes; MMA, methylmalonic aciduria; MSUD, maple syrup urine disease; OTC, ornithine transcarbamylase deficiency; PA, propionic aciduria.

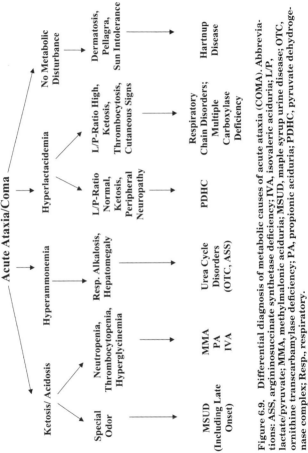

Figure 6.9. Differential diagnosis of metabolic causes of acute ataxia (COMA). Abbreviations: ASS, argininosuccinate synthetase deficiency; IVA, isovaleric aciduria; L/P, lactate/pyruvate; MMA, methylmalonic aciduria; MSUD, maple syrup urine disease; OTC, ornithine transcarbamylase deficiency; PA, propionic aciduria; PDHC, pyruvate dehydrogenase complex; Resp., respiratory.

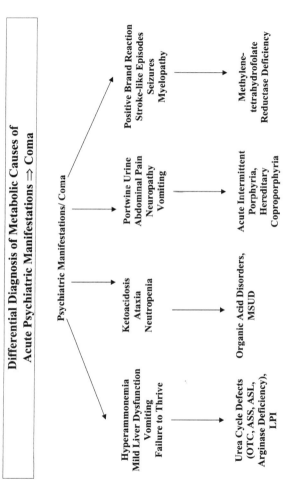

Differential Diagnosis of Metabolic Causes of Acute Psychiatric Manifestations ⇒ Coma

Psychiatric Manifestations/Coma

Hyperammonemia	Ketoacidosis	Portwine Urine	Positive Brand Reaction
Mild Liver Dysfunction	Ataxia	Abdominal Pain	Stroke-like Episodes
Vomiting	Neutropenia	Neuropathy	Seizures
Failure to Thrive		Vomiting	Myelopathy

| Urea Cycle Defects (OTC, ASS, ASL, Arginase Deficiency), LPI | Organic Acid Disorders, MSUD | Acute Intermittent Porphyria, Hereditary Coproporphyria | Methylene-tetrahydrofolate Reductase Deficiency |

Figure 6.10. Differential diagnosis of metabolic causes of acute psychiatric manifestations (COMA). Abbreviations: ASL, argininosuccinic lyase deficiency; ASS, argininosuccinate synthetase deficiency; LPI, lysinuric protein intolerance; MSUD, maple syrup urine disease; OTC, ornithine transcarbamylase deficiency.

3243A>G. Acute episodes may present initially with vomiting, headache, convulsions, or visual abnormalities and may be followed by hemiplegia or hemianopia. The morphologic correlates are true cerebral infarctions, but no evidence of vascular obstruction or atherosclerosis is seen. Strokelike episodes (metabolic stroke) are also observed in other metabolic disorders, such as the carbohydrate deficient-glycoprotein syndrome and the methylmalonic or propionic acidurias. Strokes may, of course, be absent in affected members of families with the MELAS syndrome. Some members have migrainelike headaches as the only manifestation of the disease, whereas others exhibit only diabetes or are asymptomatic. Classic cerebral strokes, as well as cardiovascular accidents, may also be caused by various metabolic disorders that cause vascular disease, such as classic homocystinuria, the thiamine-responsive megaloblastic anemia syndrome, and Fabry disease. Vascular changes resulting from altered elastic fibers are the cause of ischemic cerebral infarctions in Menkes disease. True thromboembolic events may result from defects in the anticoagulant systems, such as antithrombin III, protein C, or protein S deficiencies.

Acute ataxia and psychiatric manifestations can be the leading signs of several organic acidurias and late-onset MSUD. In these cases the metabolic derangement is most often associated with ketoacidosis. A rather confusing finding in some patients with organic acidurias is the presence of ketoacidosis combined with hyperglycemia and glycosuria, mimicking diabetic ketoacidotic coma. In the late-onset MSUD a special odor may occur, whereas in organic acidurias, such as methylmalonic aciduria, propionic aciduria, or isovaleric aciduria, moderate to severe hematologic manifestations are common. These disorders are usually characterized by neutropenia and, especially in infancy, thrombocytopenia. Recurrent infections, particularly mucocutaneous candidiasis, may be common. The diagnosis may be obtained through analyzing amino acids in plasma and organic acids in urine.

Urea cycle disorders, such as OTC deficiency, argininosuccinic aciduria, citrullinemia, arginase deficiency, or lysinuric protein intolerance, may present in childhood or adolescence with acute or recurrent episodes of hyperammonemia (see "Work-up of the Patient With Hyperammonemia," pg. 69). Clinical features may include acute ataxia or psychiatric symptoms, such as hallucinations, delirium, dizziness, aggressiveness, anxiety, or schizophrenia-like behavior. In addition, hepatomegaly, liver dysfunction, and failure to thrive may be found. The correct diagnosis will be missed unless ammonia levels in plasma are determined at the time of the acute symptoms. Hyperammonemia may be moderate or mild (150 to 250 μmol/L) even when the child is in deep coma, and the late-onset forms of urea cycle disorder, such as OTC deficiency, can easily be overlooked and misdiagnosed as schizophrenia, encephalitis, or even intoxication. Diagnostic procedures should include analyses of plasma amino acids, urinary organic acids, and orotic acid.

Mitochondrial diseases in the central nervous system manifest primarily in high-energy-consuming structures such as basal ganglia, capillary endothelium, and the cerebellum. Whereas disturbed function of the cerebellum and the basal ganglia leads to characteristic disorders of movement, disturbed capillary function results in fluctuating neurologic symptoms that range from strokelike episodes to unspecific mental deterioration and progressively accumulating damage of both gray and white matter. Acute ataxia is frequently found in association with peripheral neuropathy in patients with pyruvate dehydrogenase deficiency. Moderate or substantial elevation of lactate with a normal lactate/pyruvate ratio and the absence of ketosis supports this diagnosis. Acute ataxia associated with a high lactate/pyruvate ratio suggests multiple carboxylase deficiency or respiratory chain defects. In the latter, thrombocytosis is sometimes observed, in contrast to the thrombocytopenia associated with organic acidurias.

Finally, some inborn errors of metabolism, such as Hartnup disease, may present with clinical symptoms of recurrent acute ataxia without causing general metabolic disturbances. Typical additional symptoms, such as skin rashes, pellagra, and sun intolerance, may lead to analysis of the urinary amino acids that provides the specific diagnosis. The characteristic pattern is an excess of neutral monoamino–monocarboxylic acids in the urine with (low) normal concentrations in the plasma.

Acute intermittent porphyria and hereditary coproporphyria usually present with recurrent attacks of vomiting, abdominal pain, unspecific neuropathy, and psychiatric symptoms. These disorders must be excluded in the differential diagnosis of suspected psychogenic complaints and hysteria. Diagnosis can be made by specific analyses of porphyrins. Patients affected with disorders of the cellular methylation pathway, such as methylenetetrahydrofolate reductase deficiency, may also present with psychiatric symptoms. These often resemble acute schizophrenic episodes, but they may respond to folate therapy. Homocysteine is elevated. A positive Brand reaction may be the first abnormal laboratory finding. Other neurologic features include strokelike episodes, seizures, and myelopathy. Analyses of amino acids, especially homocysteine in plasma and CSF, provide the diagnosis. Methyltetrahydrofolate in CSF is severely reduced.

Patients with late-onset lysosomal storage disorders may present initially with psychiatric diagnoses, such as dementia, psychosis, or emotional illness. In adult-onset metachromatic leukodystrophy, psychotic changes may mirror those of schizophrenia (see Chapter 29).

EMERGENCY TREATMENT OF INHERITED METABOLIC DISEASES

Timely and correct intervention during the initial presentation of the metabolic imbalance and during later episodes precipitated by dietary indiscretion or intercurrent illness is the most important determinant of outcome in patients with inherited metabolic diseases who are at risk for acute metabolic decompensation. Patients should be supplied with an emergency card, letter, or bracelet containing instructions for emergency measures, as well as phone numbers. The specialist team should repeatedly evaluate the details of therapeutic measures with the family and the primary care physician(s).

The most critical challenge in many inherited metabolic diseases is timely and correct intervention during acute metabolic decompensation in the neonatal period or in later recurrent episodes. Fortunately, only a limited number of pathophysiologic sequences exist in the response of the infant to illness; consequently, the number of therapeutic measures is limited. Three major groups of disorders at risk for acute metabolic decompensation can be delineated and require specific therapeutic approaches in emergency situations (see Table 6.8):

- Disorders of intermediary metabolism that cause acute intoxication through the accumulation of toxic molecules;
- Disorders in which fasting tolerance is reduced;
- Disorders in which energy metabolism is disturbed.

A preliminary differentiation of these three groups should be possible with the help of basic investigations available in every hospital setting—namely, with the determination of acid–base balance, glucose, lactate, ammonia, and ketones, as discussed in previous chapters. With this information appropriate therapy can be initiated even before a precise diagnosis is made. This is especially important during the initial manifestation of a metabolic disease (i.e., when the exact diagnosis is not yet known) because therapeutic measures must be quick, vigorous, precise, and not half-hearted. Every effort must be made to obtain the relevant diagnostic information within 24 hours (e.g., results on amino acids in plasma, acylcarnitines in dried blood spots, and organic acids in urine).

In all instances provision of ample quantities of fluid and electrolytes is indispensable. Differences in the therapeutic approach relate primarily to energy requirements and methods for detoxification (Table 6.8).

Acute Intoxication

In diseases in which symptoms develop because of "acute intoxication," rapid reduction of toxic molecules is a cornerstone of treatment. In disorders of amino acid catabolism, such as MSUD, the classical organic acidurias, or the urea cycle defects, the toxic compounds are derived from exogenous, as well as endogenous, sources. After stopping the patient's intake of natural protein until the crisis is over but no longer than 48 hours, major goals of treatment are the reversal of catabolism, the promotion of anabolism, and, as a consequence, the reversal of the breakdown of endogenous protein.

In a patient known to have a disorder of amino acid catabolism who develops an intercurrent illness and subsequent manifestations of metabolic imbalance, such as ketonuria in a patient with an organic aciduria, primary emergency measures at home for 24 to 48 hours may consist of frequent feedings with a high carbohydrate content and some salt (Table 6.9) and reduction (to zero,

Table 6.8.   Emergency treatment: energy needs in infants

Disorders requiring *anabolism* (*acute intoxication*):
  60–100 kcal/kg/d
Organic acidurias, maple syrup urine disease, urea cycle disorders
  ⇒ glucose 15–20 g/kg/d
  Add fat 2 g/kg/d.
  always: Add insulin, starting with 0.05 U/kg/h.
          Adjustments are made dependent on blood glucose
          (useful combination is 1U/8g).
  early: central venous catheterization

Disorders requiring *glucose stabilization* (*reduced fasting tolerance*):
Fatty acid oxidation defects, glycogen storage disease type I,
  disorders of gluconeogenesis, galactosemia, fructose intolerance,
  tyrosinemia I
  ⇒ glucose 7–10 mg/kg/min ≈ 10 g/kg/d

Disorders requiring *restriction of energy turnover* (*disturbed energy metabolism*):
PDHC deficiency ⇒ reduce glucose supply: 2–3 mg/kg/min ≈ 3 g/kg/d
  Add fat: 2–3 g/kg/d.
Electron transport chain (Ox-Phos) abnormalities ⇒
  glucose 10–15 g/kg/d

Abbreviation: PDHC, pyruvate dehydrogenase complex.

if necessary) of the intake of natural protein. In diseases such as MSUD, the individual amino acid mixture devoid of the amino acids of the defective pathway should be continued. Detoxifying medication (e.g., carnitine in the organic acidurias; benzoate, phenylacetate, and arginine or citrulline in the hyperammonemias) should be employed. Admission to the hospital is mandatory if the intercurrent illness continues into the third day, if symptoms worsen, or if vomiting compromises external feedings.

In the hospital, therapy must be continued without interruption. In most instances an intravenous line is essential, but nasogastric administration of amino acid mixtures in MSUD can be very useful. Early placement of a gastrostomy greatly simplifies the management of many of these patients when in infancy. This can usually be discontinued after infancy.

High amounts of energy are needed to achieve anabolism (e.g., in neonates > 100 kcal/kg of body weight per day). In a sick baby this can usually be accomplished only by hyperosmolaric infusions of glucose together with fat through a central venous line. Insulin should be started early, especially in the presence of significant ketosis or in MSUD, to enhance anabolism and to prevent hyperglycemia. One approach uses a fixed combination of insulin to glucose (Table 6.8). Intravenous lipids can often be increased to 3 g/kg when serum levels of triglycerides are monitored.

Table 6.9.   Oral administration of fluid and energy for episodic acute intercurrent illness in patients with metabolic disorders

Age (years)	Glucose polymer/maltodextrin solution		
	(%)	(kcal/100 mL)	Daily amount(mL)
0–1	10	40	150–200 /kg
1–2	15	60	95 /kg
2–6	20	80	1,200–1,500
6–10	20	80	1,500–2,000
> 10	25	100	2,000

Adapted from Dixon MA, Leonard JV. Intercurrent illness in inborn errors of intermediary metabolism. *Arch Dis Child* 1992;67:1387–1391. Oral substitution should only be given during minor intercurrent illnesses and for a limited time of two to three days. The intake of some salt should also be provided. The actual amounts given have to be individually adjusted, e.g. according to a reduced body weight in an older patient with failure to thrive.

Acute episodes of massive ketoacidosis, as seen in methylmalonic or propionic aciduria, require especially vigorous supportive therapy. Large amounts of water, electrolytes, and bicarbonate and high doses of intravenous carnitine must be infused with glucose. In such instances, blood concentrations of electrolytes and bicarbonate are determined and an intravenous infusion is started before taking the time to do a history and physical examination. Following a bolus of 20 mL/kg of ringer lactate or normal saline, intravenous (IV) fluid should contain 75 to 150 mEq/L of isotonic $NaHCO_3$ (75 with massive ketosis; 150, if in coma or HCO_3^- is less than 10 mEq/L). Carnitine supplementation should be given intravenously at 300 mg/kg. Electrolytes and acid–base balance must be checked every 6 hours. Serum sodium should be ≥ 138 mmol/L. The $NaHCO_3$ content of the infusion is reduced after the serum HCO_3^- has become normal, but the same rate of infusion is continued until the ketonuria has subsided. Some children with these disorders benefit from implantation of a venous port to facilitate blood sampling and intravenous infusions.

Forced diuresis with large amounts of fluids and furosemide is successful with the methylmalonic acidurias for removing methylmalonate from the body.

Detoxification in the organic acidurias depends on the ability to form esters, such as propionylcarnitine, which are preferentially excreted in the urine, thus removing toxic intermediates. In these disorders tissue stores of carnitine are depleted. Carnitine is given to restore tissue supply, but its major utility is to promote detoxification by the formation and excretion of carnitine esters. It should be administered intravenously in doses of 200 to 300 mg/kg as it is less well tolerated enterally. Oral doses of > 100 mg/kg can be employed, but for some patients the dose may have to be reduced.

In isovaleric aciduria, adding glycine to the regimen is useful to promote the excretion of isovalerylglycine (500 mg/kg).

In MSUD the major element of therapy is harnessing the forces of anabolism to lay down accumulated leucine and other branched-chain amino acids into protein. This is done by providing mixtures of amino acids that lack leucine, isoleucine, and valine. The use of intravenous mixtures is very efficient and is essential for a patient with intractable vomiting. However, these are expensive and are not generally available. Enteral mixtures are mixed in a minimal volume of fluid and can be dripped over 24 hours in doses of 2 g/kg of amino acids. Often even a vomiting patient will tolerate a slow drip. Since concentrations of isoleucine are much lower than those of leucine, the concentrations of amino acids must be measured frequently. When the concentrations of isoleucine become low, isoleucine must be added to the enteral mixture. In many patients valine must also be added before the leucine concentration is lowered adequately.

The pharmacologic approach to the detoxification of ammonia in the urea cycle defects and in those organic acidurias that present with hyperammonemia is to provide the patient with alternative methods of waste nitrogen excretion (Fig. 6.11). Benzoate is effectively conjugated with glycine to form hippurate, which is excreted in the urine. Similarly, phenylacetate conjugates with glutamine to form phenylacetylglutamine, which also can be efficiently excreted. Administered orally, phenylbutyrate is converted to phenylacetate. In a metabolic emergency with an unknown diagnosis and a documented hyperammonemia ≥ 200 µmol/L (350 µg/dL) and in relapses of known patients, benzoate and phenylacetate–phenylbutyrate should be given intravenously (Table 6.10) with

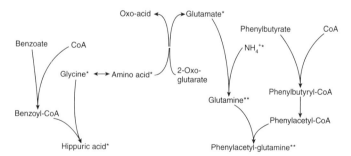

Figure 6.11.   Pharmacologic detoxification of ammonia. The asterisks represent nitrogen. Conjugation of glycine with benzoate yields hippuric acid, and conjugation of phenylacetate with glutamine results in phenylacetylglutamine as the excretable end products. Consequently, one nitrogen is excreted with each molecule of hippuric acid and two, with phenylacetateglytamine.

Table 6.10. Emergency treatment of hyperammonemic crises

Drug	Loading dose over 1 to 2 hours	Intravenous daily dose	Preparation
Na-benzoate	250 mg/kg	250(–500) mg/kg	1g in 50 mL 5% to 10% glucose
Na-phenylacetate[a]	250 mg/kg	250(–600) mg/kg	1g in 50 mL 5% to 10% glucose
L-arginine	250 mg/kg	250 mg/kg in OTC, CPS, and in as yet unknown disease; 500 mg/kg in ASS, ASL	1 g in 50 mL 5% to 10% glucose
Folic acid		0.1 mg/kg q.d.	
Pyridoxine		5 mg q.d.	

Abbreviations: ASL, argininsuccinate lyase deficiency; ASS, argininosuccinate synthetase deficiency; CPS, carbamylphosphate synthetase deficiency; OTC, ornithine transcarbamylase deficiency.
[a] In a known patient, who is not vomiting, employing oral or gastric Na-phenylbutyrate may be possible.

arginine. During combined intravenous supplementation of benzoate and phenylacetate, electrolytes must be checked regularly to avoid hypernatremia. Four hundred milligrams of sodium benzoate correspond to 2.77 mmol and therefore to 2.77 mmol of sodium. In milder episodes enteral phenylbutyrate or benzoate along with arginine may be adequate for detoxification. In urea cycle defects carnitine administration is also recommended (50 to 100 mg/kg). Zofran (0.15 mg/kg IV) appears to be especially effective against hyperemesis, which can accompany hyperammonemia.

Hyperammonemias may require extracorporal dialysis for detoxification. This should be considered with ammonia levels of more than 600 μmol/L (1,000 μg/dL). Hemodialysis has been repeatedly shown to be more effective than exchange transfusions, peritoneal dialysis, or arteriovenous hemofiltration. This supports arguments for the transport of such an infant to an appropriate facility, if the necessary logistics cannot be promptly organized locally.

In aminoacidopathies other than MSUD (i.e., phenylketonuria, the homocystinurias, or the tyrosinemias), the toxic metabolites lead primarily to chronic organ damage rather than to a metabolic emergency. Hepatorenal tyrosinemia may lead to a crisis of hepatic insufficiency. The rationale and principles of therapy remain the same as those described earlier in the metabolic emergencies, but hypercaloric treatment through central catheters is seldom indicated. Glucose should be administered with fat in accordance with endogenous glucose production rates. Oral therapy, including medication and the appropriate amino acid mixture, should be resumed as soon as possible. Patients with tyrosinemia type I should be treated with 2-(2-nitro-4-trifluoromethyl-benzoyl)-1, 3-cyclohexanedione (NTBC) as soon as possible. NTBC is a potent inhibitor of p-hydroxyphenylpyruvate dioxygenase; it blocks the genesis of the highly toxic fumarylacetoacetate and its derivatives (see Chapter 16).

In patients with galactosemia or fructose intolerance, toxic metabolites derive predominantly from exogenous sources. Once the diagnosis is suspected or made, therapy consists of the elimination of the intake of galactose or fructose respectively. However, if intravenous alimentation devoid of galactose and fructose is begun without suspicion of the underlying metabolic disorder, gradual reintroduction of oral feeding leads to protracted disease courses with varying and complicated symptoms until the diagnosis is made. Patients with galactosemia or fructose intolerance require energy to stabilize and maintain blood glucose.

Reduced Fasting Tolerance

Patients with defects of fatty acid oxidation and gluconeogenesis, such as medium-chain acyl-CoA dehydrogenase deficiency and glycogen storage disease type I, require vigorous administration of glucose in amounts sufficient for restoring and maintaining euglycemia. Frequent monitoring of blood glucose is essential if symptomatic hypoglycemia is to be avoided. The patient who is seen first in an emergency room following a convulsion and who is found to have little or no measurable glucose in the blood is usually treated first with enough hypertonic glucose to restore euglycemia. This can be followed with an infusion of 5% glucose and water, but glucose levels should be monitored and the concentration promptly changed to 10% or higher as required to keep the sugar elevated.

Supplementation of carnitine in suspected or proven defects of fatty acid oxidation currently is controversial. At a minimum, the restoration of levels of free carnitine is certainly indicated—100 mg/kg is adequate. Disorders of carbohydrate metabolism do not need detoxifying treatment.

The best long-term management of patients with disorders of fatty acid oxidation includes the avoidance of fasting. Diagnosed patients should have written instructions indicating that, if anorexia or vomiting precludes oral intake, the patient must be admitted to the hospital for the intravenous administration of glucose. Supplemental cornstarch is a useful adjunct to chronic therapy in disorders of carbohydrate metabolism and of fatty acid oxidation.

Disturbed Energy Metabolism

The "disorders of disturbed energy metabolism" include defects of PDHC, the Krebs cycle, and the respiratory electron transport chain. Chronic multisystem disease characterizes these disorders, rather than acute metabolic emergency. The occasional occurrence of life-threatening acidosis, ketoacidosis, and lactic acidemia calls for emergency treatment. Therapy in this situation necessitates vigorous treatment of the acid–base balance. Patients with PDHC deficiency are glucose-sensitive, and glucose infusions can result in a further increase in lactate. In fact, testing all patients with lactic acidemia for the lactate response to glucose is advisable. In sensitive patients intravenous glucose should be employed at rates well below the rate of endogenous glucose production (see Table 6.6). The correction of metabolic acidosis may require high amounts of sodium bicarbonate. In up to 20% of children with mitochondrial disease, the acute decompensation may be complicated by renal tubular acidosis; this may increase the requirement for sodium bicarbonate. Regardless of the cause, levels of lactate can be lowered by dialysis or by the administration of dichloroacetate. Dichloroacetate activates the pyruvate dehydrogenase complex in the brain, liver, and muscle. Although levels of lactate have been shown to improve, the overall outcome may not be altered.

In patients with mitochondrial disease, replacement of cofactors is common. Evidence in support of this is derived from the positive response to biotin in multiple carboxylase deficiency and to riboflavin in some patients with multiple acyl-CoA dehydrogenase deficiency. The prescription of a combination of coenzyme Q_{10}, vitamin E, and a balanced B-vitamin supplement called B_{50} is common. B_{50} contains a combination of thiamine, riboflavin, niacin, pyridoxine, biotin, folate, B_{12}, and pantothenic acid. If a measured deficiency in blood carnitine is found or if urinary excretion of carnitine esters is high, the patient should be treated with L-carnitine.

The ultimate goal of therapy is not simply the reversal of the metabolic emergency but the prevention of irreversible damage to the patient's brain. The diseases leading to acute intoxication, such as MSUD, the classic organic acidurias, and the urea cycle defects, carry the greatest risk of major sequelae. Additional supportive therapeutic measures are used informally in some centers to enhance achievement of this goal. These measures include mannitol for the treatment of cerebral edema, which may also enhance detoxification through increased diuresis. Increased intracranial pressure may be monitored neurosurgically. Overall supportive care, paying particular vigilance to the detection and prompt treatment of infection, is critical in patients in intensive care units.

In summary, the metabolic emergency calls for prompt diagnosis and therapeutic measures that follow the principles of adequate energy supply, the promotion of anabolism, and the use of pharmacologic and, as necessary, extracorporal detoxification. These measures are the determinants of success in handling the metabolic emergencies arising from inborn errors of metabolism.

ADDITIONAL READINGS

Ballard RA, Vinocur B, Reynolds JW, et al. Transient hyperammonemia of the preterm infant. *N Engl J Med* 1978;299:920–925.

Batshaw ML, Bachmann C, Tuchmann M, eds. Advances in inherited urea cycle disorders. *J Inher Metab Dis* 1998;21(Suppl 1):1–159.

Brusilow SW, Maestri NE. Urea cycle disorders: diagnosis, pathophysiology, and treatment. *Adv Pediatr* 1996;46:127–170.

Cornblath M, Schwartz R. *Disorders of carbohydrate metabolism in infancy.* Philadelphia: WB Saunders; 1976.

DiMauro S, Hirano M, Bonilla E, et al. The mitochondrial disorders. In: Berg BO, ed. *Principles of child neurology.* New York: McGraw-Hill; 1996:1201–1232.

Dixon MA, Leonard JV. Intercurrent illness in inborn errors of intermediary metabolism. *Arch Dis Child* 1992;67:1387–1391.

Nyhan WL, Ozand PA. *Atlas of metabolic diseases.* London: Chapman & Hall; 1998:168–177; 259–374.

Nyhan WL, Rice-Kelts M, Klein J, et al. Treatment of the acute crisis in maple syrup urine disease. *Arch Pediatr Adolesc Med* 1999;152: 593–598.

Ogier de Baulny H, Saudubray JM. Emergency treatment. In: Fernandes J, Saudubray JM, Van den Berghe G, eds. *Inborn metabolic diseases,* 3rd ed. Heidelberg: Springer; 2000:53–61.

Orho M, Bosshard NW, Buist NRM, et al. Mutations in the liver glycogen synthase gene in children with hypoglycemia due to glyocogen storage disease type 0. *J Clin Invest* 1998;102:507–515.

Saudubray JM, Martin D, de Lonlay P, et al. Recognition and management of fatty acid oxidation defects: a series of 107 patients. *J Inher Metab Dis* 1999;22:488–502.

Thoene JG. Treatment of urea cycle disorders. *J Pediatr* 1999;134: 255–256.

Wander RJA, Vreken P, den Boer MEJ, et al. Disorders of mitochondrial fatty acyl-CoA β-oxidation. *J Inher Metab Dis* 1999;22:442–487.

7 ♣ Anesthesia and Metabolic Disease

Special considerations for anesthesia and surgery were dramatized by the recognition nearly 50 years ago that genetically determined variants in *butyrylcholinesterase*, the cholinesterase found in serum, prolong the action of *succinylcholine*, the agent used in surgery to relax muscles. Patients with deficient activity of this enzyme remain paralyzed and unable to breathe long after the conclusion of surgery. Testing for these variants, of which a number exist, is done spectrophotometrically in the presence of the inhibitor dibucaine; the percentage of inhibition is called the *dibucaine number*. Management of the patient with this problem simply consists of continuing assisted ventilation until the succinylcholine is broken down. All carboxylic acid esters ultimately are hydrolyzed despite the absence of specific esterase activity.

MUCOPOLYSACCHARIDOSES

The great risk of anesthesia for patients with mucopolysaccharidosis results from instability of the atlantoaxial joint. This is a particular problem in Morquio disease, but patients with mucopolysaccharidosis (MPS) II and VI are also at risk. Deaths as complications of anesthesia have been recorded. For patients with MPS, careful positioning is required and hyperextension of the neck must be avoided. These patients should undergo general anesthesia only in centers in which anesthesiologists have experience with these diseases.

In preparation for surgery, the patient or his or her parents should be asked about previous problems with anesthesia, obstructive sleep apnea, or transient paralysis that might be an index of cervical instability. The physician should examine the patient for evidence of cord compression kyphoscoliosis and excessive upper respiratory secretions. The blood pressure should be determined, and an electrocardiogram (EKG) and echocardiogram should be done. Recent roentgenograms of the chest and the cervical spine should be reviewed. Those with kyphoscoliosis should have pulmonary function studies. Sleep studies may also be useful. Those with evidence or history of cord compression should have a magnetic resonance image of the spine performed.

Intubation and induction of anesthesia may be difficult because of limited space; therefore, smaller tubes than usual may be required. Visualization may be limited by macroglossia, micrognathia, and immobility of the neck. Immobilizing the neck with a halo brace or plaster to avoid damage to the cervical cord may be necessary. Thick secretions may lead to postoperative pulmonary problems. Recovery from anesthesia may be slow, and postoperative obstruction of the airway sometimes occurs. Whenever possible, local anesthesia is preferable. In young or uncooperative patients, however, such as those with Hunter or Sanfilippo syndromes, this may be impossible. General anesthesia is preferable to sedation, because of the need to control the airway.

RHABDOMYOLYSIS AND MYOGLOBINURIA IN DISORDERS OF FATTY ACID OXIDATION

General anesthesia and the stress of surgery have each been thought responsible for the acute breakdown of muscle that has been observed in patients with abnormalities of fatty acid oxidation. These triggers of acute attack are particularly notable with the myopathic form of carnitine palmitoyl transferase (CPT) II deficiency. However, they may do the same in any disorder of fatty acid oxidation, especially long-chain hydroxyacyl-CoA dehydrogenase (LCHAD) deficiency (see Chapter 6). Renal failure is a complication of myoglobinuria. The best answer is to precede anesthesia and surgery in these patients with an ample supply of glucose and water and the avoidance of fasting. This is accomplished by early placement of an intravenous line so that the patient is fasting no more than 6 hours. In the presence of myoglobinuria, intravenous glucose should be 10% or higher; adjunctive insulin may help to maintain euglycemia.

Surgery and anesthesia may also induce a metabolic crisis in Refsum disease via mobilization of phytanic acid in fat stores. The same preventive approaches apply.

AVOIDANCE OF HYPOGLYCEMIA

Patients with many metabolic diseases are at risk for developing hypoglycemia. For these patients the usual fasting before general anesthesia and surgery can be disastrous. The objective of management is the maintenance of euglycemia, a concentration of glucose in the blood above 4 mmol/L. Relevant disorders include the disorders of fatty acid oxidation (see Chapter 6), glycogen storage diseases, disorders of gluconeogenesis (e.g., fructose 1,6-diphosphatase deficiency), hyperinsulinism, and ketotic hypoglycemia (see Chapter 6). In each instance the patient's history and tolerance of fasting should be investigated before making plans for surgery. Most patients with disorders of fatty acid oxidation do not become hypoglycemic until they have fasted more than 12 hours, whereas some patients with glycogenosis or hyperinsulinism cannot tolerate a 4-hour fast.

Patients undergoing short or minor procedures can be scheduled for noon or later and should be given glucose. Patients receiving overnight nasogastric glucose should have intravenous glucose dispensed before the nasogastric administration is discontinued. Every patient should be receiving 10% glucose intravenously well before the time that hypoglycemia would be expected to begin; intravenous glucose should be discontinued only after the patient has demonstrated an ability to eat and retain sources of oral sugar. The canula should not be removed until the possibility of vomiting has been excluded. In general, 10% glucose should be employed at rates approximating 2,500 mL/m^2/24 hours. This would be equivalent to 150 mL/kg in infants under 1 year of age; 100 mL/kg between the ages of 1 to 2 years; 1,200 to 1,500 mL for 2 to 6 years of age; and 1,500 to 2,000 mL over the age of 6 years. Rates must be readjusted on the basis of determined levels of glucose in the blood.

ORGANIC ACIDURIAS: MAPLE SYRUP URINE DISEASE

The objective in the management of anesthesia and surgery in patients with organic aciduria is the minimization of catabolism. This objective is met best by avoiding anesthesia and surgery, if at all possible, until the patient is in an optimal metabolic state and is well over any infections. In preparation for the procedure, metabolic balance should be ascertained by checking the urine for ketones and the blood for ammonia, pH, electrolytes, and, in the case of maple syrup urine disease (MSUD), the plasma concentrations of amino acids. The administration of glucose and water in the regimen employed for hypoglycemia minimizes catabolism. In MSUD, a dose of the amino acid supplement, either one-third of the patient's daily dose or at least 0.25 g/kg, should be given as late before anesthesia as is feasible. Intravenous preparations of amino acids designed for the treatment of MSUD would be ideal at this point. Following the conclusion of the procedure, intravenous glucose should be continued until the oral administration is clearly feasible and the electrolytes are stable. A patient with MSUD may be maintained for a while with intravenous amino acids or, in their absence, with a nasogastric drip of amino acids; blood concentrations of amino acids should be monitored.

UREA CYCLE DEFECTS

In disorders of the urea cycle, the objective of care is to avoid hyperammonemia by minimizing catabolism. The approach is the same as that outlined for organic acidurias, except that the ammonia is the substance that must be carefully monitored.

In addition, patients whose usual medication includes arginine or citrulline should be given intravenous arginine. The patient's usual dose is employed, diluted 2.5 g per 50 mL of 10% glucose, and should be piggybacked via syringe pump to the glucose infusion. In patients receiving sodium benzoate, phenylbutyrate, or both, the intravenous mixture of benzoate-phenylacetate is employed in a dilution of at least 2.5 g of each per 50 mL, as before, and is given by piggyback pump. For short procedures, these medications can be started in the postoperative period. For a longer procedure, for one that is particularly likely to induce catabolism, and certainly in the presence of hyperammonemia, they can be given intraoperatively.

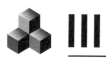

III

Investigations for Metabolic Disease

8 ♣ Biochemical Studies

Most known metabolic disorders are recognized through biochemical analyses of body fluids, predominantly blood and urine. The concentrations of physiologic metabolites in plasma or serum are usually tightly controlled, and therefore elevations or reductions of specific substances may be diagnostically relevant. Normal values for many compounds of intermediary metabolism depend on the metabolic state at the time of sampling, so adequate interpretation makes knowing whether the individual was fasting, postprandial, or postexercise crucial. Some disorders may be recognized only through specific function tests that change metabolic conditions or that expose the patient to high concentrations of specific substrates (see Chapter 11). However, some function tests may cause the accumulation of harmful substances in patients and can result in life-threatening complications. These tests should only be carried out after less dangerous diagnostic options have been exhausted.

Many inborn errors of metabolism cause the accumulation of substrates that are metabolized via alternative pathways and removed through urinary excretion. Investigations of the urine for such disorders are simpler and more sensitive than are plasma–serum analyses. Metabolite concentrations are usually measured relative to urinary creatinine levels to account for differences in fluid intake and urinary dilution. Urine analyses are also often less dependent on changes in nutrition and metabolic state as the collected urine is produced over a period of time; in addition, massive differences between normal and pathologic values can generally be recognized at all times. A spontaneous urine sample, preferably obtained in the morning when the urine is more concentrated, is sufficient for most analyses. Important exceptions are the fatty acid oxidation disorders, which frequently show urinary abnormalities only under fasting conditions or after loading with fatty acids.

Laboratory investigations for inborn errors of metabolism are often complicated and are prone to technical problems, and the interpretation of results may be difficult. To maintain acceptable standards, laboratories that perform biochemical investigations for inborn errors of metabolism should process a sufficiently high volume of samples and should participate in quality assessment schemes. National or international platforms for various metabolic tests have been established for such screens, including amino acids and organic acid analyses (e.g., European Research Network for evaluation and improvement of screening, Diagnosis and treatment of Inherited Disorders of Metabolism [ERNDIM] in Europe, College of American Pathologists [CAP] in the United States). Participation is often voluntary, so inquiring about whether the respective laboratory participates in such a program may be advisable. Adequate interpretation of the results generally requires knowledge of the clinical problems in the respective patient and a good understanding of metabolic disorders so that one can assess whether mild biochemical abnormalities are diagnostically relevant. Many commercial laboratories do not offer such specialist advice. Therefore, sending samples to an experienced specialist metabolic laboratory may be more cost-effective.

SIMPLE METABOLIC URINE TESTS

A number of simple tests that may be carried out in nonspecialized hospitals or at the bedside and that may provide important first clues for the diagnosis of metabolic disorders are available.

Sulfite Test

Method: Commercially available dipstick (e.g., Merckoquant 10013, Merck Darmstadt, Germany); fresh urine

The sulfite test recognizes increased concentrations of sulfite in the urine, which may be a marker of primary deficiencies of the enzyme sulfite oxidase or its cofactor molybdenum. Children affected with one of these disorders typically suffer from severe epileptic encephalopathy, which usually starts in the neonatal period or infancy. Testing for urinary sulfite should be a component of baseline investigations in any child with unexplained psychomotor delay, particularly when combined with severe epilepsy. The test may give a false negative if old urine samples are used. False-positive results may result from various drugs and other conditions that cause increased urinary sulfite concentrations.

DNPH Test

Method: Mix 0.5 mL urine with 0.5 mL 0.2% dinitrophenyl-hydrazine (DNPH) solution.

DNPH reacts with 2-oxoacids, such as the branched-chain oxoacids. After 5 minutes the mixture is observed for precipitate. A slight clouding may indicate a trace of 2-oxoacids. A heavy precipitate that is yellow, orange, or red indicates a positive result. The DNPH test may be used to diagnose maple syrup urine disease in a neonate with metabolic decompensation. As DNPH also reacts with physiologic ketone bodies, removing them through heating of the urine to be tested may be necessary. Another cause for a false-positive result may be glucosuria, which may also be suspected if the test for reducing substances in urine (see later) is positive.

Reducing Substances In Urine

Method: Commercially available test tablets (e.g., Clinitest, Bayer, Leverkusen, Germany)

Many disorders cause the urinary excretion of sugars and other reducing substances; Table 8.1 lists them. This excretion is easily recognized with commercially available test tablets that change from yellow to red in the presence of reducing substances.

Nitroprusside Test (Brand Reaction)

Method: Add 200 μL 5% Na cyanide to 0.5 mL urine. After 10 min add 20 μL of a saturated solution of Na nitroprusside. Mix and immediately assess the color.

Usually, the sample color is orange or bright red. A dark cherry-red or red-purple color indicates the presence of sulfur-containing

Table 8.1. Reducing substances in the urine

Substance	Disorder/origin
Galactose	Classical galactosemia, galactokinase deficiency, severe liver disease (secondary galactose intolerance)
Fructose	Fructose intolerance, essential fructosuria
4-OH-Phenylpyruvate	Tyrosinemia types I and II
Homogentisic acid	Alcaptonuria
Xylose	Pentosuria
Glucose	Diabetes mellitus, Fanconi syndrome
Oxalic acid	Hyperoxaluria
Salicylates, ascorbic acid	Drugs
Uric acid	Hyperuricosuria
Hippuric acid	Therapy of hyperammonemia with Na benzoate

acids, particularly disulfides (see Table 8.2). This may indicate homocystinuria, cystinuria, or another metabolic disorder but more frequently is caused by various drugs that contain sulfur groups. Strongly positive ketones can result in a false-positive Brand test. The test should only be conducted in a laboratory, as Na cyanide is very toxic.

An alternative method employs reduction of disulfides by nascent hydrogen, produced by reaction of HCl with Zn. Cysteine and homocysteine then react with nitroprusside to form a stable magenta ring on contact with ammonium hydroxide in sucrose.

AMINO ACIDS

Amino acids play an essential role in intermediary metabolism, not only as the building blocks of proteins but also as part of vari-

Table 8.2. Causes of a positive nitroprusside test

Substance	Disorder/origin
Cystine	Cystinuria, hyperargininemia, generalized hyperaminoaciduria
Homocystine	Classical homocystinuria, cobalamin deficiencies, cystathioninuria (bacteria in urinary tract infections)
Glutathione	Disorders of the gamma-glutamyl cycle
Drugs	N-Acetylcysteine, penicillamine, captopril, ampicillin, and others

ous other metabolic functions, such as cytosolic methylation reactions and neurotransmission. A wide range of genetic disorders either directly or indirectly affects amino acid metabolism; these disorders can be recognized through the analysis of the appropriate body fluid for amino acids.

Plasma

Sample: 1 to 2 mL ethylene diamine tetraacetate (EDTA) blood. Separate the plasma immediately and send on dry ice, if possible. Use a taxi in emergencies.

Quantitative amino acid analysis in plasma (or serum) by ion exchange chromatography or high-pressure liquid chromatography (HPLC) provides direct information on changes in amino acid homeostasis; therefore, it is one of the basic investigations indicated in most patients with a suspected metabolic disorder. Emergency analysis should be performed in patients with hyperammonemia or an acute presentation of a suspected aminoacidopathy. In such cases, samples should be sent promptly and the results should be available within a few hours. Regular (fasting) amino acid analyses are also required for patients on protein restriction or a specific metabolic dietary therapy to adjust amino acid intake and to recognize a deficiency of essential amino acids. Many amino acids can also be quantitated reliably in dried blood spots (Guthrie cards) by electrospray tandem mass spectroscopy (MS-MS) or fast atom bombardment MS. For some disorders, such as phenylketonuria and maple syrup urine disease, this test is an excellent alternative to classic chromatographic methods because it avoids a venepuncture in the patient.

Plasma amino acid concentrations are highly dependent on the metabolic status, so standard samples should be obtained 4 to 6 hours after the last meal. In addition, measuring amino acids in postprandial (and fasting) samples, particularly when a disorder of energy metabolism is suspected, is often useful. For postprandial analyses, giving a defined meal is advised so that standardized substrate intake (see Chapter 11, "Preprandial and Postprandial Analyses") is achieved. Postprandial samples show high levels of the essential amino acids; an excessive rise of alanine indicates an impairment of pyruvate metabolism and may point toward a mitochondrial disorder. In general, fasting leads to an elevation of the branched-chain amino acids; most other amino acids are low.

For optimal results separation of plasma and serum should be done as soon as possible after the sample has been taken, and samples should be shipped frozen on dry ice. Hemolysis or the shipment of whole blood results in useless values for some amino acids, either through the action of erythrocyte enzymes, such as arginase (which converts arginine to ornithine), or through greater concentrations of amino acids in blood cells (e.g., liberation of taurine from platelets). Exact arginine concentrations, for example, are essential for diagnosis and monitoring of treatment of urea cycle defects. Even after prompt separation of plasma or serum, shipment at ambient temperature results in unreliable values for glutamate and aspartate (both artificially elevated), glutamine, asparagine, cysteine, and homocysteine (reduced), among others. The concentrations of some amino acids, including phenylalanine, tyrosine, and the branched-chain amino acids (valine, isoleucine, leucine), are minimally affected by overnight shipment of plasma or serum at ambient temperature, which may be adequate for treatment control in some disorders, such as phenylketonuria and some other aminoacidopathies.

Some amino acids, notably homocysteine and tryptophan, require specific (usually HPLC) methods for exact quantification. The measurement of total homocysteine is essential for the evaluation of hyperhomocysteinemias. To obtain reliable results when samples are to be stored or sent to the laboratory, centrifuging the blood sample immediately and freezing the plasma, which should be shipped on dry ice, is necessary. In the laboratory, homocysteine is released from disulfide bonds through the addition of a reducing agent, and the total concentration is determined. Normal values of total homocysteine (fasting) in children less than 10 years of age are 3.5 to 9 µmol/L; more than 10 years, 4.5 to 11 µmol/L; premenopausal women, 6 to 15 µmol/L; postmenopausal women, 6 to 19 µmol/L; men, 8 to 18 µmol/L.

Urine

Sample: Minimum 10 mL urine; preserve with two drops of chloroform. Sample may be sent overnight at ambient temperature; a taxi should be used in emergencies.

Amino acid analysis in urine is usually less helpful than in plasma since amino acids are normally reabsorbed in the renal tubules; therefore, subtle to moderate changes in amino acid homeostasis cannot be recognized through urine analysis. Two different methods are available—standard quantitative analysis and qualitative assessment by thin-layer or paper chromatography. The qualitative analysis, which is relatively inexpensive, provides information on renal tubular function and can identify several aminoacidopathies; it is therefore often used as part of routine selective screening for metabolic disease. Quantitative urinary amino acid analysis is indicated when a renal tubular reabsorption defect, such as cystinuria, is suspected and should be used with plasma analysis in hyperammonemia when increased urinary excretion of specific amino acids (e.g., argininosuccinate) may be diagnostic for certain urea cycle defects.

Cerebrospinal Fluid

Sample: 1 mL cerebrospinal fluid (CSF); freeze immediately. The sample is sent on dry ice with a plasma sample obtained at the time of the lumbar puncture.

Amino acid analysis in CSF is indicated for patients with a suspected neurometabolic disorder, particularly in severe (neonatal) epileptic encephalopathy. (See also "Specialized CSF and Urine Analyses for Neurometabolic Disorders" later in this chapter.) Obtaining a concurrent plasma sample for amino acid analysis is important as calculation of the plasma/CSF ratio of specific amino acids may be required to diagnose some disorders, such as nonketotic hyperglycinemia (ratio of glycine in CSF to plasma > 0.06) and the serine biosynthesis defects (ratio of serine in CSF to plasma < 0.2). Elevations of the CSF-to-plasma ratio of glycine are, however, only meaningful in the presence of elevated levels, at least in the CSF. If plasma glycine is abnormally low, an isolated elevation of the CSF-to-plasma ratio caused by a normal CSF glycine does not indicate nonketotic hyperglycinemia. Also, the interpretation of CSF amino acid concentrations outside the norm is more reliable if concurrent plasma concentrations are available. Heavily blood-stained CSF samples are unusable; slightly blood-stained ones should be centrifuged immediately and the supernatant should be frozen for analysis (notify the laboratory!). Immediate deep-freezing and special analytical methods are required to determine free and total gamma-aminobutyrate (GABA).

ORGANIC ACIDS
Samples:
Urine: Minimum 10 mL random (morning) urine; preserve with two to three drops of chloroform. Sample may be sent overnight at ambient temperature; a taxi should be used in emergencies.

Plasma, CSF, vitreous fluid (only limited, specific indications): Minimum 1 mL; freeze immediately and send on dry ice.

Urinary organic acid analysis by gas chromatography–mass spectroscopy (GC-MS) provides information on a wide range of metabolic pathways and is therefore one of the main methods for selective metabolic screening. Beyond the classic organic acidurias, it is an important part of the diagnostic work-up for patients with suspected aminoacidopathies, fatty acid oxidation defects, or disorders of mitochondrial energy metabolism. Organic acid analysis should be performed in any child with clinical features of systemic intoxication, unexplained metabolic crisis, or unexplained laboratory findings of disturbed intermediary metabolism, such as metabolic acidosis, elevated lactate, high anion gap, hypoglycemia, ketonemia, neonatal ketonuria, or hyperammonemia. In addition, urinary organic acid should be analyzed in children with unclear hepatopathy or neurologic or neuromuscular symptoms, including epileptic encephalopathy, and in children with obvious multisystem disorders, particularly when the symptoms are progressive or fluctuate.

Organic acids are best analyzed in urine as they are usually well excreted via the kidneys and show much higher concentrations in urine than in other body fluids. Nevertheless, the exact quantitation of specific organic acids in plasma or CSF with isotope dilution assays may be useful in exceptional cases for the exclusion of certain disorders or the control of therapy. Examples include glutaric aciduria type I (glutaric acid and 3-hydroxyglutaric acid), cobalamin defects (methylmalonic acid), tyrosinemia type I (succinylacetone), and various cerebral organic acidurias, such as succinate semialdehyde dehydrogenase (SSADH) deficiency (4-hydroxybutyric acid) and Canavan disease (*N*-acetylaspartic acid). Stable isotope dilution assays constitute the method of choice for prenatal diagnoses. For postmortem investigations, urine should be obtained through a bladder puncture or washout; organic acid analysis in plasma, CSF, or vitreous fluid is much less informative.

ACYLCARNITINE PROFILE

Sample: Three to six dried blood spots on filter paper (Guthrie card); can be sent via normal mail. A taxi should be used in emergencies.

The analysis of the acylcarnitine spectrum in dried blood spots by MS-MS or fast atom bombardment MS allows the reliable diagnosis of most organic acidurias and fatty acid oxidation defects and is increasingly used for neonatal screening in North America and Europe. In addition, it can be employed as the primary emergency investigation in children with acute metabolic crises or hypoglycemia because it is faster than standard organic acid analysis for diagnosing classical organic acidurias and it more reliably identifies fatty acid oxidation defects. Furthermore, concentrations of many, but not all, relevant amino acids, as well as of orotic acid, that are required in a metabolic emergency of unknown cause can be quantified simultaneously by the same technique. Quantification of total and free carnitine by MS-MS from Guthrie cards is not accurate; measurement of this requires specific analysis of plasma or serum (carnitine status).

CARNITINE STATUS

Sample: 1 mL serum/plasma, ± 5 mL urine; may be sent overnight at ambient temperature.

Long-chain fatty acids are transported as carnitine esters into the mitochondrion, a process that requires transesterification of acyl-CoA compounds at the inner and outer sides of the inner mitochondrial membrane. Likewise, acyl-CoA compounds that accumulate in the mitochondrion may be converted to carnitine esters, removed from the mitochondrion, and excreted in the urine. This detoxification mechanism causes secondary carnitine depletion in most disorders that interfere with the metabolism of mitochondrial CoA-activated carboxylic acids, including organic acidurias, fatty acid oxidation defects, and respiratory chain defects. In the work-up of a suspected metabolic disorder, reduced levels of serum carnitine can be regarded as an indication of one of these disorders. Exact quantification of total, free, and esterified carnitine in serum or plasma (carnitine status) is mandatory for recognizing carnitine deficiency and monitoring carnitine supplementation in these disorders, as well as for diagnosing primary carnitine transporter deficiency.

Free carnitine is almost completely reabsorbed in the renal tubule, whereas filtrated acylcarnitine compounds are largely excreted in the urine. Carnitine analyses in urine should be performed only in conjunction with plasma analyses; these analyses may be indicated if plasma values are abnormal or when monitoring treatment. Increased urinary acylcarnitines typically occur in organic acidurias and fatty acid oxidation defects and, in conjunction with normal plasma carnitine values, suggest good detoxification capacity. High concentrations of urinary free carnitine and a reduced renal tubular reabsorption rate (< 90%) may indicate renal tubular dysfunction as a cause of systemic carnitine depletion.

LONG-CHAIN CARNITINES

Sample: 1 mL serum/plasma; if not locally available, ship on dry ice (to avoid lipolysis).

Standard carnitine status measures only short-chain carnitine esters; therefore, it is not suitable for the quantification of metabolites accumulating in long-chain fatty acid oxidation defects. The quantification of long-chain carnitines has become of limited practical relevance, as long-chain fatty acid oxidation defects are well recognized by acylcarnitine analysis and carnitine supplementation can be monitored through the analysis of plasma free carnitine. Nevertheless, quantification of long-chain carnitine compounds may be of interest for the management of some patients with long-chain fatty acid oxidation defects.

FREE FATTY ACIDS AND KETONE BODIES

Sample: 1 mL serum/plasma; ship on dry ice (to avoid lipolysis).

The analysis of free fatty acids (FFA) and ketone bodies in plasma or serum provides important information on lipid catabolism and ketogenesis; it is essential in all patients with acute metabolic coma or hypoglycemia. In addition, it is the single most important investigation at the end of a fasting test (see Chapter 11). Normal values vary greatly according to metabolic state. High insulin levels in the fed state inhibit lipolysis, resulting in low concentrations of both FFA (< 300 µmol/L) and ketones (< 100 µmol/L). Increasing lipolysis during fasting, in contrast, leads to a continuous rise of FFA levels, up to 2 to 3 mmol/L within 24 hours, and a consecutive exponential increase of ketone bodies to concentrations that should exceed those of the FFA. Interpretation of the results at an early stage of a fasting reaction may be inconclusive, as the FFA may exceed a concentration of 1 mmol/L before the ketones start to rise. A molar concentration of ketones below that of the FFA after 24 hours of fasting suggests a disorder of fatty acid oxidation or ketogenesis, whereas a molar concentration of ketones below 50% of FFA is virtually diagnostic for such a disorder. Determining FFA without ketones is useless.

MEDIUM-CHAIN AND LONG-CHAIN FATTY ACIDS

Sample: 1 mL serum/plasma; send on dry ice (to avoid lipolysis).

Some metabolic laboratories offer differentiation between medium-chain and long-chain fatty acids (C_6 to C_{18}) in plasma by GC-MS. This analysis provides information on mitochondrial fatty acid oxidation and on the accumulation of pathologic metabolites in fatty acid oxidation defects and is thus an alternative to acylcarnitine analysis where such information is unavailable. Elevations of fatty acids usually mirror the pattern of acylcarnitines except in a deficiency of carnitine palmitoyltransferase I, where the high levels of different fatty acids contrast with the reduced acylcarnitines. In addition, the exact quantification of specific compounds may be used to monitor treatment in fatty acid oxidation defects.

OROTIC ACID

Sample: Minimum 10 mL urine; preserve with two drops of chloroform. Sample may be sent overnight at ambient temperature; a taxi should be used in emergencies.

Pyrimidine biosynthesis, of which orotic acid is a major intermediary compound, is regulated at the level of carbamylphosphate synthetase II (CPS II) that catalyzes the first reaction in this pathway (see Fig. 28.1). The mitochondrial isoenzyme CPS I catalyzes the production of carbamylphosphate for nitrogen detoxification. Conditions in which mitochondrial carbamylphosphate accumulates, particularly in most urea cycle disorders, also increase cytosolic carbamylphosphate levels, pyrimidine biosynthesis, and urinary orotic acid excretion. Organic acid analysis can identify this compound, but exact quantification may require an HPLC or MS-MS. Urinary orotic acid analysis is one of the emergency investigations for children with hyperammonemia to diagnose ornithine transcarbamylase (OTC) deficiency. Latent increases in pyrimidine biosynthesis, as in heterozygous female carriers for OTC deficiency, may be recognized through elevated urinary orotic acid concentrations after the administration of allopurinol, which blocks the conversion of orotic acid to uridine monophosphate (see Chapter 11). Increased orotic acid concentrations may also be found in various other genetic disorders, including mitochondrial disorders, Rett syndrome, and Lesch–Nyhan syndrome.

PURINES AND PYRIMIDINES

Sample: Minimum 10 mL urine, preferably a morning sample or 24-hour urine collection (keep cool and dark). Preserve sample with two drops of chloroform; send at ambient temperature or on dry ice (to diagnose adenylosuccinase deficiency).

The analysis of purines and pyrimidines by HPLC of urine may be indicated, particularly in patients with renal calculi and related problems, neurologic problems, or both (see Table 28.1). Other symptoms that may be caused by genetic deficiencies in purine or pyrimidine metabolism include arthritis, muscle cramps and muscle wasting, anemia, or immunodeficiency. Diet affects purine and pyrimidine excretion, which may vary considerably during the day; a 24-hour urine collection or a morning urine specimen should be obtained for analysis. Drinks and foods that contain methylxanthines, such as coffee, black tea, cocoa, or licorice, should be avoided during urine collection and during the preceding day. When the patient has a urinary tract infection, a sample should be excluded as bacteria markedly reduce the concentrations of purines or pyrimidines in the urine. Urine for the diagnosis of neurologic disease should immediately be frozen and should be shipped to the laboratory on dry ice, since succinylaminoimidazole carboxamide ribonucleoside (SAICAR), the marker metabolite of adenylosuccinase deficiency, is unstable at room temperature. To exclude disorders of pyrimidine breakdown, urine should be examined for the presence of dihydropyrimidines by GC-MS, as in organic acid analysis, because HPLC does not detect these substances.

INVESTIGATIONS FOR DISORDERS OF GALACTOSE METABOLISM

Samples

Screening (galactose, galactose-1-phosphate uridyltransferase [GALT] activity): Three to six dried blood spots on filter paper (Guthrie card), send by normal mail.

Specific analyses (galactose, galactose-1-phosphate, enzyme studies, mutation analysis): 2 mL EDTA blood, preferentially obtained about 30 minutes after a milk feed; send at ambient temperature, if necessary (e.g., over a weekend) store at room temperature (do not refrigerate—may cause hemolysis; do not freeze—kinase is membrane-bound).

Most inborn errors of galactose metabolism can be recognized through determining galactose concentrations and GALT activity in dried blood spots (Guthrie card), which is part of neonatal screening in most Western countries. More specific analyses are required in children with pathologic screening tests, as discussed in detail in Chapter 9, and for the reliable exclusion of specific defects. Galactose is measured in plasma (normal < 3 mg/dL), whereas galactose-1-phosphate is measured in erythrocytes (normal < 0.3 mg/dL).

SUGARS

Sample: Minimum 10 mL urine; preserve with two drops of chloroform. Sample may be sent overnight at ambient temperature.

Thin-layer chromatography for the detection of pathologic urinary excretion of sugars may be valuable for the characterization of renal tubular defects and for the diagnosis of certain disorders of carbohydrate metabolism. Sugars that are routinely tested include glucose, galactose, fructose, and lactose.

GLYCOSAMINOGLYCANS

Sample: 10 mL urine; may be sent overnight at ambient temperature.

Mucopolysaccharidoses (MPS) are caused by deficient metabolism of certain glycosaminoglycans (GAG), which accumulate in the lysosomes and are excreted in the urine. They can be recognized through quantitative analysis of total urinary GAG concentration (relative to creatinine) but are more reliably diagnosed through electrophoretic separation of the different GAG fractions. Increased dermatan sulfate (associated with skeletal and organ changes) is found in MPS types I, II, VI, and VII. Increased heparan sulfate (associated with mental retardation) is found in MPS types I, II, III, and VII, whereas presence of keratan sulfate (associated with skeletal changes) is pathognomonic for MPS type IV. Chondroitin sulfate is characteristically found in MPS type VII and less consistently in MPS type IV. Quantification of total urinary GAG may give borderline or even false-normal results, particularly in patients with MPS types III (Sanfilippo) and IV (Morquio). Electrophoretic GAG separation is the method of choice if these disorders are suspected.

OLIGOSACCHARIDES

Sample: 10 mL urine; preserve with two drops of chloroform. Sample may be sent overnight at ambient temperature.

A significant proportion of lysosomal storage disorders causes accumulation of specific oligosaccharides that may be detected in the urine. These are usually recognized through separation of individual oligosaccharides by thin-layer chromatography. Quantitative analysis is available only for free neuraminic acid (sialic acid) in the diagnosis of sialic acid storage disease (Salla disease). Oligosaccharide analysis allows the diagnosis of the following disorders: fucosidosis, α-mannosidoses and β-mannosidoses, aspartylglycosaminuria, Schindler disease, sialidosis, G_{M1}- and G_{M2}-gangliosidoses, galactosialidosis, Gaucher disease, Pompe disease, and sialic acid storage disease. However, pathologic oligosaccharide patterns in thin-layer chromatography may be variable and are sometimes difficult to recognize. If the clinical picture in a patient suggests one of these disorders, performing enzyme studies may be advisable despite normal results from urinary oligosaccharide analysis. The other lysosomal disorders usually require enzyme studies for their diagnosis.

MARKERS OF PEROXISOMAL FUNCTION

Samples: 1 mL serum/plasma for very long-chain fatty acids; send on dry ice (to avoid lipolysis). 1 mL EDTA blood for the analysis of plasmalogens in erythrocytes; send overnight at ambient temperature.

Most peroxisomal disorders, particularly those of peroxisome biogenesis, cause deficient peroxisomal beta-oxidation. The examination of very-long-chain fatty acids (VLCFA) in serum or plasma is the initial method of choice for diagnosing such disorders (see Chapter 27). Follow-up studies for the exact biochemical characterization of some peroxisomal disorders may include analyses of bile acids, as well as of phytanic and pristanic acids. An isolated elevation of serum phytanic acid is found in adult Refsum disease. Disorders of etherlipid biosynthesis, such as rhizomelic chondrodysplasia punctata, or its variants require the measurement of plasmalogens in erythrocytes.

BILE ACIDS

Sample: 5 mL urine, 2 mL plasma, or 2 mL bile fluid; ship on dry ice.

Changes in bile acid concentrations may occur in various peroxisomal disorders, as well as in specific deficiencies of bile acid biosynthesis. These analyses involve quantification of specific metabolites with fast atom bombardment MS (FAB-MS) or GC-MS of various body fluids.

INVESTIGATIONS FOR CONGENITAL DISORDERS OF GLYCOSYLATION

Sample: 1 mL serum; may be sent overnight at ambient temperature.

Many enzymes, transport and membrane proteins, hormones, and so on require glycosylation in the Golgi apparatus or endoplasmic reticulum (ER) to render them functional glycoproteins. More than 30 different enzymes are involved in the build-up of the carbohydrate side chains; glycoprotein breakdown takes place in the lysosomes.

The congenital disorders of glycosylation (CDG), previously described as carbohydrate-deficient glycoprotein syndromes, result from deficiencies of enzymes required for protein glycosylation. As a group these disorders are characterized by disturbances of various physiologic functions and by a broad spectrum of symptoms. Diagnosis and differentiation for several types involves the demonstration of pathologic glycosylation patterns through isoelectric focusing of ferritin. The test as a global test of reduced glycosylation of transferrin does not detect all CDG syndromes. Secondary disturbances of glycosylation may result from chronic alcoholism, classic galactosemia, or fructose intolerance (deficient mannose-6-phosphate synthesis).

STEROLS

Sample: 1 mL serum/plasma; send on dry ice.

Sterol analysis by GC-MS is indicated for diagnosing disorders in the distal cholesterol biosynthesis pathway, particularly the Smith–Lemli–Opitz syndrome.

PORPHYRINS

Samples: 20 mL urine (random sample, no addition), 5 mL feces, 5 to 10 mL heparinized blood; no additives. Sample storage should be cool and dark; may be sent overnight at ambient temperature.

The accumulation of specific intermediary metabolites in the porphyrias causes abdominal, neurologic, and dermatologic symptoms. The various porphyrins and porphyrin precursors are usually measured in urine and/or feces. Cytosolic enzyme studies are performed in erythrocytes. The congenital erythropoietic porphyria (Günther disease) is characterized by typical discoloration of the urine (brown, red fluorescent spots in the diapers). Special screening tests for porphobilinogen in urine (Hoesch test, Watson–Schwartz test) may be used when acute hepatic porphyria is suspected. Quantifications of porphobilinogens and delta-aminolevulinic acid is preferable.

SPECIALIZED CSF AND URINE ANALYSES
FOR NEUROMETABOLIC DISORDERS

Samples:

CSF samples: Collect several samples (age < 1 year: 0.5 mL fractions, use fractions 2 to 4 for metabolic investigations; age > 1 year: 1-mL fractions, use fractions 3 to 5). Freeze samples immediately at the bedside (dry ice or liquid nitrogen), store at –70°C. The analysis of pterins requires the addition of DTE and DETAPAC as antioxidants. If samples are blood-stained, centrifuge before freezing (inform the laboratory!). The authors strongly recommend that two CSF samples (approximately 1 mL each) be stored at –70°C for follow-up analysis.

Urinary pterins: 10 mL random urine sample; keep cool and dark (dark urine collection bag); ship on dry ice. Alternatively: 5mL urine; add 6 M HCl up to pH 1.0 to 1.5; add 100 mg MnO_2 and shake for 5 minutes (ambient temperature). Centrifuge for 5 minutes (4,000 rpm); send supernatant protected against light (aluminum foil) by express mail.

In the diagnostic work-up of a suspected neurometabolic disorder, a lumbar puncture should be performed only after basic analyses have been carried out in blood and urine and after the results of neuroimaging studies have been evaluated carefully. Selective screening of CSF does not have a place. Nevertheless, a number of neurometabolic disorders can be diagnosed only by specific CSF investigations testing metabolic pathways of brain metabolism, especially of neurotransmission (Table 8.3). Whenever CSF investigations are performed, the analysis should include quantitative determination of lactate, pyruvate, and amino acids, the last by methods especially suited to CSF, in addition to cells, glucose, protein, immunoglobulin classes, specific immunoglobulins, and an evaluation of the blood–brain barrier.

Reliable results of specialized CSF investigations can be obtained only if the appropriate protocol is strictly adhered to. This should be discussed beforehand with the neurometabolic laboratory. The analyses of some substances (such as pterins, serotonin, and catecholamines) require the addition of certain chemicals to the respective sample tubes. Free GABA can only be determined in samples that have been shock-frozen at the bedside in dry ice or liquid nitrogen. Samples must be taken at a certain time of the day and must be collected in a specific order of tubes with fixed amounts of CSF, since diurnal variations and a caudocranial concentration gradient occur for many metabolites. Finally, exact labeling of the CSF samples (fractions) that are sent to the laboratory is essential.

The analysis of urinary pterins using HPLC is necessary to diagnose tetrahydrobiopterin (BH_4) cofactor deficiency in neonates with hyperphenylalaninemia (see Chapter 9). BH_4 cofactor deficiency may be restricted to the central nervous system (CNS), and pterin analysis in the CSF should be included when biogenic amines are investigated.

**Table 8.3.   Inherited metabolic diseases
requiring CSF investigations for diagnosis**

Disorder	Relevant analyte
Glucose transport protein (GLUT1) deficiency	CSF/blood ratio of glucose
Some mitochondrial encephalomyopathies	Lactate, pyruvate, and alanine in CSF
Nonketotic hyperglycinemia	CSF/plasma ratio of glycine
Serine synthesis defect	Amino acids in CSF
Cohen syndrome	β-Alanine
? Isolated pipecolic oxidase deficiency	Pipecolic acid
Defects of pathways of biogenic monoamines	Biogenic monoamine metabolites in CSF
GTP cyclohydrolase I deficiency	Biogenic amines and pterins in CSF
Cerebral dihydropteridine reductase deficiency	Biogenic amines and pterins in CSF
Folinic acid–responsive seizures	As yet unidentified CSF metabolite (analysis of biogenic amines and amino acids in CSF)
GABA transaminase deficiency	GABA in CSF
Defect of the folate binding protein	Folate in CSF
Some cases of methylenetetrahydrofolate reductase deficiency	Methyltetrahydrofolate
Some glutaric aciduria type I	Glutaric acid in CSF
Some defects in leucine catabolism	3-Hydroxyisovaleric acid in CSF

Modified from Hoffmann GF, Surtees RAH, Wevers RA. Investigations of cerebro-spinal fluid for neurometabolic disorders. *Neuropediatrics* 1998;29:59–71.
Abbreviations: CSF, cerebrospinal fluid; GABA, gamma-aminobutyric acid; GTP, guanidine triphosphate.

GLUTATHIONE AND METABOLITES

Sample: 3 mL EDTA whole blood. Centrifuge, remove, and freeze plasma. Deproteinize erythrocyte fraction with 5% sulphosalicylic acid (ratio of approximately 1:1); shake/vortex thoroughly (until homogenous brown color); centrifuge twice at 5,000 g; remove and freeze clear supernatant. Send plasma and deproteinized erythrocytes (unequivocal labeling!) on dry ice.

Disturbances of the gamma-glutamyl cycle cause a range of clinical problems, including neonatal metabolic acidosis, hemolytic anemia, electrolyte disturbances, and progressive neurologic symptoms. All four known enzyme defects are inherited in an autosomal recessive fashion. The most important disorder in this group is glutathione synthetase deficiency. Initial investigations include the analysis of organic acids (5-oxoproline), as well as quantification of glutathione and its metabolites in urine, erythrocytes, leucocytes, and/or fibroblasts. Enzyme studies are performed in erythrocytes or other nucleated cells (leucocytes, fibroblasts), but erythrocytes contain only part of the gamma-glutamyl cycle (no gamma-glutamyl transpeptidase and 5-oxoprolinase).

ADDITIONAL READINGS

Blau N, Duran M, Gibson KM, Blaskovics ME, eds. *Physician's guide to the laboratory diagnosis of metabolic diseases.* Heidelberg, Germany: Springer; 2002.

Hommes FA, ed. *Techniques in diagnostic human biochemical laboratories: a laboratory manual.* New York: Wiley-Liss; 1991.

Hoffmann GF, Surtees RAH, Wevers RA. Investigations of cerebrospinal fluid for neurometabolic disorders. *Neuropediatrics* 1998; 29:59–71.

9 ♣ Neonatal Screening for Inherited Metabolic Disease

Routine screening of all neonates for inherited disorders began in the 1960s after Horst Bickel established an effective dietary therapy for phenylketonuria (PKU) and Robert Guthrie developed a bacterial inhibition assay to detect elevated concentrations of phenylalanine in dried blood spots. Over time, neonatal screening has been expanded to several other treatable metabolic and endocrine disorders, including hypothyroidism, sickle cell disease, galactosemia, maple syrup urine disease, biotinidase deficiency, and adrenogenital syndrome. A major step in recent years has been the development of routine acylcarnitine and amino acid analysis in Guthrie cards by tandem mass spectroscopy (MS-MS). This advancement allows the detection of most aminoacidopathies, organic acidurias, and fatty acid oxidation defects, and thus, some of the most important treatable inborn errors of intermediary metabolism. MS-MS is currently being introduced in parts of the United States, Australia, Germany, and elsewhere. This chapter contains information on how to proceed when the results of neonatal screening for certain disorders are abnormal.

HYPERPHENYLALANINEMIA

Neonatal hyperphenylalaninemia results from a variety of conditions. The primary genetic deficiency is that of phenylalanine hydroxylase (PAH), the enzyme that catalyzes the conversion of phenylalanine to tyrosine and that is the site of the defect in PKU. Abnormalities in the synthesis or metabolism of the cofactor of this enzyme, tetrahydrobiopterin (BH_4), are also detected. Secondary causes of an elevated concentration of phenylalanine include prematurity, liver or kidney disease, and various drugs (e.g., trimethoprim, chemotherapeutic agents). Severe hyperphenylalaninemia above 360 to 600 μmol/L causes serious progressive damage to the developing brain, resulting in mental retardation, epilepsy, spasticity, and psychiatric problems. Early screening, diagnosis, and dietary restriction of phenylalanine intake as soon as possible after birth can prevent it.

Most neonates with consistent hyperphenylalaninemia suffer from PAH deficiency. The incidence in most Caucasian populations is between one in 4,000 and one in 12,000. For practical purposes, the authors consider two forms of PAH deficiency: PKU, which requires treatment, and mild hyperphenylalaninemia (MHP), which does not. Figure 9.1 depicts the work-up for a neonate with hyperphenylalaninemia recognized through neonatal screening. High phenylalanine values should be confirmed through quantitative analysis of plasma amino acids so that concentrations of both tyrosine and phenylalanine are known. Infants affected by PKU should immediately be admitted to a hospital with experience in the treatment of metabolic disorders. To exclude BH_4 cofactor deficiency, a BH_4 loading test (see Chapter 11) or analyses for urinary pterins and the activity of dihydropteridin reductase in blood should always be carried out if phenylalanine values are above

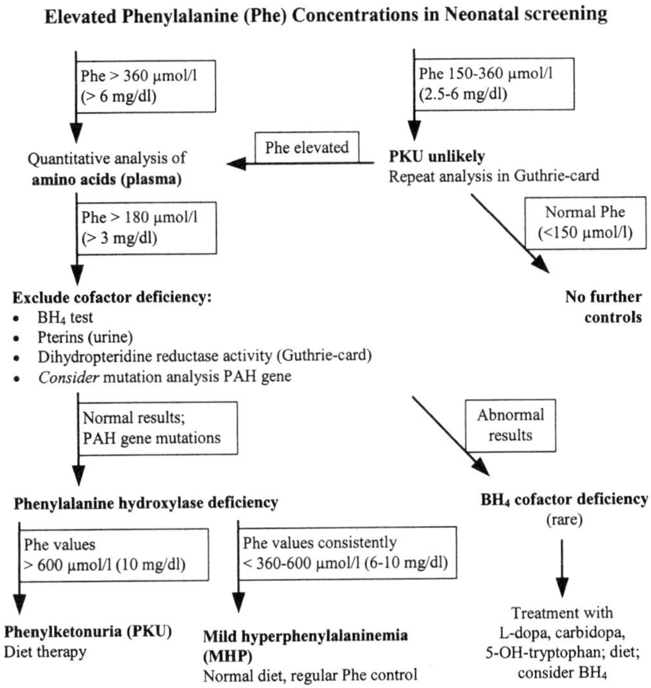

Elevated Phenylalanine (Phe) Concentrations in Neonatal screening

Figure 9.1 **Algorithmic approach to elevated phenylalanine concentrations. Abbreviations: BH$_4$, tetrahydrobiopterin; PAH, phenylalanine hydroxylase.**

360 µmol/L. A positive response to the BH$_4$ loading test is therapeutically relevant immediately. Treatment of PKU should be started instantly, with a phenylalanine-restricted diet and supplementation of essential amino acids. Recommended therapeutic phenylalanine values differ from one country to another, but they should not be above 360 µmol/L in the first 6 to 10 years of life. Most diets are more liberal for teenagers. No consensus has been reached about whether treatment is necessary in adulthood. Plasma concentrations of phenylalanine must be below 360 µmol/L before and throughout pregnancy to avoid fetal damage that can be caused by maternal PKU.

GALACTOSEMIA

The activated 1-phosphate metabolites of both galactose and fructose are highly toxic, particularly for the liver, kidneys, and brain. In classic galactosemia, galactose-1-phosphate (Gal-1-P) accumulates because of a defective transversion to uridine diphosphate-galactose (UDP-galactose) catalyzed by galactose-1-phosphate uridyltransferase (GALT). Affected children show progressive symptoms, such as vomiting, diarrhea, and jaundice, after the start of milk (lactose) feeding, usually beginning in the third to the fourth day of life. Untreated, the disease usually progresses to hepatic and renal failure and death; progressive bilateral cataracts may occur. Excluding galactose from the diet can prevent the severe acute manifestations of galactosemia. Late complications, such as ovarian failure and impaired speech and language development, may occur despite good compliance with treatment. The usefulness of neonatal screening may not be fully realized since some infants may become symptomatic before the neonatal screening results are available. Immediate start of treatment is mandatory. The incidence of classic galactosemia in neonatal screening programs in the United States ranges from one in 55,000 to one in 80,000. False-negative findings in neonatal screening may be observed after blood transfusion.

Neonatal screening ideally is carried out by measuring the activity of GALT. In some programs galactose concentrations are measured, which also detects deficiency of galactokinase. A positive screening result is followed by electrophoresis, which identifies the classic galactosemia (GG) variant and other common variants, such as Duarte (DD) and compounds (DG, duarte galactosemia). Many mutations have been identified in the GALT gene. The Duarte 2 variant has an allele frequency of 10%; it is associated with a 50% reduction in enzyme activity, which does not usually require diet modification. Even in compound heterozygotes with a severe mutation on the other allele, alteration of diet may not be required. Most children with elevated galactose concentrations found in neonatal screening have a mild form of GALT deficiency that does not require treatment. In these children galactose and Gal-1-P concentrations often normalize within a few weeks or months on an ordinary diet.

When galactose is between 15 and 20 mg/dL (0.8 to 1.1 mM), checking the general condition (feeding, vomiting, weight gain, liver size) and sending another blood spot sample (preferentially taken 60 minutes after a milk feed) to the neonatal screening laboratory for galactose measurements are sufficient.

When galactose is between 20 and 50 mg/dL (1.1 to 2.8 mM) or when the infant has a GG or DG phenotype, plasma galactose, erythrocyte Gal-1-P, and mutations should be analyzed from a 1 to 3 mL sample of ethylene diamine tetraacetate (EDTA) blood that is shipped at ambient temperature. EDTA blood may be stored at room temperature for a couple of days, if necessary. Lactose-free milk feedings are recommended until the final results are available.

Immediate hospital admission is necessary with the presence of galactose concentrations above 50 mg/dL (> 2.8 mM). Lactose-free feedings should be started as soon as the appropriate blood and urine samples have been taken to check for amino acids and reducing substances in the urine and determination of plasma galactose and erythrocyte Gal-1-P. Thorough examination of liver and kidney function should include coagulation studies and ultrasound.

The indication for long-term therapy ultimately rests on the concentration of Gal-1-P in erythrocytes, which is normally below 0.3 mg/dL (11 μM) but which may rise up to 100 mg/dL (~4 mM) in classic galactosemia. Obtaining completely normal Gal-1-P levels is impossible in most GG patients because of a substantial endogenous production of galactose. Therapeutic target concentrations of 2 to 4 (at most, 5) mg/dL are realistic. Acceptable galactose intake per day is usually 50 to 200 mg in infants, 150 to 200 mg in toddlers, 200 to 300 mg in school children, 250 to 400 mg in adolescents, and 300 to 500 mg in adults.

BIOTINIDASE DEFICIENCY

The carboxylation of 3-methylcrotonyl-CoA, propionyl-CoA, acetyl-CoA, and pyruvate is biotin-dependent. The individual apoenzymes need to be covalently bound to biotin to generate the active holoenzymes. This reaction is catalyzed by the enzyme holocarboxylase synthetase. A deficiency of this enzyme causes severe, multiple carboxylase deficiency, which usually presents in the neonatal period. Affected children show the severe metabolic decompensation typical for an organic aciduria and progressive neurologic problems; in addition, skin rashes and alopecia usually occur.

Another milder but more insidious form of multiple carboxylase deficiency is caused by an impaired release of covalently bound biotin from dietary and endogenous proteins, a reaction catalyzed by the enzyme biotinidase. The deficiency of biotinidase causes a depletion of free biotin and progressive neurologic and dermatologic symptoms, usually starting in infancy. Symptomatology includes seizures, ataxia, hearing loss, optic atrophy, spastic diplegia, and developmental delay, as well as skin rash and alopecia. These characteristic symptoms may occur in half of the affected patients, while less specific symptoms, such as hypotonia, developmental delay, and seizures, may predominate in others. Because of the insidious onset of symptoms, the diagnosis is often delayed or even missed. This is a major concern since this form of multiple carboxylase deficiency can be effectively treated with biotin. Many countries therefore include a semiquantitative colorimetric or fluorimetric measurement of biotinidase activity in dried blood spots in neonatal screening programs.

False-negative findings in neonatal screening may be observed after blood transfusion or when the neonate receives a catecholamine infusion during blood sampling. Residual biotinidase activity may vary, depending on the underlying mutations in the biotinidase gene. Mild forms of biotinidase deficiency with relatively high enzyme activity levels do occur; these forms do not cause disease and do not require treatment. Investigating other biochemical parameters like blood ammonia, plasma lactate, and urinary organic acids is advisable before commencing biotin supplementation so that the metabolic significance of possible biotin deficiency can be evaluated at this time. Nevertheless, biotin supplementation should be started immediately after the blood and urine samples for confirmatory enzymatic tests are obtained. Treatment is simple; it does not involve complicated dietary regimens as do some other disorders investigated in neonatal screening. Temporary initiation of biotin supplementation does not interfere with breastfeeding and parent–child interaction. The recommended starting dose is 10 mg per day. If reduced biotinidase activity is confirmed in the control test, the exact biotinidase activity should be determined in a 1-mL serum sample shipped on dry ice. A residual activity of 0 to 10% indicates profound biotinidase deficiency. Long-term treatment with 5 to 20 mg of biotin per day is usually sufficient to keep concentrations of lactate and ammonia in blood and of organic acids in urine in the normal range. Treatment can also be modified by determining the activity of carboxylases in lymphocytes. Biotinidase activity between 10% and 25% indicates partial deficiency, which may not necessarily require long-term treatment. Many centers recommend treatment of these children with 10 mg/day for the first year of life. Current recommendations are not yet clear on what regimens are optimal for control of late complications, particularly those involving the optic and auditory nerves.

CONGENITAL HYPOTHYROIDISM

Congenital hypothyroidism occurs in infants who are born without the ability to produce adequate amounts of thyroid hormone. Thyroid hormone is essential for normal growth and brain development. If untreated, congenital deficiency of thyroid hormone results in mental retardation and stunted growth. Infants with untreated congenital hypothyroidism may appear clinically normal up to 3 months of age, by which time some brain damage will already have occurred. When symptoms or clinical signs are present, they may include prolonged neonatal jaundice, constipation, lethargy, poor muscle tone, feeding problems, a large tongue, mottled and dry skin, a distended abdomen, and an umbilical hernia.

The most common causes of congenital hypothyroidism are total or partial failure of the thyroid gland to develop (aplasia or hypoplasia) or its development in an abnormal location (an ectopic gland). These types of hypothyroidism rarely recur in siblings. Less commonly, the hypothyroidism results from a hereditary inability to manufacture thyroid hormones, maternal medications during gestation (e.g., iodine, antithyroid drugs), or maternal antibodies.

The initial screening test is the assay of thyroid-stimulating hormone (TSH). However, in some laboratories the assay of thyroxine (T_4) is preferred. A TSH result is abnormal when it exceeds a laboratory-determined cutoff (in most laboratories > 15 μU/mL). Newborns with an excessively high TSH (> 50 μU/mL) are considered highly suspect for congenital hypothyroidism; therefore, they require immediate follow-up testing of plasma and the initiation of treatment. Those having a slightly elevated TSH should have another filter paper sample submitted for reevaluation.

Treatment includes oral L-thyroxine at a dosage that maintains blood TSH concentration of less than 4 µU /mL and T_3/T_4 in the age-related range. Dosage and follow-up should be done in consultation with a pediatric endocrinologist.

CONGENITAL ADRENAL HYPERPLASIA

Infants with congenital adrenal hyperplasia (CAH) have a deficiency of adrenal enzyme activity, resulting in limited cortisol production and, in some cases, limited aldosterone production. The pituitary gland senses the cortisol deficiency and produces increased amounts of adrenocorticotropic hormone (ACTH). The adrenal glands enlarge but continue to produce inadequate amounts of cortisol. The precursors of cortisol, some of which are virilizing hormones, accumulate and are released into the circulation. As a result of cortisol deficiency, affected infants cannot maintain adequate energy supply and blood glucose levels to meet the stress brought on by injury or illness. Lethargy and coma may finally lead to death. Because of aldosterone deficiency, sodium and water are lost in the urine, resulting in dehydration. Potassium accumulates in the blood, causing irritability or lethargy, vomiting, and muscle weakness, including cardiac muscle irritability and weakness.

Male infants with CAH usually appear normal at birth. Female infants usually show the effects of elevated virilizing hormones: an enlarged clitoris and fusion of the labia majora over the vaginal opening. Occasionally, the female infant may be so virilized that there may appear to be a male penile structure with hypospadias. Such newborns do not have a palpable gonad in the labial/scrotal sac. Their ovaries, uterus, and Fallopian tubes are normal. Both male and female babies may also exhibit symptoms of salt-wasting, which can lead to serious illness and death, within the first 2 weeks of life.

Several types of genetic defects cause the enzymatic deficiencies of CAH. All are autosomal recessive. The newborn screening test currently used is designed to detect the 21-hydroxylase deficiency. This deficiency is responsible for more than 90% of all forms of CAH. In clinical practice however, one should remember that a normal newborn screening test does not rule out other and rarer enzyme deficiencies that also cause CAH.

The screening test for CAH is a radioimmunoassay for 17-hydroxyprogesterone (17-OHP), a precursor of cortisol. If screening indicates the possibility of CAH (17-OHP > 40 nmol/L), the confirmatory test is a serum 17-OHP. CAH is almost certain if 17-OHP levels exceed 90 nmol/L. In this context, one must note that newborn screening in the first 12 hours after birth is more likely to show high 17-OHP levels than is screening done after the first day of life. 17-OHP-levels are also higher in premature babies (low weight) than in mature ones. Therefore, the importance of recording the accurate birth weight and the exact age of sampling on the collection form to assure appropriate interpretation of screening results cannot be overstressed.

Effective treatment for CAH is hormone replacement. Decisions about hormonal treatment should be made in consultation with a pediatric endocrinologist; it may include hydrocortisone and mineralocorticoids. Medications need to be adjusted as the child grows. Serum adrenal hormone levels and renin are monitored. Female infants who have virilization of the genitalia may need surgical correction. This is usually done in stages, with the first surgery occurring before the age of 2 years. Infants with CAH, if detected early and treated with appropriate doses of medication, can have normal growth, development, and intellectual potential. In addition, fertility is usually normal.

TANDEM MASS SPECTROMETRY

Tandem mass spectrometry (MS-MS) has been used to detect and to analyze acylcarnitines since the 1980s. This technique has been extended to newborn screening by the development of automated techniques of sample preparation, injection into the instrument, and analysis of results. The acylcarnitines are derivatized as methyl or butyl esters. The latter are more advantageous as many amino acids can be analyzed as butyl esters, and MS-MS analysis of amino acids can then be done on the same sample, increasing the efficiency of newborn screening.

Acylcarnitines are formed from free carnitine and are acyl-CoA moieties derived from fatty acids and organic acids (which may have been derived from amino acids) through the action of the carnitine-acyl-CoA transferases. Several enzymes are currently known, with rough specificities for C2 to C8 (carnitine acetyl-CoA transferase), C6 to C14 (carnitine octanoyl-CoA transferase), and C12 to C18 (carnitine palmitoyl-CoA transferase, CPT). CPT I, which has muscle and liver forms, occurs in the mitochondrial intermembranous space. CPT II is found in the inner mitochondrial membrane.

Acyl-CoAs (and long-chain fatty acids) do not pass directly through the mitochondrial membranes, so acylcarnitines are synthesized for transport. The result of the combined actions of CPT I, the carnitine–acylcarnitine translocase (a second form of this enzyme may occur) in the inner mitochondrial membrane, and CPT II is the availability of long-chain acyl-CoAs in the interior of the mitochondria. In the usual situation, long-chain acylcarnitines are synthesized so that fatty acids can enter the mitochondria for beta-oxidation. The carnitine acyl-CoA transferases catalyze reversible reactions so that the amount of acylcarnitine (e.g., acetylcarnitine) will reflect the availability of acyl-CoA (e.g., acetyl-CoA) and free carnitine. Short- and medium-chain fatty acids can enter the mitochondria unassisted by the carnitine–acylcarnitine shuttle.

Acylcarnitines are synthesized in the mitochondria. To be detected in the plasma, they must be transported out of the mitochondria and then out of the cells. Some, especially long-chain acylcarnitines, are absorbed onto erythrocytes. Thus, some differences are found between whole blood (or dried blood-spot) and plasma or serum levels of acylcarnitines. The short- and medium-chain acylcarnitines are filtered and are reabsorbed to varying degrees by the kidney. Abnormal amounts appear in the urine if the plasma level is extremely high, if renal synthesis is increased (as occurs in renal hypoxia), or if renal reabsorption of acylcarnitines is impaired, as occurs in the Fanconi syndromes of renal tubular dysfunction. Long-chain species do not appear in the urine but can be found in the blood and bile. Isomeric (especially branched), unsaturated, and dicarboxylic forms can be recognized and contribute to the diagnostic power of acylcarnitine analysis. Plasma, blood, or blood spots collected on filter-paper Guthrie cards are therefore the preferred samples.

Researchers at Duke University developed tandem mass spectrometry of acylcarnitines and amino acids for expanded newborn screening in the early 1990s. It allows for screening of aminoacidopathies, including PKU, organic acidurias, and disorders of fatty acid oxidation. The test is highly sensitive and highly specific and has few false-positive results. Samples are usually diagnostic by 24 hours after birth. A positive result often constitutes a metabolic emergency as infants with many of the disorders diagnosed by this technique can become critically ill in the first few days after birth.

Fully established or pilot programs are under way in many states, countries, and commercial laboratories. The newness of the technique means that some uncertainty still exists about sensitivity and specificity and costs versus benefits. However, the general consensus appears to be that sensitivity and specificity are better than those for other screening programs and that the cost benefits of presymptomatic or rapid early diagnosis justify the screening program for all disorders diagnosable by this technique.

Sensitivity is virtually 100% for medium-chain acyl-CoA dehydrogenase (MCAD) deficiency, the most common disorder. A small number of MCAD-deficient patients have significant illness, such as hypoglycemia, coma, or even sudden death, in the first 5 days before screening results are available. A metabolic disease is not always suspected or diagnosed, so the screening program serves a purpose even for these infants. For other MCAD-deficient patients, several months or years may pass before symptoms occur.

If a positive result is obtained from the test, the baby must be examined immediately, further samples as requested by the lab must be obtained, and the appropriate treatment must be started.

TECHNICAL ASPECTS
Sample Timing

For disorders of fatty acid oxidation, a suitable interval must occur between birth and collection as the fetus uses relatively little fat before birth. However, once the supply of glucose from the mother ceases, fatty acid oxidation proceeds rapidly. If fatty acid oxidation is impaired, the substrates immediately preceding the blocked reaction will accumulate; and the acylcarnitines reflecting the metabolic block will begin to appear. The exact interval is not yet established, but in the most common disorder, MCAD deficiency, an abundance of octanoylcarnitine (C8) is found by 24 hours.

At present, information on other fatty acid disorders is incomplete; disorders have gone undetected because a sample was taken too early or because the levels of diagnostic metabolites were normal. Consequently, a normal newborn screening result should not preclude retesting later if symptoms suggest a disorder already screened for. Disorders of organic acid metabolism (e.g., propionic aciduria) will result in synthesis of the relevant acylcarnitines (in this case, C3-propionylcarnitine) well before birth so that prenatal diagnosis is even possible. The best time for obtaining samples has not yet been established. Early samples have some advantages in patients with organic acid disorders, but some newborn screening tests are better done after 48 hours. In summary, as for other screening programs, a sample should be obtained before hospital discharge, no matter how young the patient. If the patient is less than 48 hours old, a second sample should be obtained at 2 weeks of age or in accordance with local policy.

Sample Collection and Handling

A standard Guthrie card is used. The card should be dried before mailing as in other newborn screening tests. Because most of the disorders detected by MS-MS can present with rapid decompensation in the newborn period, cards must be sent daily (or as close as possible to that) to the laboratory; and ideally, the laboratory should have a rapid turnaround time (1 day) for this test. Samples are generally stable for 18 months (shorter acylcarnitine species) or even longer (with longer molecules).

Method

Blood spots are punched out and eluted with a solvent to which deuterium-labeled internal standards (typically, acetyl-, propionyl-, isovaleryl-, octanoyl-, and palmitoylcarnitine) have been added. After derivatization and injection into the instrument, the acylcarnitines are analyzed by loss of a characteristic ion (m/z [mass to charge ratio] 85 or 99).

Interpretation

Both quantification (by isotope-dilution ratios) and ratios between different acylcarnitines are used. Single metabolites or a pattern may be diagnostic or suggestive of pathology and of the need for further investigation. Each laboratory must establish its own values for diagnosis or need of repeat testing. Table 9.1 presents the possible significance of abnormal values of various acylcarnitines, as well as the findings that should be expected for various metabolic disorders detected by this technique.

CONSEQUENCES

A positive result is a metabolic emergency. The laboratory must notify the physician quickly, and the infant must be evaluated at once. A repeat sample should be obtained, and confirmatory test-

(*text continues on page 122*)

Table 9.1. Acylcarnitines in the diagnosis of metabolic disorders

Analyte	Size	Disorders/comments
1A: Diagnostic relevance of acylcarnitine species		
Acetylcarnitine	C2	Quite variable, may reflect lactic acidosis or ketosis
Propionylcarnitine	C3	Propionic aciduria, methylmalonic aciduria, vitamin B_{12} deficiency (maternal/congenital), holocarboxylase synthetase deficiency, unreliably increased in biotinidase deficiency
Butyrylcarnitine	C4	SCAD deficiency, SCHAD deficiency
Isobutyrylcarnitine	C4	Isobutyryl-CoA dehydrogenase deficiency
3-Methylcrotonyl-carnitine	C5:1	3-MCC deficiency, may be detected in heterozygote infant of (asymptomatic) mother; isobutyl dehydrogenase deficiency
Methylmalonyl-carnitine	C4DC	Methylmalonic aciduria
Isovalerylcarnitine	C5	Isovaleric aciduria, 2-methyl-3-hydroxybutyryl-CoA dehydrogenase deficiency; pivaloylcarnitine derived from antibiotics containing pivoxil-sulbactam is an isomer and gives a false positive
Tiglylcarnitine	C5:1	Mitochondrial acetoacetyl-CoA thiolase (2-oxothiolase) deficiency
2-Methyl-3-hydroxybutyryl-carnitine	C5:OH	Mitochondrial acetoacetyl-CoA thiolase (2-oxothiolase) deficiency, 2-methyl-3-hydroxybutyryl-CoA dehydrogenase deficiency
Hydroxyisovaleryl-carnitine	C5:OH	3-Methylcrotonyl-CoA carboxylase deficiency, HMG-CoA lyase deficiency, methylglutaconic aciduria type I
Glutarylcarnitine	C5DC	Glutaric aciduria type I

continued

Table 9.1. *Continued.*

Species (common name when used)	Size	Disorders/comments
3-Methylglutaryl-carnitine	C6DC	HMG-CoA lyase deficiency, methylglutaconic aciduria type I
Octanoylcarnitine	C8	MCAD deficiency, valproyl-carnitine is an isomer and gives a false positive
Octenoylcarnitine	C8:1	Nonspecifically elevated with mitochondrial dysfunction, including valproate therapy
	C10:2	2,4-Dienoyl-CoA reductase deficiency
Decenoylcarnitine	C10:1	MCAD deficiency
Decanoylcarnitine	C10	Valproate therapy
	C14:1	VLCAD deficiency
	C14:2	VLCAD deficiency
	C16	CPT II deficiency, carnitine–acylcarnitine translocase deficiency
	C16:1	VLCAD deficiency
	C16OH	LCHAD/trifunctional protein deficiency
	C16DC	CPT II deficiency, carnitine–acylcarnitine translocase deficiency
Linoleylcarnitine	C18:1	CPT II deficiency, carnitine–acylcarnitine translocase deficiency
Linolenylcarnitine	C18:2	CPT II deficiency, carnitine–acylcarnitine translocase deficiency
	C18OH	LCHAD/trifunctional protein deficiency
	C18:1OH	LCHAD/trifunctional protein deficiency
	C18:DC	CPT II deficiency, carnitine–acylcarnitine translocase deficiency
	C18:1DC	CPT II deficiency, carnitine–acylcarnitine translocase deficiency

Table 9.1. *Continued.*

Disorder	Expected acylcarnitines
1B: Acylcarnitine patterns in various metabolic disorders	
Propionic aciduria	C3
Methylmalonic aciduria	C3, C4DC
3-Methylcrotonyl-CoA carboxylase deficiency	C5:1, C5OH
Isovaleric acidemia	C5
Glutaric aciduria type I	C5DC
Vitamin B_{12} deficiency	C3, C4DC
Biotinidase deficiency; holocarboxylase synthetase deficiency	C3, C4:1OHDC, C5OH. Elevations may be unreliable.
2-Methyl-3-hydroxybutyryl-CoA dehydrogenase deficiency	C5:1, C5OH
Beta-ketothiolase deficiency	C5:1, C5OH
HMG-CoA lyase deficiency	C5OH, C6DC
Carnitine transporter deficiency	Reduced concentrations of free carnitine and various acylcarnitine species
CPT I deficiency	Absence of long- and medium-chain acylcarnitines
Carnitine–acylcarnitine translocase deficiency	C18:1, C18:2, C16, C16DC, C18:2DC, C18:1DC
CPT II deficiency	C18:1, C18:2, C16, C16DC, C18:2DC, C18:1DC
VLCAD deficiency	C16:1, C14:2, C14:1
LCHAD/trifunctional protein deficiency	C18:OH, C16:1OH, C16OH
MCAD deficiency	C10:1, C8, C6
SCAD deficiency	C4
SCHAD deficiency	C4, C6, C8, C10, C10:1
Multiple acyl-CoA dehydrogenase deficiency	Multiple short- and medium-chain species
Mitochondrial oxidative phosphorylation disorders	Usually normal, occasionally elevated acetylcarnitine, increase in several medium-chain-length acylcarnitines
Congenital lactic acidosis	Usually normal, occasionally elevated C2

Abbreviations indicating structure: Cn a carbon chain of n straight or branched (the mass spectrometer does not distinguish between these possibilities); Cn:1, a single double bond; Cn:2, two double bonds; DC, dicarboxylic species; OH, hydroxy species. Other abbreviations include CPT, carnitine palmitoyl-CoA transferase; HMG-CoA, 3-hydroxy-3-methylglutaryl-CoA; LCHAD, long-chain hydroxyacyl-CoA dehydrogenase; MCAD, medium-chain acyl-CoA dehydrogenase; 3-MCC, 3-Methylcrotonyl-CoA carboxylase; SCAD, short-chain acyl-CoA dehydrogenase; SCHAD, short-chain hydroxyacyl-CoA dehydrogenase, VLCAD; very-long-chain acyl-CoA dehydrogenase.

ing initiated as follows: plasma amino acids, urinary organic acids, DNA for common mutations, and fibroblast enzyme levels, depending on the disorder suspected. If confirmatory testing will take more than a few hours, expectant therapy must be initiated, even if the infant appears healthy, while it is being carried out.

Chapter 6 discusses management of disorders that lead to metabolic emergencies.

ADDITIONAL READINGS

Chace DH, Hillman SL, Van Hove JL, et al. Rapid diagnosis of MCAD deficiency: quantitative analysis of octanoylcarnitine and other acylcarnitines in newborn blood spots by tandem mass spectrometry. *Clin Chem* 1997;43:2106–2113.

Millington DS, Norwood DL, Kodo N, et al. Application of fast atom bombardment with tandem mass spectrometry and liquid chromatography/mass spectrometry to the analysis of acylcarnitines in human urine, blood, and tissue. *Anal Biochem* 1989;180:331–339.

Naylor EW, Chace DH. Automated tandem mass spectrometry for mass newborn screening for disorders in fatty acid, organic acid, and amino acid metabolism. *J Child Neurol* 1999;14(Suppl 1):S4–S8.

Rashed MS, Ozand PT, Bucknall MP, et al. Diagnosis of inborn errors of metabolism from blood spots by acylcarnitines and amino acids profiling using automated electrospray tandem mass spectrometry. *Pediatr Res* 1995;38:324–331.

Rashed MS, Rahbeeni Z, Ozand PT. Application of electrospray tandem mass spectrometry to neonatal screening. *Semin Perinatol* 1999;23:183–193.

10 ♣ DNA Studies

In the last decade remarkable progress has been made in the molecular understanding of inborn errors of metabolism. Researchers have described the localization and structure of most genes involved in monogenic metabolic disorders and have identified disease-causing mutations. Information gained through the human genome project and reverse genetics has allowed the detection or confirmation of many "new" metabolic disorders, and with the human genome project moving into its next phase, certainly more can be expected once the function of additional human genes is known.

Mutation analyses are now frequently used for clinical purposes, including confirmation of diagnosis and prediction of disease severity. Nevertheless, how the new understanding of disorders will translate into new care for patients is uncertain, particularly in how molecular analyses can complement or replace other diagnostic methods. Many metabolic disorders are more reliably diagnosed and confirmed through biochemical and enzymatic investigations than through mutation analyses. Nevertheless, an increasing number of disorders dictate molecular studies early in the diagnostic process, usually because the disease results from prevalent mutations in particular populations or because invasive procedures are necessary to obtain samples for specific enzyme studies (e.g., liver biopsies). A collation of useful internet resources that provide molecular or metabolic information is given in Appendix D. Laboratories that offer diagnostic mutation analyses may be found through the databases GeneTests in North America (http://www.genetests.org) and EDDNAL in Europe (http://www.eddnal.com).

Physicians should only do mutation analyses in children if an important medical consequence exists. Carrier analyses in healthy siblings of children with metabolic disorders should not be performed even when requested by the parents.

SAMPLES

Sample for most applications: 5 to 10 mL ethylene diamine tetraacetate (EDTA) full blood, shipped at ambient temperature. For long distances extracting the DNA and sending that may be preferable.

Any human sample that contains cellular nuclei can be analyzed for mutation. The exact sample depends on the type of DNA to be investigated. Routine diagnostic mutation analyses are usually performed on genomic DNA, which is most conveniently extracted from 5 to 10 mL of anticoagulated whole blood (usually EDTA blood). Smaller amounts of blood (down to a few hundred microliters) may be acceptable but are less satisfactory, as DNA extraction from small samples is less reliable and the extraction method may be more expensive. The sample should not be centrifuged; it should be shipped as native whole blood by normal (overnight) mail at ambient temperature. DNA is quite stable, and the sample may be stored at room temperature or in the refrigerator for 1 or 2 days if necessary (e.g., on weekends). Alternatively, whole blood may be stored frozen for several weeks or may be sent on dry ice. Prior to sending, one should determine whether the molecular laboratory accepts frozen blood. If EDTA blood is unavailable, other materials—including dried blood spots on filter paper cards, coagulated blood, hair roots, buccal swabs, or even serum, urine, or feces—may be used for extraction of genomic DNA or for polymerase chain reaction (PCR) amplification of specific sequences, but these methods are less reliable and may be considerably more expensive.

Messenger RNA (mRNA) obtained from cells in which the target gene is expressed provides an alternative template for genetic analysis. As a single-stranded molecule, mRNA is quite unstable, and in the laboratory it is converted into double-stranded complementary DNA (cDNA), which can be stored indefinitely. cDNA analysis has certain advantages over genomic DNA. It does not have an intron–exon structure but contains the uninterrupted sequence that is translated into protein. The detection of unknown mutations may be more convenient from cDNA since larger fragments may be examined with gene scanning methods and because fewer are required for PCR-based analysis methods. Splicing mutations that cause the removal of whole exons from the translated sequence are easily recognized, thus confirming the pathologic relevance of DNA variants in the introns. On the other hand, splicing variants that are observed under physiologic or cell culture conditions sometimes do not cause disease and may be difficult to interpret. The preparation of cDNA is much more tedious than is that of genomic DNA. Although cDNA analysis in conjunction with enzyme studies may be the method of choice if organ tissue, such as liver or skin fibroblasts, is available for investigation, genomic DNA analysis remains the method of choice for most applications.

INDICATIONS

Biochemical and enzymatic analyses, when available, are generally preferable for diagnosing metabolic disorders as they reflect phenotypical parameters ("enzymatic" or "biochemical phenotype") and are therefore closer to the patient's clinical phenotype and disease expression. Nevertheless, circumstances exist in which molecular studies are cheaper, faster, and more convenient or are the only reliable method for diagnosing or confirming diagnosis of an inherited disorder. Many metabolic defects involve enzymes that are expressed only in specific organs, such as the liver or the brain, necessitating invasive procedures (if at all possible) for enzymatic confirmation. Other disorders involve structural, receptor, or membrane proteins that do not cause metabolic alterations, that are not open for enzyme testing, and that therefore may be difficult to confirm by traditional methods. Molecular studies may be fast and efficient and therefore may be the method of choice for confirming disorders caused by single prevalent mutations in the patient's population (e.g., the prevalent Caucasian medium-chain acyl-CoA dehydrogenase [MCAD] mutation 985A→G, which specifies K329E). The identification of well-characterized mutations may provide information on disease severity, prognosis, or other clinical parameters in disorders with good genotype–phenotype correlations. Common genetic variants that can influence disease course or treatment may be easily detected through specific analyses (e.g., the factor-V–Leiden mutation or the methylenetetrahydrofolate reductase [MTHFR] variant A222V). Identification of disease-causing mutations in a particular patient allows rapid, cost-efficient, and reliable testing of other family members, including prenatal diagnosis. In all cases, laboratories that offer molecular analyses for clinical purposes need to have good knowledge of the tested disorder, the genotype–phenotype correlations, and alternative diagnostic approaches, as well as the sensitivity and specificity of mutation analysis for the individual patient.

METHODS

A wide range of molecular methods, most of which are based on the polymerase chain reaction (PCR), is available for identifying mutations and other DNA variants. Different methods are used to screen for specific known variants or to examine a gene for unknown mutations. No uniform strategy that is suitable for all applications exists; consequently, a combination of methods is often used. The exact approach depends on gene characteristics, the type and frequency of mutations, and the sensitivity required to answer the clinical question. For adequate outcomes when requesting tests and interpreting their results, the clinician must be familiar with the sensitivity, specificity, and indication of the most frequently used mutation detection strategies. This chapter concentrates on PCR-based methods for the detection of point mutations or small deletions/insertions, as these are by far the most frequent causes of inborn errors of metabolism.

Several widely used *screening methods* to identify selected DNA variants exist. Most are relatively inexpensive. Commercial kits that test for several common mutations are available for some disorders, such as cystic fibrosis. The capacity for mutation detection will be greatly expanded through the introduction of DNA chips within the next decade. Nevertheless, the sensitivity of these mutation-specific screening methods for detecting relevant DNA changes is and will remain limited by definition, since rare and "new" mutations are not identified. Homozygosity or compound heterozygosity of disease-causing mutations is diagnostic in the investigated patients, but failure to identify a mutation does not exclude the disorder. Screened mutations are usually well characterized, and their clinical relevance is well known. Mutation-specific screening methods are especially useful for detecting common DNA polymorphisms that may influence multifactorial disorders (e.g., atherosclerosis), as well as for confirming inherited disorders that are caused by specific prevalent mutations in a particular population.

Examination of whole genes for mutations that may or may not have been identified previously is much more demanding with regard to both the detection and the interpretation of DNA variants. The methodological gold standard is full DNA sequencing, which is laborious, expensive, and inefficient, particularly for the examination of large genes with many exons. Most laboratories first use one of several *gene-scanning methods* to narrow down the region in which a mutation is located; they then fully characterize the exact base change by DNA sequencing. The scanning methods are sometimes difficult to interpret and may differ in their sensitivity (i.e., the reliability with which mutations are found). Failure to detect any mutation in a patient by one of the less sensitive scanning methods does not exclude the disorder in question—it just makes the disorders more unlikely. The following scanning methods are widely employed in diagnostic laboratories:

- *Single-strand configuration polymorphism (SSCP) analysis* is relatively simple and inexpensive and is widely used in many diagnostic and research laboratories. The main drawback in comparison with other scanning methods is its limited sensitivity: SSCP fails to detect 10% to 20% of mutations. Various variants are available that may improve sensitivity, but the rate of false negatives has been systematically examined only for some disorders.
- *Denaturing gradient gel electrophoresis (DGGE)* is more difficult to develop for a particular gene, but once established it is simple, sensitive, and inexpensive. It is therefore particularly well suited for mutation analysis in routine diagnostic laboratories. A well-designed DGGE system may reach a mutation detection rate of up to 100%, as in phenylketonuria mutation analysis; but this high sensitivity has not been achieved for all genes.
- *Chemical or enzymatic cleavage of DNA mismatches (CCM)* in heteroduplex molecules can be achieved by various methods. These methods work by denaturation and renaturation of non-identical DNA strands in individuals who are heterozygous or compound heterozygous for mutations or polymorphisms. The method is more complicated and laborious than are other scanning methods, and in its original version it requires toxic chemicals; however, it is well suited to analyze large DNA fragments (as in cDNA analysis) and has a high sensitivity.

The ultimate method for detecting mutations is *DNA sequencing.* Most laboratories now use semiautomated DNA sequencers that detect fluorescently labeled DNA fragments with specific laser systems. In the standard approach, the genomic target region is amplified first by PCR. Fluorescently labeled base-specific fragments are then generated through cycle sequencing with unidirectional primers and ddNTP nucleotides, either of which is labeled with a fluorescent marker dye. These fragments are then separated on conventional acrylamide gels or through capillary electrophoresis. No completely reliable system for automatically evaluating the DNA sequences generated in this fashion exists as yet, and skilled interpretation of the results is required, particularly to detect or exclude heterozygous mutations.

PITFALLS

Like any laboratory technique, mutation analysis has a certain error rate that is difficult to eliminate completely. Incorrect results or interpretations may be generated through sampling errors, methodological limitations, insufficient knowledge of the types of mutations causing a particular disease, or inadequate consideration of family or population conditions. The following factors may need to be considered in choosing mutation analysis methods and in interpreting the results:

- *What type of mutation usually causes the disease?* Different approaches should be chosen for certain mutations, such as point mutations, trinucleotide repeats, or large deletions.
- *Are certain disease-causing mutations prevalent in particular populations?* Screening for such mutations may be a cost-efficient method for confirming the disease or for reducing the likelihood of its presence in a patient. Taking the ethnic origin of a patient into consideration is essential when such an approach is chosen.
- *What is the sensitivity of comprehensive mutation analysis with PCR-based methods, such as DNA sequencing?* For some disorders it may approach 100%; for others only a proportion of mutations is recognized. PCR-based methods are usually restricted to coding exons and adjacent intron sequences of the particular gene and may fail to detect large gene deletions spanning several exons or intron mutations.
- *Could more than one mutation exist on one chromosome?* Double mutants have been identified in many genes. Although two mutations are found in a patient with a recessive disease, this finding does not necessarily mean compound heterozygosity also exists. This constellation can be assumed only when inheritance of mutations on separate chromosomes can be confirmed in samples from parents or other relatives. In addition, identifying common missense mutations through selective screening may be insufficient for predicting the phenotype in a particular patient because additional mutations affecting protein structure may be missed.
- *What is the diagnostic specificity of mutation identification?* Only some of the variants in a gene affect protein function and cause disease. Criteria that may be used to estimate pathogenetic relevance include type of mutation (e.g., missense or nonsense, predicted impact on amino acid sequence), extent of DNA analyzed, segregation with the disease in a family, prevalence of the mutation in the general population, and functional assessment through expression analysis.
- *How important are nongenetic factors of pathogenesis?* Disease penetrance may vary considerably, even within single families. Strict genotype–phenotype correlations are observed only in a proportion of metabolic disorders, and the clinical picture in a patient may be insufficiently explained by the mutations in a single gene.

11 ♣ Function Tests

Many metabolic disorders show biochemical abnormalities only intermittently when under metabolic stress, so normal findings in the interval may not reliably exclude a diagnosis in a particular patient. However, pinpointing the site or at least the area of a patient's metabolic abnormality is often possible by using a properly chosen challenge. Various *in vivo* function tests are used to create conditions that allow the assessment of metabolism in a controlled manner. Frequently this entails ingestion of specific substances that give rise to diagnostic metabolites in certain disorders. Most tests are fairly safe; many are inconvenient, but some (including the frequently performed fasting test) may lead to potentially serious complications and should be carried out only by experienced physicians after other diagnostic options have been exhausted. Planning the collection of samples carefully during the test and preparing emergency measures in case complications occur are essential.

Rapid advances in enzymatic, molecular, and other diagnostic techniques permit an increasing number of diagnoses without tests of tolerance. However, inherited metabolic diseases are serious, lifelong conditions, and functional studies will continue to have their place in diagnostic work-up and to tailor therapy.

PREPRANDIAL AND POSTPRANDIAL INVESTIGATIONS (Protein and Glucose Challenges)

Many biochemical parameters show marked variation with food intake and should be examined routinely under preprandial conditions to determine baseline values. Reduced concentrations of amino acids or other metabolites may be diagnostically relevant but are sometimes found only in preprandial samples. On the other hand, some metabolic disorders that affect substrate utilization cause abnormal metabolite concentrations only in the postprandial state. To detect relevant abnormalities reliably, examining metabolic parameters both before and after defined food intake is often necessary. In practice, this intake may be a normal meal enriched with protein and carbohydrates, the exact composition of which is less important. This test is particularly useful for diagnosing mitochondrial disorders, which typically show pathologic postprandial increases of lactate, alanine, and other small amino acids. Alanine, in contrast to lactate, is not affected by cuffing or crying, so when elevated it is a more reliable indicator of disturbed energy metabolism. This test also recognizes aminoacidemias and urea cycle defects but may trigger or aggravate acute neurologic symptoms.

Procedure

- Preprandial samples should reflect a neutral metabolic state (not a fasting reaction) and are best obtained 5 to 6 hours (up to 8 hours in older children) after the last meal. Measure blood gases, blood sugar, amino acids, lactate, and ammonia. Obtain a deproteinized blood sample (perchloric acid extraction) for pyruvate and ketone bodies in case the lactate is elevated. In urine, check for ketones (ketosticks) and measure lactate and/or organic acids and orotic acid if they were not normal previously.

- Give a normal meal enriched with protein and sugar to attain a total amount of about 1 g/kg body weight for each (protein and carbohydrate/sugar).
- Postprandial blood sample should be obtained 90 minutes after the meal; urine should be collected for 2 hours. Measure the same analytes as in the preprandial samples.

Interpretation

Blood lactate should not rise by more than 20% over baseline values and should not reach pathologic values (> 2.1 mmol/L). When lactate is elevated, measure pyruvate, acetoacetate, and 3-hydroxybutyrate in the perchloric acid extract to determine the redox ratio. Acid–base status should remain normal. Most amino acids will be elevated in the postprandial sample, but the plasma concentration of alanine should stay under 600 to 700 μmol/L and the alanine/lysine ratio should stay below 3.

GLUCOSE CHALLENGE

For aerobic generation of energy, glucose is catabolized to pyruvate, transferred into the mitochondrion, and fully oxidized via the Krebs cycle and the respiratory chain. High lactate (the reduced form of pyruvate) is the most valuable diagnostic marker of disturbed mitochondrial energy metabolism in respiratory chain defects and in other disorders that affect cellular respiration. However, frequently lactate is elevated only after intake of glucose or glucogenic amino acids; single normal lactate values do not exclude a primary mitochondriopathy (see Chapter 6, "Work-up of the Patient with Lactic Acidemia"). A controlled glucose challenge is useful for assessing cellular respiration in patients with suspected disorders of energy metabolism in whom lactate values have been repeatedly normal. It is relatively inexpensive because all general and pediatric hospitals can measure lactate, but it may require frequent venepunctures; in addition, lactate concentrations may be affected by cuffing or crying. Measuring pyruvate when lactate is normal is unnecessary, but deproteinized blood samples (perchloric acid extraction) should be obtained to determine the redox ratio (lactate/pyruvate) when lactate is high. A glucose challenge should not be carried out when lactate has been consistently elevated or when a significant postprandial increase of lactate has already been demonstrated because it may cause acute metabolic decompensation. In such cases, appropriate enzyme studies (muscle biopsy) and molecular analyses should be undertaken immediately upon completion of the basic biochemical analyses. Other indications for the glucose challenge include unclear hypoglycemic episodes and suspected glycogen storage disease (see Chapter 6, "Work-up of the Patient with Lactic Acidemia").

Preparations

- Basic investigations, including those of amino acids and organic acids, should be complete; blood lactate should be normal in repeated measurements before and after meals at different times of the day.

- Glucose challenge should be carried out in the morning after overnight fasting (in younger infants at least 4 to 5 hours after the last meal).
- Secure intravenous access. An established line avoids frequent venepuncture and potential effects on lactate levels.

Procedure
- Measure baseline blood lactate, blood sugar, and acid–base status; obtain 10 mL urine for lactate and/or organic acids before test.
- Give glucose, 1.75–2 g/kg (maximum of 50 g), as a 10% oral solution. The solution may be administered through a nasogastric tube (flush with water) in small children. For older children the solution should be stored in the refrigerator because it is more pleasant to drink when cool.
- Measure blood lactate, blood sugar, and acid–base status at 15, 30, 45, 60, 90, 120, and 180 minutes after the test; collect urine for 2 hours to assess lactate and/or organic acids. Obtain deproteinized blood samples (perchloric acid extraction) for pyruvate and ketone bodies in case lactate is elevated.

Interpretation

Blood sugar should be elevated after the test, but lactate should not rise by more than 20% over baseline values and should not reach pathologic values (> 2.1 mmol/L). Acid–base status and urine measurements should remain normal.

FRUCTOSE CHALLENGE

The major indication for use of the fructose tolerance test is a suspicion of hereditary fructose intolerance. Evaluation of the response to fructose loading can also provide valuable diagnostic information for patients with suspected defects of gluconeogenesis, such as fructose-1,6-diphosphatase deficiency. It provides no additional information in patients with glycogen storage disease. It may be useful in guiding therapy in those patients with defects of oxidative phosphorylation in whom fructose administration leads to a major elevation of lactic acid. The test may cause potentially life-threatening hypoglycemia and should be performed with great care only after other diagnostic options, including mutation analysis of the aldolase B gene, have been exhausted. Close clinical observation is essential, and resuscitation facilities must be available. The test may cause severe nausea and/or abdominal pain from 15 to 90 minutes after oral fructose intake. Intravenous fructose challenge is preferable as nausea and vomiting are less common (occurring 15 to 50 minutes after intravenous administration), but these preparations are currently unavailable in most countries.

Preparations
- The child should be placed on a fructose-free diet for at least 2 weeks before the test, and liver function tests should have become normal.

- Explain the potential risks (hypoglycemia, nausea, vomiting) to the parents and obtain informed consent.
- Blood sugar before the test should be in the upper normal range to reduce the risk of life-threatening hypoglycemia.
- An intravenous line should be maintained with 0.9% NaCl to allow sampling of specimens and rapid infusion of glucose as necessary.
- Prepare an intravenous glucose solution (20%) for emergency administration in case of onset of hypoglycemia.

Procedure: Oral Fructose Challenge
- Establish basal values. Measure blood sugar, phosphate, magnesium, uric acid, and lactate; determine fructose if possible.
- Give oral fructose, 1 g/kg, as a 20% solution over 5 to 7 minutes.
- Obtain blood samples after 15, 30, 45, 60, 90, and 120 minutes; measure the same analytes as in the basal sample.

Procedure: Intravenous Fructose Challenge
- Establish basal values: measure blood sugar, phosphate, magnesium, uric acid, and lactate; determine fructose if possible.
- Give intravenous fructose, 0.25 g/kg, as a 10% solution over 2 to 4 minutes.
- Obtain blood samples after 5, 10, 15, 30, 45, 60, and 90 minutes; measure the same parameters as in the basal sample.
- Optionally, measure sugars (including fructose) and amino acids in a baseline urine sample, as well as in urine samples collected over the 6 to 12 hours after the load.

Treatment of Adverse Reactions
In cases of hypoglycemia (blood glucose < 40 mg% or 2.3 mmol/L) or if the patient becomes symptomatic with irritability, sweating, and drowsiness, give 2 mL of 20% or 4 mL of 10% glucose per kilogram of body weight intravenously as a bolus and follow with 3 to 5 mL 10% glucose per kilogram of body weight per hour until normoglycemia is restored and the patient can take and retain oral food and fluid.

Interpretation
In hereditary fructose intolerance fructose loading leads to profound metabolic disturbances. Progressive hypoglycemia dominates the picture. An even sharper fall of inorganic phosphate occurs within a few minutes. A slight rise of magnesium follows a sharp rise in fructose and uric acid. Levels of transaminases may increase, and a slight fall in serum potassium may occur. Lactate, pyruvate, alanine, free fatty acids, glycerol, ketone bodies, and growth hormone may also rise. Fructose may be found in the urine in amounts that depend on the level of hyperfructosemia. The renal threshold is 20 mg/dL. Transitory renal tubular dysfunction may lead to mild aminoaciduria and proteinuria. The fall in glucose and phosphate along with the rise in urate are sufficient to diagnose hereditary fructose intolerance.

A hypoglycemic response to fructose administration is also observed in fructose-1,6-diphosphate deficiency. This disorder may be differentiated from fructose intolerance by a history of fasting hypoglycemia and lactic acidemia and by an absence of aversion to fruits and sweets. Enzyme assay of biopsied liver provides the definitive diagnosis in both.

MONITORED PROLONGED FAST

Monitored fasting is a powerful tool for unraveling the nature of metabolic disorders of energy metabolism. However, one must remember that fasting is potentially dangerous and should therefore be conducted only after other, less risky investigations have failed to provide a clear diagnosis. Fasting can cause life-threatening cardiac complications, particularly in patients with long-chain fatty acid oxidation defects. Sudden cardiac arrest may occur even under controlled conditions in an intensive care unit. Therefore a fasting test is contraindicated in almost all patients with cardiomyopathy. However, following a careful selection of patients and under careful observation, it can be carried out safely.

Fasting results in a series of hormonal and metabolic responses to ensure an endogenous supply of energy after exogenous intake ends. After each feeding, nutrients are supplied via gastrointestinal absorption. Depending on the amount and composition of the food, this absorption period can last for up to 6 hours in adults. It often lasts less than 4 hours in infants and small children. With diminishing exogenous supply of glucose, plasma glucose concentrations fall and insulin levels decrease in a parallel fashion. The decrease of insulin and the increase of counteracting hormones diminish glucose consumption in muscle and peripheral tissues. The body begins to utilize glycogen reserves by glycogenolysis.

In principle, hypoglycemia may result from endocrine or metabolic disease. Therefore measuring insulin, cortisol, and growth hormone, as well as metabolic parameters, in patients who develop hypoglycemia is necessary. Patients with hyperinsulinism become hypoglycemic after a very short period of fasting.

After 8 to 10 hours of fasting, free fatty acids begin to substitute for glucose as the primary energy source in muscle, whereas depleting ordinary stores of glycogen may take 17 to 24 hours. Two central metabolic adaptations to prolonged fasting are initiated in the liver. Glucose is synthesized via glyconeogenesis from alanine and oxaloacetate derived from amino acids, as well as from glycerol resulting from fatty acid oxidation. More important, fatty acid oxidation funnels into ketone body production, providing an alternative source of energy.

Patients with defects of glycogenolysis (glycogen storage disorders) often become hypoglycemic directly after the absorption period. Patients with defects of glyconeogenesis may become hypoglycemic after 10 to 20 hours of fasting, whereas those with defects of ketogenesis or ketolysis develop hypoglycemia between 15 to 24 hours. Infants and small children may have a shorter tolerance of fasting. In prolonged fasting the body finally draws selectively on its lipid resources to spare vitally needed proteins. Depending on his or her nutritional state, an adult with a defect in fatty acid oxidation may not become symptomatic until fasting has been prolonged for 36 hours. In general, hypoglycemia after a short period of fasting signifies disordered carbohydrate metabolism; hypoglycemia that occurs only after prolonged fasting signifies disordered fatty acid oxidation or ketolysis. Some patients with electron transport defects follow the prolonged pattern because fatty acid oxidation may be impaired secondarily.

Free fatty acids can be oxidized as an energy source in most body tissues. As they do not cross the blood–brain barrier, homeostasis of the brain energy supply depends on the adequate production of ketone bodies. Defects of fatty acid oxidation, in which ketone production may be impaired and toxic intermediates are produced, may cause acute encephalopathy that is accompanied by hepatocellular dysfunction, producing a Reyelike syndrome.

The fasting test has lost some importance with the advent of acylcarnitine analysis in dried blood spots and is now largely irrelevant, if not contraindicated, for the diagnosis of fatty acid oxidation defects. These disorders frequently show clinical symptoms only at times of fasting, when hypoketotic hypoglycemia and massive excretion of dicarboxylic acids without appropriate ketones in the urine may occur. The single most important investigation is the determination of free fatty acids (elevated) and ketone bodies (not sufficiently elevated) in a serum or plasma sample at a time of symptomatic hypoglycemia. Diagnostic problems arise when the acute hypoglycemic illness is treated without prior collection of a serum sample because biochemical abnormalities may disappear completely with restoration of glucose homeostasis.

Fatty acid oxidation defects should be ruled out before a diagnostic fast by urinary organic acids and acylglycine excretion patterns, as well as by analysis of plasma free and total carnitine and especially of acylcarnitine profiles in dried blood spots. The last usually remain abnormal in the nonfasting state. Phenylpropionic acid loading may reveal either medium-chain acyl-CoA dehydrogenase (MCAD) deficiency or an increased excretion of phenylhydracrylic acid as a marker of long-chain hydroxyacyl-CoA dehydrogenase (LCHAD) deficiency, but again acylcarnitine analysis has largely supplanted this test. Fatty acid oxidation enzymes may be analyzed in leukocytes or fibroblasts. Analyzing for the common mutation K329E in the ACADM gene confirms the diagnosis of MCAD deficiency in most patients of European descent. Early analysis of the common HADHA gene mutation E510Q is indicated if LCHAD deficiency is suggested by the clinical and biochemical symptoms—progressive or episodic myopathy or cardiomyopathy and specific acylcarnitine pattern with or without bouts of hypoketotic hypoglycemia and hydroxydicarboxylic aciduria.

Determination of fasting tolerance through a monitored fast is indicated in patients with recurrent episodes of apparently fasting-related symptoms, such as episodes of decreased consciousness, or especially with recurrent documented hypoglycemia or Reyelike disease in whom other analyses (including acylcarnitines) have been inconclusive. In particular, patients with a deficiency of mitochondrial 3-hydroxy-3-methylglutaryl-(HMG)-CoA synthase, an isolated disorder of ketogenesis, show a normal acylcarnitine profile even during hypoglycemic episodes. A fasting test may reveal the typical hypoketotic hypoglycemia and a unique spectrum of urinary organic acids. Enzymatic confirmation of this disorder requires a liver biopsy as this enzyme is not expressed in other tissues and is problematic because of the cytosolic enzyme. Primary mutation analysis may be the best way to confirm the diagnosis.

In patients with lactic acidemia, a fasting test is also useful to distinguish those with disorders of gluconeogenesis from those with defective oxidation of pyruvate (see Chapter 6, "Work-up of the Patient with Lactic Acidemia"). Other indications for controlled fasting include the following:

- Recurrent episodes of symptomatic ketonemia;
- Recurrent cyclic vomiting;
- Recurrent intermittent metabolic acidosis;
- Suspicion of fluctuating neurometabolic disease;
- Controlled determination of fasting tolerance to fine-tune the therapy of metabolic disorders, as in patients with glycogen storage diseases and nesidioblastosis. Also to judge the duration of safe intervals between feedings (e.g., in patients with mitochondrial disorders).

Preparations

A fasting test should be performed only if the patient is in a stable, steady-state condition. Caloric intake for the last 3 days should have been adequate for age. The test must be postponed in the case of even minor intercurrent illness. Especially important is a detailed history with respect to the individual fasting tolerance and events and time courses of adverse reactions to previous fasting. With this information and that of the presumptive diagnoses, the timing of the fast can be optimally planned. The duration of the fasting period may be scheduled according to the age of the child (Table 11.1), unless the clinical history indicates a shorter period. In general, allowing a fast at night for as long as the patient usually goes without eating is usually safe, but the period beyond should take place during the daytime. If hypoglycemia occurs, it should be at a time of optimal staffing.

Table 11.1.   Suggested time periods for fasting in different age groups

Age	< 6 Months	6–8 Months	8–12 Months	1–7 Years	> 7 Years
Starting time	4 A.M.	Midnight	7 P.M.	3 P.M.	1 P.M.
Duration	8 h	15 h	20 h	24 h	24 h

A monitored fast should be undertaken only in settings in which the entire staff is experienced in the procedure and with close clinical supervision and well-set-out guidelines for response to hypoglycemia or other adverse events. Necessary details must be explained in advance to everybody involved. Special care must be taken to ensure complete collection of samples. Filling out the forms and assembling and labeling all tubes, including day and timing of the samples, before starting the test are advisable.

The aim, nature, and possible adverse effects of the fasting test must be explained in detail to the patient and family to ensure optimal cooperation, as well as early notification of symptoms. Informed consent must be obtained from the parents before the test.

An intravenous line must be established to provide immediate access for treating hypoglycemia. It may be maintained with 0.9% NaCl or a heparin lock.

Procedure

After baseline studies of plasma free fatty acids and ketone bodies (acetoacetate and 3-hydroxybutyrate), blood sugar, and urinary organic acids, fasting is conducted with careful bedside monitoring of the concentrations of glucose in blood and ketones in urine. The patient is allowed to drink water and unsweetened tea but no juices or soft drinks, including "diet" beverages. Heart rate may be monitored by electrocardiogram.

Table 11.2 provides an example of a fasting test of 24 hours. Under normal conditions, ketogenesis is brisk; concentrations of acetoacetate and 3-hydroxybutyrate rise sharply, especially after 15 to 17 hours, and gluconeogenesis occurs, which preserves normoglycemia. The fast is stopped with the development of hypoglycemia at any time; with close monitoring, avoiding symptoms of hypoglycemia is usually possible.

Blood samples should be obtained at 15, 20, and 24 hours, and always at a time of hypoglycemia, when the fast is stopped. The following basic laboratory analytes should be measured: blood sugar, free fatty acids and ketone bodies (acetoacetate, 3-hydroxybutyrate), lactate, electrolytes, blood gases, transaminases, and creatine kinase. In addition, dried blood spots must be obtained in order to analyze the acylcarnitine profile. Serum carnitine status and amino acids may be considered, and a spare serum sample should be obtained in case additional tests are indicated. Hormone studies, including insulin, glucagon, and growth hormone, must be carried out during hypoglycemia. Urine should be collected in 8-hour aliquots for the quantitative determination of organic acids. Glucose levels are evaluated hourly after the first missed feeding and are assessed more frequently if the blood sugar falls below 50 mg/dL. All urine passed should be checked for ketones. Comprehensive investigation of intermediary metabolites and hormones in blood and urine is especially important at the scheduled end of the fast or at the time of developing hypoglycemia when the fast is terminated.

Table 11.2.   Twenty-four-hour fast in a 6-year-old child

Protocol and specimens

Begin fast at time T = 0 at 4 P.M.

T(ime) = 0 (4 P.M.): End of last meal with intake documented.

T = 1 (5 P.M.): **Serum glucose**, electrolytes, transaminases, creatine kinase. Blood gases. Lactate, pyruvate, **3-hydroxybutyrate**, acetoacetate from perchloric acid tube. **Plasma amino acids, free fatty acids**, and carnitine. Acylcarnitines on Guthrie card. Start collection of urine in 8-hour aliquots. Monitor ketones in urine at the bedside.

T = 1 until T = 12: Blood glucose concentration is monitored q 3 h at the bedside.

From T = 12 (4 A.M.) onward collect glucose levels hourly. Heart rate may be monitored by ECG.

T = 15 (7 A.M.): Serum glucose, electrolytes. Blood gases. Lactate, pyruvate, 3-hydroxybutyrate, acetoacetate. Plasma amino acids, free fatty acids.

T = 20 (noon): Serum glucose, electrolytes. Blood gases. Lactate, pyruvate, 3-hydroxybutyrate, acetoacetate. Plasma amino acids, free fatty acids.

T = 24 (4 P.M.) or at the time of hypoglycemia: **Serum glucose**, electrolytes, transaminases, creatine kinase. **Insulin, cortisol, growth hormone**, and additional specimen for follow-up hormonal investigations. Blood gases. Lactate, pyruvate, **3-hydroxybutyrate**, acetoacetate. **Plasma amino acids, free fatty acids. Acylcarnitines.** Collect first urine sample after the end of the test separately.

Quantitative analysis of organic acids is performed on the first and last aliquots. The middle collection is to ensure a sample for analysis in a patient developing hypoglycemia during that period.

Abbreviation: ECG, electrocardiogram.
Parameters that are indispensible for evaluation and interpretation are highlighted in bold (see also Table 11.3).

In investigating lactic acidemia, fasting helps to distinguish disorders of gluconeogenesis from defects of oxidative phosphorylation (see Chapter 6). For this purpose, giving glucagon at 6 hours into the fast is useful. This may provide a presumptive diagnosis in a patient with glycogen storage disease type I. In addition, doing so depletes the liver of glycogen derived from exogenous glucose so that, as the fast continues, gluconeogenesis is required to prevent hypoglycemia. Table 6.5 shows a schedule. If the suspicion of a defect of oxidative phosphorylation is especially high, the fasting test can be combined with a glucose and/or protein load as the last feed.

Treatment of Adverse Reactions

The fasting test must be terminated if the intravenous line is lost and cannot be immediately replaced or if the patient develops symptoms caused by hypoglycemia or ketoacidosis, such as irritability, sweating, and drowsiness. It should also be discontinued at any sign of cardiac arrhythmia or if hypoglycemia (blood glucose < 40 mg/dL or 2.3 mmol/L) or significant metabolic acidosis (bicarbonate < 15 mmol/L) is documented.

For treatment of hypoglycemia, 2 mL of 20% or 4 mL of 10% glucose per kilogram of body weight are given intravenously as a bolus and should be followed by 3 to 5 mL 10% glucose per kilogram of body weight per hour until normoglycemia is restored and the patient retains oral food and fluid.

Interpretation

If the patient develops hypoglycemia, the fasting test is abnormal. Accurate interpretation requires knowledge of age-dependent hormonal and metabolic responses to fasting, as well as reference values from control individuals. Table 11.3 is based on experience with nearly 100 control subjects from two published series and on additional control subjects, selected after extensive metabolic investigations failed to give any indication of an inherited metabolic disease.

In older children and adults, ketone body production may not be maximal until the second or third day of fasting because of greater capacities for storage of glycogen and because of efficient gluconeogenesis. Prolonged fasting (extended up to 36 or even 48 hours) may be justified in adults. Infants and small children have much lower glycogen stores and higher capacities for forming and utilizing ketone bodies. Significant ketone body production occurs before 24 hours. Interestingly, infants show an intermediate response to fasting as compared with toddlers and older children. This is explained by larger glycogen stores in infants as a result of high-calorie meals at regular intervals. Ketone body production for children more than 7 years of age varied and, in some, was only moderate, even after 24 hours (Table 11.3). Even with these children, metabolic defects of ketogenesis or ketolysis should, however, be diagnosable after a 24-hour fast.

Reliable quantification of acetoacetate and pyruvate is difficult. For evaluating the fasting response, ketone bodies (particularly 3-hydroxybutyrate) may be measured in a plasma or serum sample. However, the ratio of 3-hydroxybutyrate to acetoacetate is important in the work-up of a suspected defect of pyruvate metabolism or oxidative phosphorylation, and analysis should be carried out in deproteinized blood samples (perchloric acid extraction) if such a disorder is suspected. Additional clues to a defect of pyruvate carboxylase are bouts of hyperammonemia and elevated levels of citrulline and lysine on amino acid analysis.

A good indicator of blood pyruvate concentrations is the simultaneously determined level of alanine in plasma. An alanine level of 450 µmol/L corresponds to a blood pyruvate concentration of 100 µmol/L (i.e., the upper limit of the normal range). Other amino acids to be evaluated at the end of a fasting test are the branched-

Table 11.3. Control ranges of metabolites of energy metabolism in response to controlled prolonged fasting

	Glucose mmol/L (mg %)	Ketones mmol/L	3-OH-BA mmol/L	3-OH-BA/ acetoacetate	FFA mmol/L	FFA/ ketones	FFA/ 3-OH-BA	Glucose X ketones	Lactate	L/P
Infants										
15 h fasting	3.8–5.3 (68–95)	0.1–1.6	0.1–1.0	1.4–2.7	0.4–1.6	0.6–5.4	0.9–4.4	0.5–6	0.9–2.3	11–21
20 h fasting	3.5–4.7 (63–85)	0.6–3.5	0.4–2.5	1.7–3.1	0.6–1.4	0.3–1.7	0.5–2.1	3–12	0.8–2.0	12–19
24 h fasting	2.6–4.6 (47–83)	1.4–4.1	1.0–2.9	2.2–2.9	1.1–1.7	0.3–0.7	0.5–0.9	7–12	0.8–2.1	11–20
1–7 years										
15 h fasting	3.5–5.1 (63–92)	0.1–2.2	< 0.1–1.0	1.2–3.2	0.6–1.8	0.6–4.0	0.9–11	0.7–8	0.6–1.7	12–18

20 h fasting	2.8–4.5 (50–81)	1.0–3.8	0.6–2.9	2.3–3.3	0.8–2.6	0.4–1.7	0.4–2.1	4–12	0.5–1.8	10–19
24 h fasting	2.8–3.9 (50–70)	2.1–6.1	1.5–3.4	2.5–3.5	1.0–2.9	0.4–0.9	0.4–1.3	8–13	0.6–1.8	10–18
7–18 years										
15 h fasting	3.8–5.3 (68–95)	<0.1–0.8	<0.1–0.5	0.5–2.6	0.2–1.3	1.7–8	3.3–22	0.2–2.1	0.6–1.0	11–15
20 h fasting	3.5–4.7 (63–85)	0.1–1.5	<0.1–1.2	1.3–3.0	0.6–1.4	0.7–4.1	1.5–7.8	0.4–5.1	0.6–1.1	10–17
24 h fasting	2.6–4.6 (47–83)	0.7–4.1	0.5–1.6	1.5–3.1	0.9–1.8	0.5–2.0	1.1–2.4	2.4–8.1	0.4–1.0	8–18

FFA, free fatty acids; Ketones, sum of 3-hydroxybutyrate and acetoacetate; L/P, lactate/pyruvate ratio; 3-OH-BA, 3-hydroxybutyrate. Glucose concentrations are converted from mg% into mmol/L by division by 18 and vice versa.
The table is modified from Bonnefont et al. (1990) following the grouping of subjects and analytes considered and expanding the ranges from experiences with an additional 25 control subjects studied at the authors' departments.

chain amino acids isoleucine, leucine, and valine, which are physiologically elevated during acute starvation. However, if the increase becomes excessive and allo-isoleucine is detectable, a variant of maple syrup urine disease may be the cause of recurrent episodes of hyperketotic hypoglycemia.

Table 11.4 provides a diagnostic algorithm of differential metabolic responses to fasting in disorders of carbohydrate and energy metabolism. In general, a high level of free fatty acids and low levels of 3-hydroxybutyrate and acetoacetate indicate a disorder of fatty acid oxidation or of ketogenesis. In defects of ketolysis, an elevated product of blood glucose times ketones during fasting is the most suggestive parameter. Table 11.5 gives a summary of metabolic and hormonal disorders in which pathologic responses are elucidated by fasting.

Congenital hyperinsulinism, previously described as nesidioblastosis or persistent hyperinsulinemia of infancy and the most common cause of persistent symptomatic hypoglycemia in neonates and small infants, leads to hypoketotic hypoglycemia with low levels of free fatty acids. This disorder can be due to defects of the sulfonylurea receptor. The same constellation of neonatal hypoglycemia and impaired lipolysis can result from hyperproinsulinemia. In such patients insulin levels are low and proinsulin levels are grossly elevated.

Diagnosis of hormonal disorders depends on the correct collection of specimens during fasting and on interpretation in connection with the blood glucose concentrations. Diagnosis needs to be ascertained by repeated determinations of insulin or by detailed studies of pituitary function and additional investigations in patients with insufficiency of one or more of the counteracting hormones. Single growth hormone determinations in response to hypoglycemia are of little value for diagnosing growth hormone deficiency, and different provocative tests should be employed if the diagnosis is clinically suspected. Catecholamine deficiency on the basis of dopamine-β-hydroxylase deficiency or tyrosine hydroxylase deficiency is an exceedingly rare condition with a tendency to hypoglycemia. Analyses of catecholamines in urine and of biogenic amines in cerebrospinal fluid (CSF) can reveal it in patients suffering from severe orthostatic hypotension.

Significant hepatomegaly and repeated bouts of hypoglycemia usually lead to a presumptive diagnosis of glycogen storage diseases before the diagnostic fast. Fatty acid oxidation requires the coordinated action of at least 17 different enzymes and one additional transport protein. In each metabolic center, patients with definitive diagnoses of defective fatty acid oxidation are found in whom the exact enzymatic defect could not be determined. In addition, a number of enzymes for which no human defects have been discovered are involved in fatty acid oxidation and ketolysis.

Otherwise completely healthy children can develop severe metabolic decompensation with excessive ketosis, with or without hypoglycemia, during intercurrent illnesses. In these children, pro-
(*text continues on page 144*)

Table 11.4. Response to fasting in disorders of carbohydrate and energy metabolism

Presumptive diagnosis	Glucose	Blood ketones	3-OH-butyrate/ acetoacetate	Free fatty acids	FFA/ketones	Lactate	L/P
Glycogenosis I	⇓⇓	N–⇓	N	N	N–⇑	⇑⇑⇑	N
Glycogenosis III, VI & 0	⇒⇓	⇑	N	N	N	N	N
Defects of gluconeogenesis	⇓⇓	N–⇓	N	N	N–⇑	⇑⇑⇑	N
Defects of fatty acid oxidation	⇓⇓	⇓⇓	N–⇓	N	⇑⇑⇑	⇑	N
Defects of ketolysis	N–⇓	⇑⇑⇑	N	N	⇒	N	N
Defects of pyruvate carboxylase	⇒	⇑	⇒	N	N	⇑⇑⇑	⇑
Defects of pyruvate dehydrogenase	N	N–⇓	N	N	N	⇑–⇑⇑⇑	**N**
Defects of oxidative phosphylation	N–⇓	⇑	⇑–⇑⇑⇑	N	N	**N–⇑⇑⇑**	⇑–⇑⇑⇑

FFA free fatty acids; L/P, lactate/pyruvate ratio; N, normal values (see Table 11.3); ⇑, pathologically elevated values; ⇓, pathologically decreased values (which may mean insufficient elevation [e.g., of blood ketones]).
Parameters of specific diagnostic value are highlighted in bold or are larger (arrows).

Table 11.5. Differential diagnosis of pathological responses to fasting

Disorder	Response to fasting	Diagnostic markers (in addition to hypoglycemia)
Disorders of fatty acid oxidation or ketogenesis	Hypoketotic hypoglycemia	Free fatty acids/ketones > 2. Carnitine deficiency, except for CPT I with elevated free carnitine. Dicarboxylic aciduria. Variable elevations of lactate. Acute illness—increased creatine kinase and uric acid.
Glycogenoses I, III, and VI	Hypoglycemia	Massive hepatomegaly. Variable elevations of lactate, urate, cholesterol, triglycerides, creatine kinase, and transaminases. Hypophosphatemia.
Defects of gluconeogenesis	Hypoglycemia	Hepatomegaly. Elevations of lactate.
Defects of ketolysis	Hyperketotic hypoglycemia	Persistently elevated free fatty acids and ketones. Ketones × glucose > 15 (fasting).
Mitochondrial disease	Hyperketotic hypoglycemia	Multisystem disease. Elevations of lactate and ketones as well as of L/P and 3-OH-BA/acetoacetate ratios.

Condition	Findings
Maple syrup urine disease (intermittent variant)	Hyperketotic hypoglycemia	Maybe ataxia. Elevations of branched-chain amino acids, including allo-isoleucine.
Congenital hyperinsulinism (nesidioblastosis)	Hypoketotic hypoglycemia	Increased insulin levels > 5 mU/L at glucose < 30 mg% or > 8 mU/L at glucose < 40 mg%. Insulin (mU/L)/ glucose (mg%)>0.3. Low free fatty acids and ketones.
Hypocortisolism, growth hormone deficiency, panhypopituitarism	Hypoketotic hypoglycemia, but sometimes significant ketosis is found in patients with Addison disease	Cortisol < 400 nmol/L. Deficiency of growth and/or thyroid hormone.
Catecholamine deficiency	Hypoketotic hypoglycemia	Decreased catecholamines.
Cyclic vomiting (diminished glycogen and protein stores)	Hyperketotic hypoglycemia	No specific abnormalities.

CPT I, carnitine palmitoyl transferase I; ketones, sum of 3-hydroxybutyrate and acetoacetate; L/P, lactate/pyruvate ratio; 3-OH-BA, 3-hydroxy-butyrate.

longed fasting can provoke similar reactions. Although this is not a homogenous group of patients, an exaggerated, uncoordinated production of ketone bodies and significant metabolic acidosis leading to nausea and protracted vomiting appear as common factors. Susceptibility to these reactions slowly diminishes with age but may persist into adolescence and young adulthood. True hypoglycemia is uncommon in these children, who appear to have a defect in using ketones. Distinguishing this condition from abdominal migraine is difficult. Relatively low stores of fat and glycogen appear to be another common denominator for such exaggerated ketogenesis. Affected children are often slim, with relatively low muscle mass. Children with pathologic muscular wasting, such as patients with spinal muscular atrophy, who have severely diminished glycogen and protein stores are at an especially high risk for metabolic decompensation during fasting.

OIL CHALLENGE

The oil challenge test examines the oxidation of fatty acids without generating a catabolic state and can identify beta-oxidation enzyme defects through the accumulation of specific metabolites. It does not necessarily reflect the biochemical changes during fasting and may be less reliable for the diagnosis of ketogenesis defects, such as HMG-CoA synthase deficiency. This test has been largely superseded by acylcarnitine analyses, which should be completed with other metabolic investigations, such as serum carnitine status, urinary organic acids, and fatty acid analysis in serum. Complications of the oil challenge test include abdominal pain and vomiting, diarrhea for up to 2 days after the test, and other nonspecific symptoms, such as muscle pain.

Preparations

The patient should be in a stable metabolic state without episodes of decompensation, such as coma or Reye syndrome, for at least 3 months. Nutritional state should be good with a balanced, normal diet for at least 3 days before the test. Patients are allowed a normal supper on the evening before the test, which is carried out after overnight fasting of at least 10 hours. Informed consent should be obtained from the parents.

Procedure

Intake of unsweetened fluids (tea, mineral water) does not need to be limited throughout the test.

- Baseline studies should include blood sugar, acylcarnitines (dried blood spots), electrolytes, liver enzymes, creatine kinase, triglycerides, free fatty acids, ketone bodies, blood gases (pH, anion gap), and lactate, as well as urinary ketones (ketosticks) and organic acids. As an alternative or addition to acylcarnitine profiling, organic acids in plasma can be investigated.
- Pure sunflower oil, 1.5 g/kg (which equals approximately 1.5 mL/kg), is administered through a nasogastric tube in small children (rinse with water) or as a drink with older children.

- Blood samples for measuring the same analytes as those in the baseline samples should be obtained after 30, 60, 90, 120, and 180 minutes. Collect urine for 3 hours to measure urinary ketones (ketosticks) and organic acids.

Interpretation

Fatty acid oxidation defects are recognized through elevations of specific acylcarnitines and urinary dicarboxylic acids.

PHENYLPROPIONIC ACID LOADING TEST

Phenylpropionic acid (PPA) is a nontoxic substance that, through a single round of beta-oxidation, is normally converted to hippuric acid, which is excreted in the urine. PPA oxidation is catabolized by enzymes that are specific for medium-chain acyl-CoA compounds, and the PPA loading test is traditionally performed to confirm MCAD deficiency. Like the other tests of beta-oxidation function, the PPA loading test has now been largely superseded by acyl-carnitine analysis in conjunction with enzyme studies or mutation analysis. The PPA loading test can be normal in mild MCAD deficiency, which is still picked up by acylcarnitine analysis in dried blood spots.

Procedure

The test is usually carried out in the morning (fasting).

- Obtain a urine sample before PPA administration for organic acid analysis.
- Give phenylpropionic acid orally in a dose of 25 mg/kg. The substance is not licensed as a medical drug but may be obtained from metabolic laboratories. It has an unpleasant cinnamon taste and should be mixed with a substance (e.g., with jam) or should be administered in 50 to 100 mL of tea through a nasogastric tube. The child should be encouraged to drink generously after ingestion of PPA and can have normal meals.
- Collect urine for 6 to 12 hours after PPA administration for organic acid analysis.

Interpretation

Excessive excretion of hippuric and benzoic acids in urine indicates normal activity of medium-chain beta-oxidations. Marked excretion of phenylpropionylglycine and insufficient hippuric acid suggests MCAD deficiency. Increased excretion of phenyl-hydracrylic acid is another pathologic response characteristic of LCHAD deficiency. However, the diagnostic sensitivity for LCHAD is far lower than in MCAD deficiency. Insufficient rise of hippuric acid without other abnormalities indicates insufficient PPA intake and thus invalidates the test results.

ALLOPURINOL TEST

Various genetic disorders, especially urea cycle defects, show increased urinary excretion of the pyrimidine uridine or its precursor orotic acid. In the case of urea cycle defects, the cause is undoubtably the mitochondrial accumulation of carbamoylphosphate that has been transferred into the cytosol and channeled into pyrimidine biosynthesis, thus bypassing the rate-limiting first step in the pathway catalyzed by the cytosolic enzyme carbamoylphosphate synthase II (CPS II) (see Figs. 6.6 and 28.2). CPS II is different from the mitochondrial isoenzyme CPS I, which is required for the detoxification of ammonia. Orotic aciduria is a diagnostic feature, particularly in ornithine transcarbamylase (OTC) deficiency, which lacks specific amino acid changes. Nevertheless, orotic acid may be normal in the interval in mild forms of OTC deficiency, particularly in heterozygous carrier women. In these cases, demonstrating an increase in pyrimidine biosynthesis may be possible with allopurinol-mediated blockage of uridine monophosphate synthase, the enzyme that converts orotic acid to uridine monophosphate, leading to an excessive rise of orotic acid and its metabolite orotidine. The allopurinol test may be used for the diagnosis of heterozygous or mild OTC deficiency in cases of unclear transient or intermittent hyperammonemia, unclear comatose or encephalopathic episodes in both sexes, or stepwise regressing neurodegenerative disease in girls or women, especially when epilepsy and ataxia are prominent symptoms.

Procedure

The patient should avoid caffeine in tea, coffee (decaffeinated coffee is acceptable), cocoa, chocolate, chocolate biscuits, any cola drink, or benzoate-containing beverages for 24 hours before the test. Otherwise, a special diet before or through the test is not needed. For women, the test should be performed 7 to 12 days after their last menstrual period, if possible. The test is usually started in the morning.

- Collect 10 mL urine for baseline measurement of orotic acid and orotidine, which should be done by high-pressure liquid chromatography (HPLC), not by a colorimetric method.
- Give allopurinol orally in a dose of 100 mg for preschool children, 200 mg for children between 6 and 10 years of age, or 300 mg for older children and adults.
- Collect urine over 24 hours in four 6-hour fractions (0 to 6 hours, 7 to 12 hours, 13 to 18 hours, 19 to 24 hours); send 10 mL of each fraction for analysis. The samples should be sent together either frozen or, after conservation with three drops of chloroform, at ambient temperature by express mail. Labeling sample tubes accurately and informing the laboratory of all medication taken during the test, as well as in the preceding days, are important.

Interpretation

Excessive rise of orotic acid and/or orotidine indicates increased throughput in pyrimidine synthesis as is typically caused by mild (heterozygous) OTC deficiency. However, both false-positive and false-negative test results have been reported. Positive tests can also be found in other genetic disorders, including Rett syndrome, amino acid transport defects, creatine synthesis disorders, and mitochondrial disorders. A negative allopurinol test (normal orotic acid after protein challenge) does not fully exclude heterozygous OTC deficiency, as mosaicism in the liver (lyonization) may be skewed in favor of normal hepatocytes to a degree that renders the detection of metabolic effects impossible. OTC gene mutation analysis should be considered if OTC deficiency remains a possibility.

PHENYLALANINE CHALLENGE

The hydroxylation reactions of phenylalanine, tyrosine, and tryptophan require tetrahydrobiopterin (BH$_4$) as a cofactor. A deficiency in the biosynthesis or recycling of BH$_4$ may cause reduced synthesis of monoamine neurotransmitters. Frequently, this is not noticeable in plasma amino acid concentrations but can be demonstrated in the kinetics of phenylalanine hydroxylation after an oral challenge. The phenylalanine challenge test may be useful in patients with unclear dystonic movement disorders, particularly when Segawa syndrome is suspected. It may also be performed in conjunction with a BH$_4$ test in mild hyperphenylalaninemia.

Procedure

The phenylalanine challenge should be carried out at least 1 hour after a light breakfast (minimal protein). No food is permitted until the end of the test. Obtain two separate samples of 1 mL ethylene diamine tetraacetate (EDTA) blood to determine basal values of phenylalanine, tyrosine, and plasma pterins. For pterin analysis, centrifuging the samples immediately and freezing the plasma in two portions is important. Plasma should be stored at $-70°C$ or should be sent on dry ice to the metabolic laboratory.

- Give 100 mg/kg L-phenylalanine in orange juice; if necessary, use a nasogastric tube. Do not mix with drinks containing aspartame or protein. Phenylalanine does not dissolve well, so stir the mix just before the patient drinks it and rinse the residual phenylalanine with additional juice.
- Obtain blood samples 1, 2, and 4 hours after phenylalanine ingestion; again centrifuge and freeze plasma immediately in two portions for the analyses of phenylalanine, tyrosine, and pterins.

Interpretation

Plasma phenylalanine levels should rise sharply after ingestion, with a maximum at around 60 minutes, and should then decline continuously through conversion of phenylalanine into tyrosine. Biopterin concentrations should rise several-fold above baseline. Plasma concentrations of phenylalanine should not exceed tyrosine by more than fivefold after loading. A protracted rise and a slow decrease of phenylalanine combined with a delayed rise of tyrosine indicate a reduced hydroxylation capacity, which may be caused either by a mutation in the phenylalanine hydroxylase gene or by reduced availability of BH$_4$.

Further differentiation is possible by examining pterins in the blood and urine, by analyzing mutation of the phenylalanine hydroxylase gene, or by repeating a modified phenylalanine challenge. This time BH_4 (20 mg/kg) is administered 1 hour before or 2 hours after phenylalanine (100 mg/kg). If the availability of BH_4 is reduced, administering it before phenylalanine results in a complete normalization of the test. If BH_4 is given during the test, phenylalanine immediately decreases and tyrosine rises, leading to normalization of metabolite levels (see later). In the latter setting, plasma amino acids are determined after another 1, 2, 4, and 8 hours (i.e., amino acids are determined before and 1, 2, 3, 4, 6, and 10 hours after phenylalanine loading).

BH_4 TEST

Elevated plasma phenylalanine (hyperphenylalaninemia), which in most Western countries is detected in routine neonatal screening, usually results from phenylalanine hydroxylase deficiency (phenylketonuria, PKU) but occasionally is due to a deficiency of the cofactor tetrahydrobiopterin (BH_4). The BH_4 test is intended to differentiate between the two conditions. Oral administration of BH_4 does not significantly reduce plasma phenylalanine concentrations in newborns with PKU but may rapidly normalize phenylalanine in patients with a primary defect of pterin synthesis or recycling. As this is of immediate therapeutic relevance, a BH_4 test should be considered in all neonates with plasma phenylalanine concentration above 400 μmol/L (6.5 mg/dL). For the reliable exclusion of cofactor deficiency, measuring dihydropteridine reductase activity with a filter paper card (Guthrie card), which is usually sent with the samples of the BH_4 test to the metabolic laboratory, is also necessary. The BH_4 test is not reliable when phenylalanine levels are below 400 μmol/L, as the therapeutic effect is more difficult to recognize. In such cases carrying out a BH_4 test in conjunction with phenylalanine loading (100 mg/kg 2 hours before administering BH_4) can be useful.

Procedure

- Collect 5 to 10 mL of urine for pterin analysis, protect against light (urine may need to be collected in a dark bag), and freeze. Obtain 2 mL EDTA whole blood, centrifuge, and freeze plasma for amino acid analysis. Samples should be sent on dry ice to the laboratory. Alternatively, urine may be oxidized with MnO_2 and may be sent at ambient temperature by express mail (for this purpose, acidify 5 mL urine with 6 M HCl up to a pH of 1.0 to 1.5; add 100 mg MnO_2; shake for 5 minutes at ambient temperature; centrifuge for 5 minutes at 4,000 rpm; and mail supernatant protected against light by aluminum foil or in a dark container).
- Give 20 mg/kg BH_4 diluted in water 30 minutes before a normal meal. Beware of the photosensitivity of BH_4 (protect against light).

- Obtain plasma 1, 4, and 8 hours after BH_4 administration for amino acid analysis. Collect urine 4 to 8 hours after administering BH_4 for pterin analysis. (Samples should be prepared in the same way as the baseline samples.)

When the test is carried out in conjunction with phenylalanine loading, determine plasma amino acids before, as well as at 1 and 2 hours after phenylalanine loading (100 mg/kg). BH_4 (20 mg/kg) should be administered 2 hours after phenylalanine, and plasma amino acids are measured after another 1, 2, 4, and 8 hours (i.e., amino acids are determined before and 1, 2, 3, 4, 6, and 10 hours after phenylalanine loading). The infant or older patient may be fed or may eat regularly throughout the test.

Interpretation

A marked decrease of the phenylalanine concentrations together with a rise of tyrosine after BH_4 administration indicates cofactor deficiency. Phenylalanine and tyrosine concentrations remain largely unchanged in PKU.

LEUCINE CHALLENGE

Insulin secretion from the pancreas is controlled by a complex system involving several enzymes and transmembrane carriers. In some people food intake and, more specifically, the ingestion of large amounts of leucine (leucine-sensitive hypoglycemia) release inappropriate insulin. The leucine challenge test examines the insulin reaction to food intake and the function of the blood sugar–insulin feedback mechanism and may help in patients with postprandial hypoglycemia or suspected hyperinsulinism–hyperammonemia (HI-HA) syndrome. One must appreciate, however, that some patients with hyperinsulinism syndrome suffer severe, life-threatening hypoglycemia after quite small amounts of leucine, so appropriate emergency measures must be prepared before the test is started. A leucine challenge is not suitable for diagnosing maple syrup urine disease. If that condition is suspected, alloisoleucine should be used, which will not cause severe symptoms in affected patients.

Procedure

The test is carried out in the morning after overnight fasting. Insert an intravenous cannula and prepare a 20% glucose solution for emergency application in case of severe hypoglycemia.

- Obtain blood samples for baseline measurements of blood sugar, insulin, and ammonia.
- Give L-leucine orally in a dose of 150 mg/kg or intravenously in a dose of 50 to 75 mg/kg.
- Determine blood sugar, insulin, and ammonia at 15, 30, 45, 60, and 90 minutes after leucine challenge.

Interpretation

Patients with leucine-sensitive hyperinsulinism usually develop hypoglycemia caused by excessive insulin secretion (> 3 mU/L at blood sugar < 2.0 mmol/L) approximately one-half hour after leucine administration. Concomitant hyperammonemia indicates a defect of glutamate dehydrogenase.

METHIONINE CHALLENGE

Cytosolic methyl group transfer from serine to S-adenosylmethionine via the folate cycle is required for a wide range of cellular methylation reactions. This pathway involves the vitamin B_{12}-dependent remethylation of homocysteine to methionine. Deficiencies of the folate cycle or cobalamin (vitamin B_{12}) metabolism, including common genetic variants such as the A222V variant of the enzyme methylenetetrahydrofolate reductase (MTHFR), may disturb the regeneration of methionine and may lead to an increase in plasma homocysteine concentration. In some patients a tendency toward elevated homocysteine, which is a risk factor for various disorders, including premature thromboembolic vascular diseases, is only recognized after oral loading with methionine.

Procedure

The test should be carried out in the morning after overnight fasting. The patient does not need to be on a special diet before or during the test.

- Obtain fasting blood samples for the analysis of homocysteine, folic acid, and vitamin B_{12}. For homocysteine analysis, 1 to 2 mL of EDTA blood should immediately be centrifuged, and the plasma should be analyzed or frozen and sent on dry ice to the metabolic laboratory. In some cases obtaining an additional EDTA whole blood sample for DNA analysis, such as testing for the MTHFR variant A222V, is advisable.
- Give L-methionine orally at a dose of 100 mg/kg. For improved taste the methionine may be dissolved in orange juice or another suitable drink.
- Obtain an EDTA blood sample after 6 hours for homocysteine analysis.

Interpretation

Normal values of homocysteine after the methionine challenge should be as follows:

Women, premenopausal	18 to 51 µmol/L
Women, postmenopausal	25 to 69 µmol/L
Men	25 to 54 µmol/L

An excessive rise of homocysteine indicates a reduced remethylation capacity, which may be caused by vitamin B_{12} deficiency or a disturbance of the folate cycle, such as presence of the MTHFR variant A222V.

GLUCAGON STIMULATION

Glucagon is a counterregulatory hormone whose secretion is normally stimulated by hypoglycemia. It acts to stimulate hepatic glycogenolysis by stimulating phosphorylase; however, glucose-6-phosphatase activity is required for release of free-glucose into the blood. Thus the glucagon stimulation test is an excellent provocative test for von Gierke disease, glycogenosis type I, in which the hepatic activity of this enzyme is in most patients absent or nearly absent (see also Chapter 6, "Hypoglycemia").

The test is usually done after a fast of at least 6 hours. An overnight fast is usually employed in normal individuals. The duration of fasting for an infant with glycogenosis I depends on tolerance and may have to be 4 hours or less. The dose of glucagon that the authors generally employ is 0.5 mg intramuscularly. Doses from 0.03 to 0.1 mg/kg up to a maximum of 1 mg have been used. Blood concentrations of glucose should be measured at time zero, at 15-minute intervals after injection for 60 minutes, and then at 90 minutes and 120 minutes. Lactate and alanine may also be measured in each sample if the patient is not anemic or too small (e.g., a tiny baby). In a young infant these determinations could be done on every other sample.

In control individuals glucagon administration is followed by a prompt glycemic response, and the concentrations of lactate and alanine do not increase. In a patient with glycogenosis I, the curve for glucose may be flat or a decline may occur. In some patients a small elevation of glucose concentration in the blood may be found because 6% to 8% of the glucose residues of glycogen are released as free glucose by the debranching enzyme. However, the increase is usually not prompt and does not exceed 50% of the fasting level within 30 minutes. In glycogenosis type I, levels of lactate and alanine increase after glucagon. The level of lactate rises rapidly and may go very high, even above 15 mmolar.

In glycogenosis type III or debrancher deficiency, reaching a presumptive diagnosis is possible by determining the response to glucagon in the fed and fasted state. Administration of glucagon after a 12- to 14-hour fast is followed by little or no increase in blood glucose. The patient is then fed, and the glucagon test is repeated 2 to 6 hours later; the glycemic response is then normal. These patients do not have lactic acidemia, and concentrations of lactate do not increase following glucagon. Their concentrations of alanine are low.

In patients with glycogen synthase deficiency, glucagon administration in the fasting state causes no elevation of glucose, lactate, or alanine. In the fed state, glucagon causes a glycemic response. Similar to patients with glycogenosis III, elevation of lactate occurs with a glucose tolerance test.

FOREARM ISCHEMIA TEST

Adequate functioning of glycolysis is necessary for energy production during muscle exercise. With sufficient oxygen supply, glucose-6-phosphate is fully oxidized in the mitochondrion, whereas anaerobic glycolysis results in the production of lactate. The purine nucleotide cycle, which involves the deamination of adenosine monophosphate (AMP) to inosine monophosphate and the release of ammonia, is also required for adequate muscle function. The forearm ischemia test examines both systems through measurement of lactate and ammonia concentrations both before and after anaerobic exercise. It may be useful in patients with muscle cramps or other muscular symptoms on exertion. Normally, a marked increase in the concentration of both analytes occurs after anaerobic exercise. An adequate rise of ammonia with an absent rise of lactate indicates a deficiency in the breakdown of glycogen or in glycolysis, as in glycogen storage disease types V (McArdle), III (Cori), or VII (Tauri). In contrast, an absence in the rise of ammonia with normal lactate production indicates a deficiency in the purine nucleotide cycle, such as muscle–AMP deaminase deficiency. The test is invalid if neither lactate nor ammonia is elevated as this implies insufficient muscle work. Significant increase in creatine kinase after the test may indicate that different metabolic disorders are affecting the muscle (e.g., a long-chain fatty acid oxidation defect).

Procedure

- Obtain a urine sample 20 to 30 minutes before the test to determine myoglobin; the patient should rest in bed.
- Insert a large, intravenous cannula into the cubital vein of the test arm, which should be the right arm in right-handed patients, just before the test. A blood sample is taken to measure lactate, ammonia, and creatine kinase.
- Attach an inflatable cuff for blood pressure measurements to the upper test arm and pump it to a pressure of 250 mmHg or to 20 mmHg above the systolic blood pressure of the patient. The palmar vessels may be blocked with a small cuff across the wrist. Then ask the patient to exert the forearm and hand muscles as strenuously as possible. This may require strong encouragement as it is difficult to achieve, particularly for children; but insufficient exercise makes the test invalid. A standardized approach may involve a dynamometer, which is best set at 80% maximum strength. Alternatively, a hand-powered torch may be used, which also gives feedback (brightness of the light) on muscle work. Squeezing a firm roll, such as a towel, as hard as possible every 2 seconds does not usually cause a sufficient rise of lactate and ammonia and therefore is not a good alternative. After the end of muscle exercise, release the cuffs.
- Obtain blood samples from the intravenous line immediately after muscle exercise and then at 1, 3, 5, and 7 minutes for measuring lactate, ammonia, and creatinine kinase. Myoglobin is determined in the first urine produced after muscle exercise.

Interpretation

Normally, lactate should rise by more than 2 mmol/L, and ammonia should increase by more than 50 µmol/L above basal values. Unsatisfactory rise of both lactate and ammonia indicates insufficient muscle activity and makes the test invalid. Inadequate rise of lactate indicates deficient glyco(geno)lysis, whereas deficient rise of ammonia suggests muscle-AMP-deaminase deficiency. Elevations of creatine kinase or myoglobin may reflect muscle cell damage, which may result from metabolic disorders, such as a long-chain fatty acid oxidation defect, or from electron chain disorders.

ADDITIONAL READINGS

Bonham JR, Guthrie P, Downing M, et al. The allopurinol test lacks specificity for primary urea cycle defects but may indicate unrecognized mitochondrial disease. *J Inher Metab Dis* 1999;22:174–184.

Bonnefont JP, Specola NB, Vassault A, et al. The fasting test in paediatrics: application to the diagnosis of pathological hypo- and hyperketotic states. *Eur J Pediatr* 1990;150:80–85.

Cahill GF. Starvation. *Trans Am Clin Climatol Assoc* 1982;94:1–21.

Fernandes J, Saudubray JM, Huber J. Diagnostic procedures: function tests and postmortem protocol. In: Fernandes J, Saudubray JM, Van den Berghe G, eds. *Inborn metabolic diseases,* 3rd ed. Heidelberg: Springer; 2000:43–51.

Hyland K, Fryburg JS, Wilson WG, et al. Oral phenylalanine loading in dopa-responsive dystonia: a possible diagnostic test. *Neurology* 1997;48:1290–1297.

Morris AAM, Thekekara A, Wilks Z, et al. Evaluation of fasts for investigating hypoglycaemia or suspected metabolic disease. *Arch Dis Child* 1996;75:115–119.

12 ♠ Biopsies

Biopsies are performed in order to make a diagnosis and to have material for a later diagnosis. In some instances, the histologic or ultrastructural appearance of the tissue may provide a diagnosis. The sample may also serve as a source of both DNA and enzyme.

DIAGNOSTIC ASSAYS FROM BIOPSIES

Enzymes and Mitochondrial DNA

The enzymes defective in inherited disorders of metabolism are expressed in many different tissues. Enzymatic diagnosis can often be done on leukocytes or cultured fibroblasts. Blood samples are the easiest to obtain, and many enzymes are quite stable in anticoagulated blood, which is brought or shipped (unfrozen) to the laboratory. Most of the lysosomal enzymes discussed in Chapter 29 are included in this category.

In some diseases the responsible enzyme has limited tissue distribution; biopsies must be performed on one of the tissues in which the enzyme is expressed in order to obtain samples suitable for testing. For example, glycogen debrancher enzyme deficiency is the basis of type III glycogen storage disease, which affects the liver and often muscle as well, so a biopsy of one of those tissues for enzyme and glycogen assays and microscopic examination is usually performed to establish the diagnosis. If the diagnosis is already suspected, a DNA-based approach using leukocytes or cultured fibroblasts might be suitable.

The diagnosis of nonketotic hyperglycinemia is primarily made by a simultaneous analysis of amino acids from blood and cerebrospinal fluid. A more definitive diagnosis requires demonstration of deficient catalytic activity of the glycine cleavage complex in a liver biopsy. This is also the prerequisite for a prenatal diagnosis in chorionic villi. In addition, if a DNA-based diagnosis is to be attempted, the deficient protein of the glycine cleavage complex must first be identified from a liver biopsy. Only then is a search for pathologic mutations in the DNA practical at present.

The gold standard for the enzymatic diagnosis of mitochondrial disorders resulting from defects of the electron transport chain usually involves extended biochemical and histologic analysis of fresh skeletal muscle or sometimes of the liver or other tissues. Testing can include the determination of oxygen consumption, pyruvate oxidation rates, ATP plus phosphocreatine production rates, and determination of activities of the pyruvate dehydrogenase complex, the citric acid cycle enzymes, and oxidative phosphorylation (OXPHOS) complexes (see Chapter 6).

The assessment of mtDNA mutations often also requires mutation analysis in different tissues, including muscle. Qualitative abnormalities of mtDNA include point mutations, deletions, deletion/duplications, and rearrangements. Pathogenic relevant mutations are mostly heteroplasmic. Heteroplasmy describes the coexistence of mutant and wild-type mitochondrial DNA within cells and tissues. The fraction of mutant mitochondrial DNA may vary from less than 1% to more than 95% in tissues of patients with mitochondrial disease. Heteroplasmy occurs both within and between cells and between organs in patients with mitochondrial disease. Finding heteroplasmy strengthens the argument that a mutation is pathogenic, as heteroplasmy is relatively rare in normal individuals. One must also keep in mind that many mitochondrial functional defects are due to mutations in nuclear DNA, not in the mitochondrial genome.

In some other situations a diagnosis of an inherited metabolic disease is certain, but further testing to demonstrate the enzymatic defect is still desirable. This occurs, for example, in preparation for prenatal diagnosis in most disorders where one needs to demonstrate that differences can be shown between the affected individuals and heterozygotes, so that enzyme activity in chorionic villus cells or amniocytes can be interpreted accurately. Reliable prenatal diagnosis for respiratory chain disorders using enzyme analysis is often impractical; if the molecular basis for the problem is known, a DNA-based approach can be attempted. Unfortunately, reliable prenatal diagnosis is impossible for mtDNA mutations.

Molecular Analysis: Nuclear DNA

The rapid increase in our knowledge of the molecular biology of metabolic disorders is leading to direct DNA diagnosis in an increasing number of situations (see Chapter 10). In some cases this is because only a limited number of mutations need to be sought (e.g., hemochromatosis where two pathologic mutations account for most cases). In other instances efficient techniques allow searching for a larger number of mutations quickly. The eventual goal of searching for a very large number of mutations, perhaps using DNA microarray ("DNA chip" technology), is likely to be realized within a few years. At that time characterization of enzyme deficiencies may be bypassed in favor of direct mutational analysis. Such an approach will make testing of relatives and prenatal diagnosis much simpler than the current enzyme-based diagnosis.

Nucleated cells are the usual source of DNA for molecular diagnosis. Leukocytes from a blood sample are the easiest to obtain, and DNA may be separated and stored. Lymphocytes can also be separated and transformed to become an ongoing source of genetic material. In some situations, DNA adequate for limited testing can be obtained from a brush sample of buccal mucosa squamous cells or saliva.

Sometimes a blood sample has not been obtained or is no longer available. Occasionally, a patient has died, and later a test is developed that permits diagnosis. Fibroblasts obtained from a skin biopsy are an important source of material, as they may be grown and then frozen for future studies. The original neonatal Guthrie cards are sometimes the last resource for material from a patient that allow postmortem analytical or molecular diagnosis. Many diagnoses have been made years after a patient has died, yielding accurate information regarding recurrence risk to parents and relatives and reproductive options.

Histochemistry and Ultrastructure

The histochemical or ultrastructural appearance of many tissues can be a good guide to the final diagnosis, but it is usually not specific. Skin biopsy has been used to diagnose Batten disease (now several different disorders), for example, but special care must be taken to include the deeper layers, which contain the characteristic curvilinear bodies or fingerprint profiles. Conjunctival biopsy is used at some centers when a neurodegenerative disorder is being investigated, as peripheral nerve tissue is usually visible in the same sample; rectal biopsy for histology of Batten disease has been used in the past.

Muscle biopsy is often done when evaluating muscle weakness or cardiomyopathy. Both light and electron microscopy may be needed. Lipid inclusions suggest altered fatty acid oxidation or impaired mitochondrial function. Excess glycogen, determined by staining or quantitative analysis, suggests altered glycogen metabolism. Increased lipids are also present in some glycogen storage diseases. Increased membrane-bound (i.e., lysosomal) glycogen is typical of Pompe disease.

Disorders of oxidative phosphorylation often lead to changes in mitochondria. Abnormalities of number, size, morphology, and distribution may occur. Clusters of abnormal mitochondria may be present just beneath the cell membrane, creating the appearance called *ragged-red fibers* when seen by light microscopy in cross-section. In comparison to adults, ragged-red fibers are uncommon in children with mitochondrial disorders. Inclusions within the mitochondria are often found in OXPHOS disorders.

Cardiac biopsy is similar to muscle biopsy, but the samples are usually very small. If abnormalities are not uniformly distributed, a chance of being misled by a normal result exists. Obtaining enough skeletal muscle for diagnostic enzymology, mitochondrial oxidative phosphorylation studies, and histochemistry is usually possible; obtaining enough material by cardiac biopsy for all these purposes is difficult. Thus one must be very selective, and well prepared, when doing a cardiac biopsy.

Lysosomal storage diseases characteristically result in obvious evidence of membrane-bound, stored material in many tissues, with some limitations due to the particular enzyme deficiency. A few disorders are confined to the central nervous system, so for these peripheral biopsies are not helpful. For the most part, liver and bone marrow cells show similar inclusions. In the past, a biopsy was generally performed before doing enzyme assays on leukocytes or other tissues. Now, enzyme assays (or DNA tests) are generally available, so a tissue biopsy is not always necessary.

TISSUE BIOPSIES: SKIN, MUSCLE, LIVER, AND HEART
Skin

Skin biopsies are usually performed to obtain fibroblasts for culture and, sometimes, for direct light or electron-microscopic examination. A skin biopsy can be performed by several different methods; the most common employs a standard dermatologic punch. The sample is stable, easy to transport, and versatile. As with all procedures, informed consent must be obtained.

Equipment

Isopropyl alcohol wipes or alcohol and sterile gauze or cotton
Sterile gloves
2-mL syringe with 27G needle, 1% injectable lidocaine *or* Lidocaine-prilocaine (EMLA) cream
Sterile drape (optional)
3-mm sterile skin biopsy punch *or* scalpel
Sterile scissors and forceps
Sterile gauze for dressing
10-mL container for sample transport, containing tissue transport medium, viral culture medium, or normal saline *without preservative*

Site

Skin biopsy is typically performed in a location where a small scar is not likely to be a problem. In infants the middle back is often used, as it is a site away from fecal contamination that is not easily reached with fingers. Have an assistant hold the infant on the examining table to stabilize the site. In older individuals the skin over the scapula or deltoid or on the inner surface of the forearm is commonly used, depending on the subject's (or parent's) preference. A sliver of skin or a subcutaneous tissue biopsy can be taken from the area of a surgical incision made for other purposes, such as when muscle and nerve biopsies are also done, or during an unrelated surgical procedure, such as circumcision (foreskin), as long as no iodine-containing antiseptics are used (see later).

Preparation

The skin must be thoroughly cleansed to avoid bacterial or fungal overgrowth, as well as infection, in the culture. Many choose isopropyl alcohol as the cleaning agent. Some use hexachlorophene. Standard alcohol wipes may be used, but sterile gauze or cotton that has been soaked in alcohol is preferable. The biopsy site is prepared at least three times, using a new wipe each time. Start over the site and proceed in widening circles to a diameter of at least 5 cm. Iodine-containing antiseptics should be avoided, as they will interfere with cell growth in the culture.

Sterile gloves should be used, as this procedure involves some blood exposure. A small sterile drape may be used if desired.

Anesthesia

One percent lidocaine, with or without epinephrine, is suitable. A volume of 1 to 2 mL is sufficient. The anesthesia is typically administered by infiltration of the dermis and subcutaneous tissues using a syringe fitted with a 27G needle. Always draw back on the syringe before injecting to ensure that a vessel has not been entered inadvertently. The anesthesia works within a minute.

Lidocaine-prilocaine (EMLA) cream also works well, but it must be applied an hour before doing the biopsy. The cream is applied to the biopsy area, and an occlusive patch is placed over it. After an hour the patch is removed and the skin is cleaned as above. The biopsy site should be pricked gently and then firmly with a sterile needle to be sure the anesthetic has worked.

Procedure

The biopsy is taken after cleaning and anesthesia. The best method is to use a sterile 3-mm circular skin biopsy punch. Single-use disposable punches made for this purpose are convenient. The punch is twisted with gentle force into the skin until it penetrates the subcutaneous tissue. The skin piece is then lifted up with forceps, and the tissue directly underneath is cut with sterile scissors.

An alternative method is to make two cuts with a sterile scalpel, cutting a sliver of skin roughly 1 cm long and 3 mm wide. The piece of skin is then lifted and detached with the scalpel blade or scissors.

A third method is to elevate a small bleb of skin with the injected anesthetic. Then pass a 23G needle under the bleb, and use a straight-edged scalpel blade to shave off the top of the bleb.

The 3-mm punch biopsy site or the site of a bleb biopsy can be dressed with sterile gauze and tape. A larger biopsy site made using a scalpel or a circular punch larger than 3 mm may require a single suture. The wound, which will heal in a week, should be kept protected and dry.

Sample Handling

The sample should be placed in the transport medium provided by the laboratory and the screw cap should be securely fastened. (Culture medium alters the appearance of the cells, so it should not be used if microscopic examination is planned.) Viral culture medium, which contains antibiotics, or sterile normal saline *without preservative* may be used in a sterile container; a 10-mL tube is satisfactory. The sample should be sent to the laboratory quickly. If it is to be shipped, the container must be completely filled with saline or transport medium so that tipping does not expose the sample to air and the risk of drying out. *Be careful not to ship a sample that should not be frozen (e.g., skin or whole blood) in the same container as a frozen specimen. Use a different container.*

The sample may be immediately cultured in the laboratory and then analyzed. If the fibroblasts are to be studied in a different laboratory, some of the original culture should be retained and stored in the sending laboratory in case of mishap en route or in the receiving laboratory. If the importance of the biopsy is unclear, as in a postmortem examination where other tests are pending, some laboratories prefer to freeze the sample directly using a cryoprotective agent and then to thaw it for later growth, if needed. The primary culture of the sample should be postponed only if the laboratory is confident that the cells can be revived. A sample that was directly frozen can be revived only for a few months, whereas frozen cultured fibroblasts can be revived after many years.

Complications

Anesthetic reaction, bleeding, and site infection are possible. All are extremely rare.

Muscle

Muscle biopsies can be obtained by needle or through an incision. Surgeons usually perform open biopsies, so close cooperation among the metabolic specialist, the surgeon, the pathologist, and the laboratory scientist is necessary. Careful communication will ensure that the sample is obtained and handled properly. The metabolic specialist or specialist nurse may need to go into the operating room with the patient to attend to the critical details.

Site

A muscle biopsy can sometimes be performed in conjunction with a nerve and skin biopsy. In this situation the nerve chosen for biopsy is usually the sural nerve, and the muscle biopsy is taken from the adjacent gastrocnemius. The skin biopsy is taken from the margin of the incision. If a nerve biopsy is not needed, the vastus lateralis, quadriceps femoris, or deltoid is commonly chosen, depending on both the size of the patient and the size of sample needed. Before taking a biopsy from a different site, the anatomic pathologist and enzymologist should be consulted. Biochemical studies are independent of the site of the biopsy; however, histology may differ between sites. If mitochondrial heteroplasmy exists, it too may differ from one site to another and may determine the histologic appearance. Some progressive diseases, including mitochondrial disorders, may present with patchy involvement, so choosing a muscle that is clinically involved but that has not been replaced completely by fat or connective tissue is wise. A muscle biopsy should not be done where an electromyogram has been performed in the past 2 weeks because of changes in the muscle from the electrode.

A needle muscle biopsy can be done when only a small sample is needed, as for metabolic testing, and when the distortion present in the biopsy sample (which will contract immediately) does not interfere with the histologic interpretation.

Anesthesia

Muscle biopsy can be done readily under local anesthesia. In the operating room general anesthesia may be required. The possibility of malignant hyperthermia in any person with a myopathy must be kept in mind, so low-risk anesthetics should be used. Many metabolic myopathies, including mitochondrial myopathies, cause heightened susceptibility to muscle damage, including malignant hyperthermia, from anesthesia. Therefore, avoiding the drugs most likely to cause this reaction (halothane and nondepolarizing muscle relaxants) and monitoring body temperature and pCO_2 carefully are crucial.

Sample Handling

A muscle biopsy is usually taken for several reasons, including light and electron microscopy, staining for enzymes, mitochondrial enzyme analysis, and mitochondrial DNA extraction and analysis. Typically, a section of muscle is taken while using a clamp to keep the muscle extended and is placed in glutaraldehyde after excision for ultrastructural analysis and light microscopy. A second section (clamping is not necessary) is placed in saline or transport medium for biochemical analysis and mitochondrial studies or is frozen directly.

Muscle to be frozen for later biochemical analysis should be sliced to a thickness no greater than 5 mm and should be wrapped with a small piece of aluminum foil. The foil package is then surrounded immediately by dry ice until the sample is thoroughly frozen and is brought to the laboratory while in the ice. The samples in foil should be stored at −70°C in airtight screw-cap vials or sealed plastic bags that have been labeled with indelible ink. Alternatively, the sample can be frozen instantly by placement in isopentane in a liquid nitrogen bath

Samples for mitochondrial studies must be organized in close consultation with the laboratory as only fresh samples are suitable for functional studies. They should be obtained at the institution where the histologic and enzymatic studies are performed as the delay caused by shipping inevitably complicates the interpretation of results. Frozen samples can be used for enzymatic studies and can be shipped.

In needle muscle biopsy two or three cores are usually taken for biochemical and enzymatic analysis, light and electron microscopy, and metabolic studies. Samples for light and electron microscopy are placed in glutaraldehyde. (*Do not freeze.*) Samples for immediate biochemical analysis should be processed in accordance with local lab practice; samples for later studies should be frozen as described earlier.

Complications

Anesthetic reactions (see above), bleeding, and infection may occur. Anyone with muscle weakness may need prolonged ventilatory support. This commonly is found in patients with mitochondrial myopathies.

Heart Biopsy: A Specialized Muscle Biopsy

Heart biopsy is often considered when evaluating cardiomyopathy, especially when inflammatory disease (viral myocarditis) is possible. Certain disorders of heart muscle, including heteroplasmic mitochondrial disorders confined to heart muscle by somatic mutation or segregation of mutant mitochondria during development, can be diagnosed by heart biopsy only during life. An experienced specialist must perform this procedure. The sample size obtained is small, so misleading results are possible. A diagnosis is rarely obtained using electron microscopy, but the concentric cristae of Barth syndrome can be seen only in this way.

Liver

Biopsy of the liver, like that of muscle, may be done either as an open procedure or by using a biopsy needle to obtain smaller samples. The choice depends on the clinical situation and the laboratory doing the analysis. If a mitochondrial disorder is suspected, the possibility of complications resulting from anesthesia must be kept in mind.

Despite recent advances in DNA analysis, a liver biopsy specimen is necessary to establish or to confirm an enzyme deficiency in many inborn errors of metabolism. Such disorders include the following: glycogen storage diseases (e.g., types 6 and 9), fructose 1, 6-diphosphatase deficiency, nonketotic hyperglycinemia, tyrosinemia type 2 (tyrosine aminotransferase deficiency), some urea cycle disorders (e.g., deficiency of ornithine transcarbamylase or N-acetylglutamate synthase), lysinuric protein intolerance, primary hyperoxaluria type I (alanine–glyoxylate aminotransferase deficiency), and Menkes or Wilson disease. Sometimes, a disorder of lipid metabolism, such as Wolman disease or Niemann-Pick disease type C, is suspected first after examining a liver biopsy. Before the development of very-long-chain fatty acid analysis, the first suspicion of peroxisomal disorders was often from liver histology and ultrastructure.

If a needle biopsy is done, cores can be taken for light and electron microscopy, enzymology, biochemical analysis, and mitochondrial studies, depending on the situation. If an open biopsy is done, a 1-cm^3 sample can be obtained and can then be cut in pieces no thicker than 0.5 cm. Processing is similar to that for muscle tissue.

POSTMORTEM BIOPSIES

Skin and other biopsies may be done after death. The tissue sample obtained may prove to be essential for establishing or confirming a diagnosis so that subsequent genetic counseling can be confidently done. A family that has decided not to permit an autopsy may allow postmortem biopsies. Unless an autopsy is going to be conducted immediately, biopsies of internal organs for enzyme analysis, especially those for respiratory chain assays, should be done soon after death.

Skin fibroblasts remain viable for 2 to 3 days after death and, in some cases, up to a week. Fibroblasts from other tissues (e.g., the tendon) have also been used in this situation. The biopsy should be taken from a site that will not be visible when the body is clothed, so that the appearance of the body is not disturbed if a viewing of the body is to occur later. A small suture or tape can be used to minimize fluid leakage afterward.

Liver and other internal tissues autolyze quickly after death. Changes occur in mitochondria within 2 hours, and respiratory chain enzyme activity deteriorates rapidly. Consequently, liver, heart, and muscle biopsies must be done promptly if accurate results are to be obtained. Small open muscle, open liver, and skin biopsies are easily obtained. If only a single incision is permitted, rectus abdominis muscle, liver, and skin can be obtained. Needle biopsies may not yield as much information, but sometimes they are all that the family will permit. Many enzymes of intermediary metabolism are relatively stable, so liver, muscle, heart, kidney, and even brain samples may provide essential diagnostic or confirmatory information even when obtained a day or two after death during a routine autopsy. However, obtaining tissue for metabolic diagnosis as soon as possible is always best. As for any procedure, someone with the appropriate skills must perform it after obtaining informed consent. Even when the preferred samples have not been obtained, a late diagnosis can sometimes be made from fixed tissue, using DNA extracted from preserved tissue (paraffin blocks or even tissue in formalin), or by other methods, such as staining for certain enzymes.

13 ♣ Neuroradiologic and Neurophysiologic Investigations

New and advanced neuroimaging and functional imaging techniques have revolutionized our approach and understanding of inherited metabolic diseases, especially of neurometabolic and neurodegenerative disorders. Important information can be obtained by greatly improved techniques of cerebral ultrasonography; however, the breakthrough for visualizing cerebral pathology and even pathophysiology *in vivo* came with the availability of computerized tomography (CT) and the development of magnetic resonance imaging (MRI) and localized magnetic resonance spectroscopy (MRS) of brain disorders.

Many patients with inherited metabolic diseases present initially or even exclusively with neurologic disease; as a consequence, neuroimaging techniques are often employed early in the diagnostic work-up. As inherited metabolic diseases often cause suggestive patterns of visible neuropathology, a suspicion of an underlying inherited metabolic disease sometimes is initially raised after the first neuroradiologic examination. In addition to the predominantly affected cerebral structures listed in Table 13.1, any unexplained fluctuating or progressive, symmetric, pathologic changes that are independent of defined regions of vascular supply are highly suspicious for disorders of small-molecule intermediary metabolism.

Modern imaging techniques are complex and are developing at a speed comparable to techniques of DNA analysis. Although a thorough understanding of the physics is not necessary for the metabolic physician, some basic parameters of the images and their consequences should be able to be interpreted (Table 13.2). Because metabolic brain disease can be as confusing to the neuroradiologist as imaging parameters can appear to the metabolic physician, maximum information is obtained by using an interdisciplinary approach. Ideally, the images should be jointly evaluated. One should always ask that the original images, not just the written interpretation, be brought along with the patient when he or she comes for a second opinion. If in any doubt, the images together with clinical notes and specific questions should be passed on to a third colleague with experience in especially tricky areas, such as the developmental state of different brain areas and the interpretation of white matter changes.

In planning the diagnostic work-up of an unclassified encephalopathy with a high suspicion of a primary neurometabolic disorder, the first choice of neuroimaging beyond early infancy, when excellent ultrasonographic images can be easily obtained, is MRI. Sagittal, T1-weighted MRI sequences will be performed in all patients, allowing the best assessment of the midline structures. Special attention should be paid to the corpus callosum and the cerebellum.

Structural abnormalities possibly suggesting an inherited metabolic disease include defects of the corpus callosum, the basal

Table 13.1.   Indicators of possible inherited metabolic diseases on neuroimaging

(Progressive) cerebellar atrophy

White matter abnormalities
  Leukodystrophy (centrum semiovale)
  Spongiform encephalopathy (arcuate fibers)
  Predominant white matter involvement in generalized brain disease

Prominent basal ganglia involvement
  Bleeding/infarcts
  Necroses
  "Holes"
  Calcifications
  Atrophy

Vascular insults (unilateral atrophy)

Chronic recurrent subdural effusions and/or hematomas[a]

Transient germinaloid cysts at the caudothalamic pit

Frontotemporal atrophy

Agenesis of corpus callosum

Abnormalities of gyral formation and neuronal migration

Generalized cerebral atrophy

---

[a] May be misinterpreted as child abuse.

ganglia, and the cerebellum. The cerebellum is especially susceptible to metabolic and toxic injuries but is relatively resistant to hypoxia and ischemia. Coronal sections are necessary in order to evaluate the cerebellum in detail and may reveal regional atrophies better than do standard sections. Neuroimaging should be performed early in the evaluation of ataxia. Follow-up investigations may be needed to differentiate progressive disorders from nonprogressive ones (Table 13.3).

MRI images during the first 18 months of life depict enormous developmental processes. Thereafter, the brain is mature by MRI standards. If an MRI was obtained in infancy, a follow-up investigation in the third or fourth year of life often provides valuable additional information in children suffering from an unclassified encephalopathy.

In contrast to older children and adults, white matter maturation in young infants is best visualized on T1 images. The intensity of the white matter quickly increases, and gray and subcortical white matter will normally become isointense on MR images some time later during the first year of life. Because this phenomenon may obscure structural details, especially around the gyri and sulci, these need to be examined on both T1- and T2-weighted sequences. Therefore, in patients younger than 18 months of age, T1-weighted images, as well as T2-weighted images, should be obtained in the axial planes. In older children, obtaining T2- weighted images in

Table 13.2.   Nuclear magnetic resonance imaging

	T1	T2
Imaging parameters		
TR (repetition time)	500–600 msec	2,500–3000 msec
TE (echo time)	11–20 msec	30–60 msec/ 70–120 msec
Slice thickness	3–5 mm	4–5 mm
SE (spin echo): TR/TE	Short	Long
Normal findings (mature brain)		
	White matter = white	White matter = dark
White matter pathology		
	Getting dark	Getting white
Gray matter pathology		
Relaxation time- (acute stage)	Prolonged	Prolonged
Relaxation time- (chronic stage)	Shortened	Shortened

the axial planes is usually sufficient. The administration of contrast agents in the investigation of neurometabolic disorders is generally not indicated.

The appraisal of whether a disease involves principally the gray matter, the white matter, or both is one of the most important and most difficult questions in assessing neuroimaging of patients with possible neurometabolic disorders (Table 13.4). The answer may require serial MR images because of the developmental changes in the young brain. Nevertheless, these investigations are most useful in the early stages of the diseases, independent of the age, as the end stages of neurometabolic disorders are often almost indistinguishable, even if different areas and structures were initially affected. Progressive neurometabolic diseases will result in severe diffuse loss of brain tissue (i.e., gray matter), as well as in increased water content in the remaining tissue, including the white matter. Many neurometabolic diseases do not show a preponderance of gray over white matter but affect both in their disease processes, which are reflected in the neuroimaging findings. This can be also true for patients suffering from diseases listed in Table 13.4, which have been shown to involve primarily either gray matter or white matter (e.g., mitochondrial disorders, organic acidurias, and peroxisomal disorders). To add to the confusion, variant and atypical patterns are sometimes observed. Nevertheless, a systematic evaluation of myelination and gray matter can provide important clues for the diagnosis of neurometabolic diseases.

**Table 13.3.   Metabolic disorders
of the cerebellum causing ataxia**

Nonprogressive	Progressive
Joubert–Boltshauser syndrome	Abetalipoproteinemia
	Ataxia telangiectasia
Ritscher–Schinzel syndrome	Friedrich ataxia
	G_{M2}-gangliosidosis (late-onset)
Congenital disorders of glycosylation (CDG)	Hartnup disease
	4-Hydroxybutyric aciduria
	L-2-Hydroxyglutaric aciduria
	Infantile neuroaxonal dystrophy
	Kearns–Sayre syndrome
	Mevalonic aciduria
	Mitochondrial disorders
	Leukodystrophy (metachromatic)
	Myelinopathia centralis diffusa
	Niemann–Pick type C
	Neuronal ceroid lipofuscinosis
	Refsum disease
	Primary vitamin E deficiency
	Spinocerebellar degeneration
	Thiamine deficiency
	Wilson disease

Although both gray and white matter pathologies are usually better visualized by MRI than they are by CT, the latter may provide identical, although usually less striking, information. Furthermore, MRI has the advantage of avoiding radiation. However, one should remember that CT is still more readily available in some places and that the need for and intensity of sedation is reduced with CT because of shorter times of investigation. Finally, if involvement of the basal ganglia is clinically suspected, a CT may visualize calcifications that MRI may not recognize.

A special mention of neuroimaging findings is warranted for the "cerebral" organic acidurias. Organic acid analysis should be performed in any patient with an unexplained encephalopathy, especially if it is accompanied by suggestive imaging findings (Table 13.1). N-acetylaspartic aciduria (Canavan disease) and L-2-hydroxyglutaric aciduria are both characterized by a progressive loss of myelinated arcuate fibers, a spongiform encephalopathy. The neuroimaging results are especially unique in L-2-hydroxyglutaric aciduria, with the loss of arcuate fibers, severe cerebellar atrophy, and signal changes of the basal ganglia. Frontotemporal atrophy and corresponding reduced opercularization, germinal cysts,

Table 13.4. Pathology of cerebral gray versus white matter in metabolic disorders

Gray matter involvement	White matter involvement
Deep (striatum) Juvenile Huntington disease Leigh disease MELAS	**Complete lack of myelination** Pelizaeus-Mertzbacher disease Trichothiodystrophy
Deep (Pallidum) Hallervorden–Spatz disease Methylmalonic aciduria Propionic aciduria	**Peripheral (arcuate fibers)** Alexander disease Canavan disease Galactosemia L-2-Hydroxyglutaric aciduria Van der Knaap disease
Cortical Ceroid lipofuscinosis Mucolipidoses G_{M1}–gangliosidosis	**Centrum semiovale** Disorders of cytosolic methyl group transfer (B_{12} and folate cycles) Krabbe disease Lowe disease Maple syrup urine disease Metachromatic leukodystrophy Peroxisomal disorders Phenylketonuria
	Diffuse 3-Hydroxy-3-methyl-CoA lyase deficiency Nonketotic hyperglycinemia Urea cycle disorders Unspecific end stage of white matter disease

Adapted from Barkovich AJ. *Pediatric neuroimaging*, 3rd ed. New York: Lippincott Williams & Wilkins; 2000.
Abbreviation: MELAS, mitochondrial encephalomyelopathy, lactic acidemia, and strokelike episodes.

and delayed myelination are characteristic findings in glutaric aciduria type I caused by glutaryl-coenzyme A dehydrogenase deficiency during the first months of life that precedes the onset of irreversible neurologic sequelae. Similar findings are also observed in other organic acidurias and mitochondrial disorders, although not as regularly as in glutaric aciduria type I. In D-2-hydroxyglutaric aciduria, neuroimaging reveals disturbed and delayed gyration, myelination, opercularization, ventriculomegaly, cysts over the head of the caudate nucleus, and more pronounced occipital horns. Chronic subdural effusions or hematomas following relatively mild or even absent traumas are also common in "cerebral" organic acidurias and may be mistaken for indicators of child abuse.

Over the last decade localized MRS of the brain has increasingly been used to study brain metabolism in children with both known and unclassified metabolic diseases. This has led to the detection of three "new" neurometabolic disorders: creatine deficiency due to defective guanidinoacetate methyltransferase, a disturbance in polyol metabolism associated with a leukoencephalopathy, and a total lack of N-acetylaspartate in a patient with an as yet undefined defect. In other disorders MRS can provide valuable diagnostic clues such as demonstration of elevations of substances, including N-acetylaspartate in Canavan disease, glycine in nonketotic hyperglycinemia, branched-chain amino acids in maple syrup urine disease, succinate in succinate ubiquinone oxidoreductase deficiency, lactate in children with mitochondrial disorders, and glutamine in the hyperammonemias.

The diagnostic potential of MRS should not be overestimated, however. It provides a relatively narrow window to brain metabolism. Robust techniques are available mainly for proton resonances, where sensitivity for metabolites is in the low millimolar range. Spectral findings, expressed as peak height or area ratios, must be converted into absolute concentrations by calibrating *in vivo* resonance areas with those of model solutions. In control brains values can be obtained for N-acetylaspartate, lactate, some amino acids, inositols, choline-containing compounds, and total creatine. For a meaningful interpretation of MRS data, a thorough understanding of neurochemistry of various brain regions, as well as experience with the enormous maturational, nutritional, and functional influences, is a prerequisite. For example, one must know that N-acetylaspartate is located almost exclusively in neurons; that myoinositol is located in primary glia cells; and that the concentration of choline-containing compounds roughly parallels myelination (Table 13.5).

Information from MRS must be interpreted in a fashion that is complementary to morphologic information from the MRI. In addition, detailed clinical and biochemical evaluations should be available before planning the investigation. Patients who can be considered for MRS are those in whom focal or generalized lesions have been demonstrated on MRI or those presenting with distinct neurologic or biochemical abnormalities. The time required for investigation is usually from 1 to 2 hours and necessitates sedation, as well as cardiopulmonary monitoring.

MRS has been shown to be more sensitive than MRI in detecting early pathologic changes in X-linked leukodystrophy; therefore, it has a place in monitoring these patients, as well as those with guanidinoacetate methyltransferase deficiency. Its greatest potential, however, lies in pathophysiologic studies of neurometabolic as well as neuroimmunologic diseases (e.g., white matter disorders and multiple sclerosis).

Table 13.5. *In vivo* **neuropathology by magnetic resonance spectroscopy**

Neuronal Damage	⇓ *N*-Acetylaspartate ⇓ Glutamate ⇑ Choline
Demyelination	⇑ Free lipids ⇑ Creatine =/⇑ Lactate ⇓ Phosphodiester[a]
Gliosis	⇑ Inositols ⇑ Glutamine
Cystic degeneration	⇓ All regularly observed metabolites ⇑ Glucose and lactate

[a]All changes are demonstrated by proton magnetic resonance spectroscopy except for the evaluation of phosphodiester, which requires phosphor spectroscopy.

In comparison to the diagnostic information provided with relative ease by neuroimaging and functional imaging techniques, the contribution of neurophysiologic methods may appear limited at first glance, especially in pediatric patients. Of major clinical importance are electroencephalography (EEG), nerve conduction velocity, evoked potentials, and electroretinography. Electromyography is performed in patients in whom a primary myopathy is suspected or in whom myopathic symptoms predominate. It differentiates between muscular and neural pathology. A specific repetitive pattern can be demonstrated in patients with glycogenosis type 2 and a subform of β-galactosidase deficiency.

The EEG is valuable in demonstrating β-activity and/or diffuse slowing in conditions of metabolic intoxication. Many disorders lead predominantly to slowing of the background activity to various degrees. The burst-suppression pattern is detected in nonketotic hyperglycemia, as well as in acute neonatal encephalopathies from disorders of organic acid metabolism (e.g., propionic aciduria). In two entities of the neuronal ceroid lipofuscinoses, the EEG findings can be very specific throughout certain periods of the disease course. Posterior polyspikes after single flashes are seen at an early stage in the late infantile form (Jansky-Bielschowsky), and a flat (isoelectric) curve is found at 3 to 4 years of age in the infantile form (Santavuori-Hantia).

A reduced nerve conduction velocity distinguishes demyelination of the peripheral nerve from axonal degeneration. Important information results in the diagnosis and clinical follow-up of patients with disorders of lipid metabolism (e.g., abetalipoproteinemia and Tangier disease), congenital disorders of glycosylation (CDG) syndromes, porphyrias, peroxisomal disorders, storage disorders, neuropathies due to defective DNA repair (e.g., ataxia teleangiectasia), and defects of the methylation pathways (i.e., cobalamin [vitamin B_{12}], the folate, and the methionine-homocysteine cycles). A peripheral neuropathy also develops in organic acidurias (e.g., 3-hydroxyacyl-CoA dehydrogenase deficiency and pyruvate dehydrogenase deficiency) as a result of defective energy metabolism.

Brainstem auditory evoked potentials (AEP), visual evoked potentials (VEP), and somatosensory evoked potentials (SSEP) are often abnormal in patients with neurodegenerative and neurometabolic disorders. These patients may consequently suffer from loss of hearing and vision to different degrees. Visual evoked potentials can help detect preclinical degeneration of the optic nerve in some patients with mitochondrial disorders or spinocerebellar degeneration. Hearing problems can be differentiated between lesions of the auditory nerves, as in Friedreich ataxia, or peripheral neuropathies and central abnormalities, as in leukodystrophies and peroxisomal or mitochondrial disorders. The authors believe that neurophysiologic investigations should be performed more widely in patients with suspected or proven inherited metabolic diseases. Although neurophysiologic testing may not have the same power in the differential diagnosis as the imaging techniques, it does provide complementary functional information and has an important place in the clinical work-up and follow-up of patients.

ADDITIONAL READINGS

Barkovich AJ. *Pediatric neuroimaging,* 3rd ed. New York: Lippincott Williams & Wilkins; 2000.

Frahm J, Hanefeld F. Localized proton magnetic resonance spectroscopy of brain disorders in children. In: Bachelard H, ed. *Advances in neurochemistry: resonance spectroscopy and imaging in neurochemistry,* Vol. 8. New York: Plenum Press; 1997:329–402.

Hoffmann GF, Gibson KM. Disorders of organic acid metabolism. In: Moser HW, ed. *Handbook of clinical neurology: neurodystrophies and neurolipidoses,* Vol. 66. Amsterdam: Elsevier; 1996:639–660.

Kohlschütter A. Neuroradiological and neurophysiological indices for neurometabolic disorders. *Eur J Pediatr* 1994;153(Suppl. 1):S90–S93.

Steinlin M, Blaser S, Boltshauser E. Cerebellar involvement in metabolic disorders: a pattern recognition approach. *Neuroradiology* 1998; 40:347–354.

14 ♣ Postmortem Investigations

If a patient with suspected metabolic disease dies, storing adequate amounts of biological fluids and available tissues for further diagnostic procedures is important. The use of these samples should be carefully planned in accordance with advice from specialists in the area of inborn errors of metabolism.

With sudden infant death syndrome (SIDS), recognizing that defects of fatty acid oxidation may be responsible, particularly long-chain defects that can lead to respiratory arrest and heart block or arrhythmias, is important. In most cases, autopsy reveals an excess of fat droplets in the liver or heart, but even in the absence of steatosis, blood spots should always be collected on filter paper for analysis for the common medium-chain acyl-CoA dehydrogenase (MCAD) mutation A985G and of acylcarnitines by electrospray tandem-mass spectrometry. With the exception of the mitochondrial fatty acid oxidation defects, most inborn errors of metabolism, such as urea cycle defects, organic acidurias, congenital lactic acidosis, and carbohydrate disorders, do not cause SIDS. Instead they cause an acute illness with obvious clinical symptoms that precedes death by hours or days.

When a child dies, a diagnosis is still important for genetic counseling and for studies on siblings, as well as on those that are as yet unborn. In general, the following specimens should be taken for postmortem investigations if an inborn error of metabolism has to be ruled out or confirmed:

- *Plasma.* Heparinized plasma (approximately 5 mL) should be separated and deep-frozen (–80°C).
- *Blood spots.* Blood should be dropped on filter paper (Guthrie cards) for analysis of acylcarnitines.
- *Blood.* Whole blood (10 to 15 mL) anticoagulated with ethylene diamine tetraacetate (EDTA) should be deep-frozen for later extraction of DNA for studies of molecular biology.
- *Urine.* Urine samples should be collected in different tubes and should be deep-frozen.
- *Cerebrospinal fluid (CSF).* CSF (1 mL) should be collected in a tube and deep-frozen (–80°C).
- *Vitreous humor.* This can be useful in reaching a diagnosis. It should be collected in a tube and deep-frozen.
- *Skin.* Skin for fibroblast culture must be taken with sterile precautions into the medium, and the cell culture must be established. Fibroblasts are best cultured premortem.
- *Liver.* Three or more samples of 1 cm³ each should be snap-frozen in liquid nitrogen and should be stored on dry ice at –80°C or in liquid nitrogen for histochemistry and enzymology.
- *Muscle (skeletal or heart) and other tissues.* These should be taken as indicated for liver tissue.

Specific investigations of these samples depend on the history, clinical symptoms, and routine laboratory data. The spectrum of specific analyses to be done on postmortem samples is broad; it most often includes analyses of amino acids, organic acids, carnitine, and the profile of acylcarnitines. These studies may lead to specific enzymology and molecular studies, or clinical and laboratory data may suggest these studies directly.

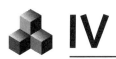

IV

Organ Systems
in Metabolic Diseases

15 ♣ Cardiomyopathy and Cardiac Failure

Errors of metabolism are associated with a wide variety of cardiac manifestations, including hypertrophic or dilated cardiomyopathy, dysrhythmias and conduction disturbances, and valvular disease. Most metabolic cardiomyopathies result from disorders of energy production and generally involve other organs, particularly skeletal muscle and liver. Taken as a group, the disorders of fatty acid oxidation and of oxidative phosphorylation are the most common of the metabolic cardiomyopathies; disorders of glycogen metabolism, especially Pompe disease, are also important. The cardiac manifestations in some metabolic disorders may be late, subtle, or as a result of metabolic derangements in other organs. Valvular dysfunction and infiltrative cardiomyopathy occur as late complications in many of the lysosomal storage disorders. Myocardial dysfunction is common in hemochromatosis, the metabolic cardiomyopathy that is most easily prevented. Peripheral vascular disease is prominent in homocystinuria.

Perhaps 15% of cardiomyopathies in children result from named or suspected disorders of intermediary metabolism. These conditions constitute a lower proportion of cardiomyopathy among adults, where ischemic heart disease and diabetic cardiomyopathy are two of the major causes in developed countries.

Metabolic disorders with cardiac manifestations can be conveniently divided into those in which the cardiac manifestations are primary or prominent (Table 15.1) and those in which they are less common or less significant (Table 15.2). Pompe disease (severe lysosomal type II glycogen storage disease) usually presents in infancy. Problems of fatty acid oxidation are likely to present in infancy; mitochondrial disorders may present at any age.

SPECIAL ASPECTS OF CARDIAC METABOLISM

The major fuels for the heart under nearly all circumstances are glucose and fatty acids. The heart, like skeletal muscle, maintains a reserve of high-energy phosphate compounds (e.g., phosphocreatine), as well as of glycogen. Before birth the heart uses fatty acids less and glycolysis more and tolerates anaerobic metabolism more readily than after the first few weeks following birth. This transition period sometimes leads to the appearance of a cardiomyopathy that has previously been clinically silent. After this period of a few weeks, the metabolism of the heart relies on both fatty acids and glucose for fuel; if glucose becomes the limiting substance (during hypoglycemia), the heart can function well, whereas hypoglycemia in the newborn period may lead to significant impairment of cardiac function and dilatation of the heart. During times of increased energy demand and greater cardiac output, use of fatty acids and glucose increases. Long-chain fatty acids, which require carnitine for transport into the mitochondria, are the usual forms present in the blood. Medium-chain fatty acids, which enter the mitochondria
(*text continues on page 181*)

Table 15.1. Metabolic disorders with cardiomyopathy as a presenting or early symptom

Disorder	Hyper-trophic	Dilated	Dys-rhythmia	Heart block	Organic acids	Carnitine level	Acylcarnitine species	Diagnostic tissues	Comments
I. Fatty acid oxidation									
Carnitine transporter deficiency	++	+	+		+	↓↓		F,M,K,W	
Carnitine–acylcarnitine translocase deficiency	++	+	++		+	→	++	F	
CPT II deficiency	++	+	++		+	→	++	F,W,M,L	Heterozygote may have symptoms and may be vulnerable to malignant hyperthermia.
VLCAD deficiency	++	+	+		++	→	++	F,W	
LCHAD/trifunctional enzyme deficiency	++	+	+		++	→	++	D,F	HELLP syndrome in pregnant heterozygotes.

							Comments
II. Mitochondrial disorders							
Numerous disorders	+	‡	‡	+	+	D,F,H,L,M,W	Heart block or sudden death may occur. May have lactic acidosis and increased lactate/pyruvate ratio.
MAD deficiency	‡	+	‡	‡	+	F,M	
III. Organic acidurias							
Propionic aciduria; methylmalonic aciduria, Cbl C defect	+	+	‡	‡	‡	F,L,W	Cardiomyopathy unrelated to metabolic decompensation or nutritional status; may be presenting symptom.
IV. Infiltrative disorders							
Lysosomal glycogen storage disease (severe form—Pompe)						W	Macroglossia, severe cardiomyopathy and skeletal myopathy. Characteristic EKG.

continued

Table 15.1. *Continued.*

Disorder	Hyper-trophic	Dilated	Dys-rhythmia	Heart block	Organic acids	Carnitine level	Acylcarnitine species	Diagnostic tissues	Comments
V. Disorders of glycogen/glucose metabolism									
GSD Type IV (brancher deficiency)	++							D,M,L	Severe liver disease. Neuropathy, dementia in adult form.
Phosphorylase b kinase deficiency	++							H	Rapidly fatal. Very rare cardiac glycogenosis.
Triosephosphate isomerase deficiency			++					E	Hemolytic anemia. Sudden death.
VI. Hemo-chromatosis	+	+	+	+				P,D	Restrictive cardiomyopathy occasionally.

VII. Nutrient deficiency

				Diagnostic tissues	Clinical features
Secondary carnitine deficiency	+		+	P,M	
Selenium deficiency		++		E	
Thiamine deficiency/dependency				P,E,U	Hyperkinetic heart, CHF, edema, lactic acidosis
Congenital disorders of glycosylation (CDG) especially type 1a		→		F	Pericardial effusion, tamponade.

+, Mildly abnormal. ++, Usually and prominently abnormal.

Diagnostic tissues commonly used. Abbreviations: D, DNA (leukocytes and other tissues); E, erythrocytes; F, fibroblasts; H, heart; L, liver; M, skeletal muscle; P, plasma; U, urine; W, white blood cells (leukocytes).

Other abbreviations: Cbl, cobalamin; CHF, congestive heart failure; CPT II, carnitine palmitoyltransferase II; EKG, electrocardiogram; GSD, glycogen storage disease; HELLP, hemolysis, elevated liver enzymes, and low platelets; LCHAD, long-chain hydroxyacyl-CoA dehydrogenase; MAD, multiple acyl-CoA dehydrogenase; VLCAD, very-long-chain acyl-CoA dehydrogenase.

Table 15.2.   Disorders in which cardiac involvement is usually mild or late (symptoms recognized after systemic illness or involvement of other organs)

Disorder	Comments, special issues
MAD deficiency (mild, including SCHAD deficiency)	Biochemically similar to severe forms, but later onset and milder or intermittent symptoms. Cardiomyopathy similar to fatty acid oxidation defects (Table 15.1).
Friedrich ataxia	Mitochondrial damage may be due to iron accumulation. Diabetes common.
Mucopolysaccharidoses—general pathology	Myocardial thickening, especially septum and LV wall. Aortic and mitral valve thickening and regurgitation, narrowing of aorta and coronary, pulmonary, and renal arteries
MPS I-S, I-H	Infiltration, thickening of septum, LV wall
MPS II	EFE, MS, AS, AR, MR, infarction
MPS VI	MV, AV calcification, stenosis
Gaucher disease	Myocardial thickening due to infiltration
Fabry disease	Infiltration leading to LVH; MV prolapse, thickening
Fucosidosis	Cardiomegaly
Mannosidosis	Short PR interval
Sialidosis	Cardiomegaly, MR, CHF; pericardial effusion
Mucolipidosis II, III	Aortic regurgitation, cardiomegaly
Aspartylglycosaminuria	MR, aortic thickening
Homocystinuria	Hypercoagulability, strokes; mitral valve prolapse

Abbreviations: AR, aortic regurgitation; AS, aortic stenosis; AV, arteriovenous; CHF, congestive heart failure; EFE, endocardial fibroelastosis; LV, left ventricle; LVH, left ventricular hypertrophy; MAD, multiple acyl-CoA dehydrogenase; MPS, mucopolysaccharidoses; MR, mitral regurgitation; MS, mitral stenosis; MV, mitral valve; SCHAD, short-chain hydroxyacyl-CoA dehydrogenase.

directly, can be used to provide fuel to the heart and other organs if a problem with long-chain fatty acid oxidation exists. Furthermore, during times of metabolic stress, the myocardium switches and uses more glucose than at other times, so provision of continuous glucose during times of cardiac dysfunction can be beneficial.

The heart, because it relies more than other tissues on fatty acid oxidation, may be particularly vulnerable to disturbances of its major energy source. Disturbances of cellular function that affect only a small group of cells can have a devastating impact if the region influenced is part of the cardiac conduction pathways or a stimulus on them.

PATTERNS OF METABOLIC CARDIAC DISEASE

Hypertrophy and Dilation

The functional categorization of cardiomyopathies as hypertrophic or dilated does not help the clinician much in discovering the etiology, whereas knowing the etiology does help predict the course and plan therapy. Hypertrophy can result from accumulated material stored in the myocardium (e.g., glycogen), from the heart's response to poor functioning of the contractile apparatus (abnormalities of structural proteins), or from impaired energetics (mitochondrial disorders). Dilatation results when the abnormal or poorly functioning heart cannot contract adequately and begins to stretch out of shape. This occurs in the disorders of carnitine availability, and it may occur in the late stages of disorders of fatty acid oxidation and oxidative phosphorylation and in some of the organic acidurias. Dysrhythmias and conduction defects are particular features of some mitochondrial disorders but can occur in any cardiomyopathy.

Endocardial Fibroelastosis

Endocardial fibroelastosis describes a condition peculiar to infants and young children in which significant thickening and stiffening of the endocardium occurs. The basis for this response is unknown. It can occur in disparate conditions, ranging from viral myocarditis to carnitine transporter deficiency, Barth syndrome, severe mucopolysaccharidoses (MPS) I (Hurler syndrome), and MPS VI (Maroteaux–Lamy syndrome).

FATTY ACID OXIDATION DISORDERS: CARDIOMYOPATHIES

Disorders of fatty acid oxidation that involve long-chain fatty acids often present as cardiomyopathy. Sometimes the onset is abrupt or overwhelming, particularly in the newborn period. Sudden death may occur, presumably reflecting arrhythmia. Liver involvement (manifesting as fasting hypoketotic hypoglycemia, hyperammonemia, or a Reyelike syndrome) and skeletal muscle involvement are common. Very-long-chain acyl-CoA dehydrogenase (VLCAD) and carnitine palmitoyl-CoA transferase (CPT) II deficiencies are probably the most common; long-chain hydroxyacyl-CoA dehydrogenase (LCHAD) and trifunctional protein and carnitine-acylcarnitine translocase deficiencies present similarly. Chapter 19 discusses the metabolic pathways and the skeletal muscle aspects of these conditions. Medium-chain acyl-CoA dehydrogenase (MCAD) deficiency, the most common disorder of fatty acid oxidation (and a cause of carnitine depletion), is unusual for a fatty acid oxidation disorder because cardiomyopathy is an extremely uncommon feature, but dysrhythmia and sudden death are real concerns.

Carnitine-Acylcarnitine Translocase Deficiency

Most patients with translocase deficiency have had severe disease in infancy, including acute cardiac events (shock, heart failure, and cardiac arrest). Arrhythmias can be prominent. Ventricular hypertrophy may also be found. Significant hepatic and skeletal muscle dysfunction (hyperammonemia, weakness) occur. Total blood carnitine level, especially the free fraction, may be low. Acylcarnitine analysis shows mainly long-chain species, reflecting their synthesis by carnitine palmitoyltransferase (CPT) I and subsequent accumulation. Emergency management includes the provision of glucose, restriction of long-chain fats, and supplementation with medium-chain lipids (see also Chapter 6, "Emergency Treatment of Inherited Metabolic Diseases"). Despite these measures, neonatal fatality is common.

Carnitine Palmitoyl-CoA Transferase II Deficiency

The severe infantile form of CPT II deficiency leads to severe cardiac, skeletal muscle, and liver dysfunction, resulting in circulatory shock, heart failure, hypoketotic hypoglycemia, hyperammonemia, and coma. Renal dysgenesis, reminiscent of the cystic malformations that occur in glutaric aciduria type II (see Chapter 23), may be present.

Plasma and tissue carnitine levels are low, especially that of free carnitine. Acylcarnitine analysis shows long-chain species $C16:0$, $C18:1$, $C18:2$, as occurs in translocase deficiency.

Arrhythmias represent a common feature of CPT II deficiency. Long-chain acylcarnitines, long-chain acyl-CoAs, and long-chain free fatty acids all have detergent effects on membranes; therefore, an accumulation might have disruptive effects. On the other hand, the relative deficiency of free carnitine adversely affects the ratio of free coenzyme A (CoASH) to acyl-CoA, and the plasma and tissue deficiency of carnitine impairs fatty acid oxidation. The true magnitude of the contribution of long-chain acylcarnitines to arrhythmias in CPT II deficiency (and related disorders) is unknown, as is the true risk of carnitine administration in a desperately ill child with this disorder.

Mild CPT II deficiency, among the most common fatty acid oxidation disorders, is typified by recurrent rhabdomyolysis; it does not present with significant cardiac involvement. Residual enzyme activity in these patients is higher than is that in the severe infantile form.

Very-Long-Chain Acyl-CoA Dehydrogenase Deficiency

Very-long-chain acyl-CoA dehydrogenation is the first step of beta-oxidation (see Fig. 19.1) in the mitochondria after synthesis of the acyl-CoA (e.g., palmitoyl-CoA) is catalyzed by CPT II. Understanding why impairment of this step can lead to severe organ dysfunction, especially in heart, liver, and skeletal muscle, is easy. Patients with VLCAD deficiency were thought to have long-chain acyl-CoA dehydrogenase (LCAD) deficiency until about 1993. Since then, a greater understanding of the enzymatic processes has led to the condition being renamed.

Cardiac symptoms (feeding difficulties, tachypnea, and congestive failure), if they occur, are likely to be seen in infants and young children; concurrent liver dysfunction may exist. This is the common presentation of this disorder. Cardiac hypertrophy, especially of the left ventricle, is common. Electrocardiogram (EKG) may show increased voltages. Urinary organic acids may show increased dicarboxylic acids; plasma or blood spot acylcarnitine analysis shows elevated C14:1 species. Enzyme assay can be done on fibroblasts and other tissues.

Treatment involves avoiding fasting, limiting essential long-chain fats to the amount needed for growth, and providing medium-chain lipids and other foods as calorie sources in place of long-chain fats. Although the total plasma carnitine level is often low, chronic carnitine supplementation has not led to dramatic improvement. Supplementation restores levels of free carnitine.

Long-Chain Hydroxyacyl-CoA Dehydrogenase/ Trifunctional Enzyme Deficiency

Many infants with LCHAD deficiency present with cardiomyopathy, sometimes in the newborn period. This is one of the more common disorders of cardiac fatty acid oxidation. Liver dysfunction may be severe, including cirrhosis, and significant skeletal muscle involvement may occur. Plasma carnitine level may be low; acylcarnitine analysis shows increased hydroxy forms of C16:0, C18:1, and C18:2. Findings that are unusual for a disorder of fatty acid oxidation include lactic acidosis, pigmentary retinopathy (in older children and adults), and peripheral neuropathy. Absent deep tendon reflexes and toe walking have also been reported.

In the late-onset form, dominated by intermittent muscle symptoms, asymptomatic ventricular hypertrophy may occur.

Carnitine Transporter Deficiency

A deficiency of the carnitine transporter leads to severe carnitine depletion by a few months to several years of age. In the most extreme cases, it can present as neonatal hydrops. Thickening of the left ventricle, hepatomegaly with hepatic dysfunction (hypoglycemia, hyperammonemia, increased transaminases), hypotonia, and developmental delay occur. The EKG may show high, peaked T waves and left ventricular hypertrophy. The plasma total carnitine level is exceedingly low, often less than 5 µmol/L; and the acylcarnitine profile shows no abnormal species. In contrast to specific elevations in other disorders of fatty acid oxidation, the quantities of all acylcarnitines may be very low, which suggests the diagnosis. The urinary organic acids may show dicarboxylic aciduria. Endocardial biopsy, if performed (not needed for diagnosis), can show lipid infiltration and endocardial fibroelastosis.

The milder, later onset form may present with cardiac dilatation, abnormal EKG, and hepatomegaly. Skeletal muscle strength may appear to be normal on static testing, but endurance is poor. Muscle biopsy shows lipid storage. Urinary organic acids are usually unremarkable.

In this autosomal recessive condition, the fractional excretion of carnitine in the urine approaches 100% because the defective transport of carnitine into tissues, such as cardiac or skeletal muscle, also prevents its renal tubular reabsorption. Accordingly, carnitine must be provided frequently. During an acute crisis, intravenous carnitine can be given in a dose of 300 mg/kg/d as a continuous infusion. Oral carnitine should be given four times daily. The oral dose for children is 100 to 200 mg/kg/d; for adults, it is 2 to 4 g/d, but some patients have required much more to maintain satisfactory plasma levels. The maximal oral dose is usually set by intestinal tolerance; diarrhea does not occur with parenteral use. Following treatment the cardiomyopathy improves dramatically, and the heart size returns to normal. Skeletal weakness may also improve, although muscle carnitine levels remain low (2% to 4% of normal).

Secondary Carnitine Deficiency

Secondary carnitine deficiency occurs in a large number of settings, as discussed in Chapter 19. Even with low plasma levels the cardiac uptake of carnitine is usually sufficient to avoid symptoms. However, premature infants occasionally receive long-term total parenteral nutrition (TPN) without carnitine supplementation and become profoundly depleted after a few months. The need for carnitine in infants may exceed the synthetic capability, as an infant needs sufficient carnitine for the increasing mass of muscle and other tissues, whereas adults need only to replace what is lost. A lower renal threshold for carnitine in a sick infant may also become pathophysiologically relevant.

Infants with carnitine depletion may have poor cardiac output and dilated cardiomyopathy. The plasma carnitine level may be less than 10 μmol/L. One would expect hypoglycemia from liver carnitine depletion, but this does not occur because of the continuous high-dose glucose of the TPN. Carnitine supplementation (15 to 30 mg/kg/d intravenously, given with the TPN infusion) leads to rapid improvement in blood levels and cardiac function.

Severe carnitine depletion can occur in the setting of renal Fanconi syndrome (as in cystinosis and mitochondrial dysfunction) or of treatment with valproate or the antibiotic pivampicillin. Although very low plasma carnitine levels are found for a short time during episodes of illness in a patient with MCAD deficiency and glutaric aciduria type I, they are not usually associated with cardiomyopathy.

MITOCHONDRIAL CARDIOMYOPATHIES

Chapter 6 discusses the mitochondrial disorders in general terms. Many patients with mitochondrial disorders and cardiomyopathy fit a general pattern of dysfunction, such as Kearns–Sayre syndrome or mitochondrial encephalomyelopathy, lactic acidemia, and stroke-like episodes (MELAS). However, many others do not. Involvement of other organs, especially the brain, eye (and eye movements), skeletal muscle, liver, and kidney, is common. Lactic acidosis with an increased ratio of lactate to pyruvate is common. Disturbances of cardiac rhythm, such as complete heart block or bundle branch block, are frequent; and sudden death may occur, sometimes as the first indication of a mitochondrial disorder. A diagnosis in this situation may be possible if tissues (especially a heart sample) for mitochondrial studies are acquired rapidly after death.

The Kearns–Sayre syndrome is the prototypical mitochondrial disorder in which disturbance of conduction is progressive. Most patients represent nonfamilial heteroplasmic deletions of mitochondrial DNA. Cardiac symptoms include hypertrophic or dilated cardiomyopathy, atrial or ventricular arrhythmias, Wolf–Parkinson–White syndrome, and other preexcitation syndromes. Progressive heart block necessitates pacemaker placement. Major noncardiac symptoms include retinitis pigmentosa, ophthalmoplegia, ataxia, myopathy, and increased cerebrospinal fluid (CSF) protein, with onset before 20 years of age. Many other manifestations may occur, including deafness, seizures, diabetes or other endocrinopathy, renal and gastro-intestinal symptoms, and lactic acidosis. Similar manifestations with later onset are typical of chronic progressive external ophthalmoplegia-plus (CPEO-plus).

Another mitochondrial disorder likely to have cardiac involvement is MELAS. Most manifestations of this are due to mutation A3243G in the mitochondrial tRNA^{Leu} gene. Benign infantile myopathy and cardiomyopathy (BIMC) results from mutations in complex I, including the ND3 subunit.

Multiple Acyl-CoA Dehydrogenase Deficiency

Infants with the severe form of multiple acyl-CoA dehydrogenase (MAD) deficiency, especially the form without malformations, often have cardiomyopathy. Hypotonia, encephalopathy, overwhelming acidosis, and metabolic derangements resulting from impairment of multiple pathways are common. The diagnosis is usually established by analysis of urinary organic acids or plasma/blood acylcarnitines and is confirmed by enzyme analysis or Western blot of fibroblasts. Carnitine depletion is common. Survival is uncommon as treatment is difficult, but provision of abundant carnitine, riboflavin, and calories (as carbohydrates) can be beneficial to the patient.

The mild form of MAD, which has been referred to as ethylmalonic-adipic aciduria, usually does not involve the heart.

Barth Syndrome

Barth syndrome is an X-linked recessive condition that is similar to many mitochondrial oxidative phosphorylation diseases. Neutropenia, dilated cardiomyopathy, and increased urinary excretion of 3-methylglutaconate, 3-methylglutarate, and 2-ethylhydracrylate, acids suggestive of mitochondrial dysfunction, occur. The onset typically occurs in infancy, but spontaneous improvement may appear in later childhood. Biopsy of skeletal muscle or the heart shows abnormal mitochondria, which may be abnormal in shape and which may contain inclusion bodies and dense, tightly packed concentric cristae. Lactic acidosis may be prominent. At least one patient has had a dramatic and sustained response to treatment with pantothenic acid, a precursor of coenzyme A. Pantothenol has been ineffective. The molecular defect in Barth syndrome is in a protein called G4.5, or tafazzin, whose function is not yet known.

Friedreich Ataxia

Friedreich ataxia presents with slowly progressive spinocerebellar dysfunction in children and young adults. Cardiomyopathy and diabetes are common. The genetic defect is a trinucleotide expansion in the frataxin gene. The mechanism of cellular injury appears to be related to iron accumulation within mitochondria. Cellular damage leading to apoptosis may be due to peroxidative damage to mitochondrial membranes.

CARDIOMYOPATHIES OF ORGANIC ACIDURIAS

Two common organic acid disorders, propionic aciduria and methylmalonic aciduria, which are part of the branched-chain amino acid catabolic pathway, may present with a cardiomyopathy from birth to a few years of age. The onset may be subtle or sudden. Cardiac failure with dilatation, poor contractility, and rhythm disturbances, including ventricular irritability or bradycardia, may occur. The basis for this cardiomyopathy is unknown. In some cases it has occurred in children being treated successfully for the metabolic disorder, and in others it has been the presenting symptom. Suggested causes include viruses, nutritional deficiency of carnitine or of some other nutrients, and primary toxicity of metabolites accumulating as a result of the underlying enzymopathy. Treatment is directed at correcting the metabolic derangement and at providing appropriate supportive care. Cardiomyopathy may also occur in β-ketothiolase deficiency and in a newly described disorder of valine catabolism, isobutyryl-CoA dehydrogenase deficiency.

INFILTRATIVE CARDIOMYOPATHIES

Glycogen Storage Disease II (Pompe Disease, Lysosomal Acid Maltase Deficiency)

Pompe disease is the most common lysosomal disorder with severe cardiac manifestations. Pompe disease is among the most common metabolic myopathies, and involvement of the heart and skeletal muscles is primary. Symptoms appear in early infancy, and the disorder progresses rapidly. Weakness, floppiness, and macroglossia may be apparent within a few months. Cardiac manifestations include shortness of breath and poor feeding. Chest x-ray shows cardiomegaly; echocardiography shows concentric symmetric hypertrophy; EKG shows left axis deviation, short PR interval, high QRS voltages, and inverted T waves. Peripheral blood leukocytes may show vacuoles, and often, pathologic excretion of oligosaccharides in the urine is found. Enzyme assay can be performed on leukocytes, fibroblasts, and muscle. Muscle biopsy shows a major accumulation that is stainable with periodic acid-Schiff (PAS) reagent; electron microscopy shows membrane-bound (i.e., in lysosomes) accumulation of glycogen. Infants with Pompe disease often succumb in a few months but may survive for 2 or 3 years. Trials of enzyme replacement therapy are under way and, so far, have demonstrated encouraging results.

Patients with milder forms of acid maltase deficiency do not have cardiac symptoms. They present with progressive weakness (see Chapter 19).

Other Infiltrative Cardiomyopathies

The myocardium may become thickened because of accumulated material, particularly within lysosomes. In Fabry disease thickening of the left ventricle may be found. This can also occur in heterozygous women of this X-linked disorder, perhaps reflecting skewed lyonization, as well as in hemizygous men. Coronary artery disease is also common in Fabry disease. The mucopolysaccharidoses and fucosidosis may be complicated by storage in the septum and posterior wall of the left ventricle. Lysosomal storage in the heart may also occur in Gaucher disease.

CARDIOMYOPATHIES DUE TO OTHER DISORDERS OF GLYCOGEN/GLUCOSE METABOLISM

Glycogen Storage Disease Type III (GSD III) Debrancher Deficiency (Cori or Forbes Disease)

In type IIIa GSD, the liver and skeletal or cardiac muscle are involved; in the less common type IIIb, only hepatic disease, manifesting as fasting hypoglycemia, increased transaminases, and rarely, mild lactic acidosis occur. The cardiomyopathy in type IIIa usually does not cause symptoms, but obstruction to blood flow and heart failure occasionally occur. Ventricular hypertrophy may be present on EKG.

Glycogen Storage Disease Type IV (GSD Type IV) Brancher Deficiency (Anderson Disease)

The usual form of glycogen brancher deficiency manifests as hepatomegaly and cirrhosis. The deficiency of the branching enzyme activity leads to the accumulation of an amylopectin-like glycogen, which incites an inflammatory response. Severely affected patients, who are rare, may have heart involvement with dilatation in infancy. Liver transplantation is curative for the liver disease. The heart condition may be ameliorated as well, as shown by improvement in cardiac function and the lessening of storage.

HEMOCHROMATOSIS

Hemochromatosis is among the most common autosomal recessive conditions in many parts of the world, occurring as often as one in 300 persons. The incidence of symptomatic hemochromatosis is not truly known because of underrecognition. Two mutant alleles of the HFE gene account for essentially all cases. Homozygotes for C282Y are at highest risk; compound heterozygotes C282Y/H63D are at less risk; and homozygotes for H63D are at minimal risk for iron overload.

Hepatomegaly and hepatic dysfunction, manifest by elevation of transaminases, are common (see Chapter 16). Pancreatic dysfunction may lead to diabetes, and adrenal dysfunction may lead to Addison disease. Darkening of the skin from iron may be mistaken for the effects of Addison disease. Arthropathy is common. Cardiomyopathy has an insidious onset and may be attributed to diabetes. The cardiomyopathy usually results in biventricular dilatation. Ventricular thickening is an early finding; a restrictive form occurs occasionally. Arrhythmias (e.g., ventricular ectopic beats, tachycardias, ventricular fibrillation, and heart block) may occur.

Transferrin saturation, serum iron concentration, and ferritin levels are the usual tests for iron overload; definitive diagnosis, formerly done by liver biopsy, is now generally done by molecular testing, although biopsy may be needed to assess the degree of liver injury.

Hemochromatosis is treated by phlebotomy (as blood donation if the donor is otherwise suitable), so early diagnosis is essential. Tissue damage, such as cardiomyopathy and hepatic fibrosis, may not be reversible. As hemochromatosis is a recessive disease, all siblings must be tested. Parents and children should also be tested, as pseudodominant pedigrees, which are a consequence of the high frequency of the mutant alleles, are frequent. Molecular methods are best for cascade testing, once the mutations of the proband are known, to avoid the problem of false-negative results of iron testing.

A distinct disorder is juvenile hemochromatosis, with similar findings, but its onset is in childhood. It does not map to the HFE locus of hemochromatosis.

NUTRIENT-DEFICIENCY CARDIOMYOPATHIES

Thiamine

Thiamine (vitamin B_1) in the form of thiamine pyrophosphate is essential for the function of several decarboxylases of 2-oxoacids, including pyruvate, the branched-chain oxoacids, and 2-oxoglutarate. Severe thiamine deficiency leads to beri-beri, a form of cardiac and peripheral vessel dysfunction characterized by loss of peripheral vascular tone, edema, tachycardia, cardiac dilatation, and heart failure. Brain damage (Wernicke encephalopathy) reminiscent of Leigh disease may occur, and other organs may be damaged. Thiamine deficiency can occur in patients with organic acidurias who are receiving limited diets. In this setting lactic acidosis is the presenting feature, reflecting impaired activity of pyruvate decarboxylase, the first step in the pyruvate dehydrogenase complex. Deficiency of thiamine resulting from autosomal recessive thiamine transport defects typically results in anemia (usually megaloblastic but may be sideroblastic or aplastic), sensorineural deafness, and diabetes. Tachycardia and edema may occur in the most severely affected infants. Diagnosis is made by measuring blood or urine thiamine content.

Selenium

Selenium in selenomethionine is a component of proteins. Free selenium also serves as an essential cofactor in the activity of various metalloenzymes, such as glutathione peroxidase. Selenium deficiency, especially with vitamin E deficiency, impairs the antioxidant function of various pathways. An increased vulnerability to cardiotropic enteroviruses may result. Selenium deficiency is a common cause of cardiomyopathy in the Keshan district of China, where insufficient selenium is found in soil and foods. Manifestations include cardiac dilatation, dysrhythmias, and ultrastructural changes. The condition may be fatal unless treated. Pancreatic insufficiency may also develop.

Selenium deficiency may also occur in developed countries. It has been observed following prolonged parenteral nutrition and in patients with small bowel disease. Patients with many forms of heart disease, including ischemic heart disease and human immunodeficiency virus (HIV) cardiomyopathy, have lower selenium levels than do controls, raising the possibility that selenium depletion may be playing a role in the heart disease. Selenium deficiency is diagnosed by measurement of erythrocyte selenium along with glutathione (total and reduced) and glutathione peroxidase; it is treated with sodium selenite, 60 to 100 μg/d.

METABOLIC DISORDERS AND VALVULAR ABNORMALITIES

Several metabolic disorders are associated with valvular dysfunction late in the course of the disorder. Thickening of the valves, especially the mitral and aortic, sometimes with calcification, occurs in several lysosomal storage disorders, including Hurler (MPS I-H), Scheie (MPS I-S), Hunter (MPS II) and Maroteaux–Lamy (MPS VI) syndromes. Pulmonary hypertension may also develop. Mitral stenosis and mitral valve prolapse with regurgitation can occur in MPS IV (Morquio). In MPS IIIB mitral valve stenosis occasionally occurs.

The mucolipidoses, especially mucolipidosis I (sialidosis), can be complicated by mitral regurgitation. The lipidoses, especially Gaucher disease and Farber disease, may show storage in the connective tissues of the valves, causing thickening of the aortic and mitral valves and the development of nodules. The chordae tendineae may develop similar deposits. Functionally, aortic or mitral stenosis or regurgitation may be present. Stiffening of the valves occurs in alkaptonuria, a disorder of tyrosine catabolism that causes darkening (ochronosis) and stiffening of cartilaginous tissues.

ABNORMALITIES OF THE VESSELS

Abnormalities of blood vessels occur in several metabolic disorders and are discussed in greater detail elsewhere. Tortuosity of vessels is particularly prominent in Menkes syndrome. Angiokeratomata of the umbilicus, buttocks, and genitalia are a feature of X-linked Fabry disease; they appear in adolescence. In fucosidosis (autosomal recessive), they appear in the first few years of life.

Hypercoagulability, which can lead to major occlusions of cerebral vessels or to multiple small cerebral infarcts, is a prominent aspect of homocystinuria or the congenital disorders of glycosylation (CDG) syndromes. Strokes are also a frequent feature in mitochondrial disorders, perhaps as a consequence of dysregulation of vascular function. Sudden occlusions, gradual occlusion (resulting in moya-moya, a proliferative vascular response), migraine with stroke, and strokelike episodes without residua may all occur in mitochondrial disorders, particularly MELAS.

Atherosclerosis, a major feature of the hyperlipidemias, leads to myocardial infarction and cerebrovascular disease. It is accelerated in Fabry disease, including some heterozygous females, and in some mucopolysaccharidoses.

INVESTIGATIONS

Laboratory tests to investigate a suspected metabolic cardiomyopathy should focus initially on obtaining information rapidly to determine if a specific treatment for the disorder exists. At the same time, supportive care to ease myocardial workload should be instituted; and preparations should be made for invasive testing, if needed.

Initial tests include plasma pyruvate and lactate, amino acids, carnitine, and acylcarnitine profile. Consideration should be given to determining thiamine, selenium, vitamin E, and glutathione levels. Creatine kinase with fractionation may be useful.

Lactate is often elevated in patients with cardiac failure; this may simply be due to poor perfusion. In such a setting, the lactate/pyruvate ratio is likely to be elevated and is not, per se, suggestive of disturbed oxidative phosphorylation (see Chapter 6, "Work-up of the Patient with Lactic Acidemia"). Renal tubular function can be assessed by checking for wasting of amino acids, phosphate, and bicarbonate, indicating the presence of a Fanconi syndrome or isolated renal tubular acidosis. Urinary organic acids with increased Krebs cycle intermediates and lactate may be suggestive of mitochondrial dysfunction. 3-Methylglutaconic acid indicates Barth syndrome. Hepatic dysfunction may be reflected by increases in transaminases and ammonia and by hypoglycemia.

Second-order tests include the enzymes of fatty acid oxidation that can be assayed in fibroblasts or lymphocytes. Mitochondrial function and DNA are assessed in blood leukocytes and other tissues, especially muscle. Heteroplasmy may not be detected in peripheral blood cells (see Chapters 6 and 19).

ADDITIONAL READING

Böhles HJ, Sewell A, Hofstetter F. *Metabolic cardiomyopathies.* Stuttgart: Wiesenmeier; 1998.

16 ♣ Approach to the Patient with Hepatic Disease

Disease of the liver is a common and an important sequel to inherited metabolic disease. Defects in the degradation of amino acids, fatty acids, fructose, galactose, glycogen, and ketone bodies, as well as defects of gluconeogenesis, ketogenesis, ammonia detoxification, or oxidative phosphorylation, can lead to significant liver disease. Specific symptoms of these disorders reflect response to the demand on the pathway affected; they include pathologic alterations of blood ammonia, glucose, lactate, ketone bodies, and pH. Specific symptoms are often obscured by the consequences of nonspecific responses of the liver to injuries that lead to hepatocellular damage, decreased liver function, cholestasis, and hepatomegaly. Other inherited diseases interfere primarily with hepatic cell integrity; these include Wilson disease, α_1-antitrypsin deficiency, and deficiencies of biosynthetic pathways, such as those in cholesterol biosynthesis, peroxisomal disorders, congenital disorders of glycosylation (CDG), and defects in the synthesis of bile acids. Very striking physical involvement of the liver with relatively little functional derangement is seen in lysosomal storage disorders.

In contrast to the complex, interrelated functions of the liver in intermediary metabolism, the hepatic clinical response to inherited metabolic disease is limited and is often indistinguishable from reactions to acquired causes, such as infections. The diagnostic laboratory evaluation of liver disease must therefore be rather broad, especially in neonates. Careful evaluation of the history and clinical presentation should include a detailed dietary history, as well as a list of all medications, the general appearance of the patient, somatic and psychomotor development, organomegaly, neurologic signs, and ophthalmologic examination. When combined with the results of routine clinical chemical investigations (Table 16.1), this should lead to the suspicion of an inborn error of metabolism, a provisional grouping into one of four main groups of presentation (Table 16.2), and initiation of specific metabolic tests (Table 16.3).

The family and personal history of the patient can help in acquired, as well as inherited, liver disease. Routes of infection may become obvious. Linkage of symptoms to oral intake of food or drugs may be almost diagnostic in fructose intolerance, paracetamol intoxication, or accidental poisoning.

Another important key to diagnosis is the age at presentation. During the first 3 months of life, most patients with liver disease, including those with inherited metabolic diseases, present with conjugated hyperbilirubinemia. Only a few well-defined inherited diseases cause unconjugated hyperbilirubinemia; these are the hemolytic anemias or impaired conjugation of bilirubin resulting from a recessive deficiency of uridine diphosphate (UDP)-glucuronyl transferase in Crigler–Najjar syndrome or due to a dominantly inherited mild reduction of UDP-glucuronyl transferase in Gilbert syndrome. The latter is a benign condition manifesting in neonates only if they are afflicted with a second

Table 16.1. First-line investigations in disease of the liver

Alanine and aspartate aminotransferases (transaminases)
Cholinesterase
Bilirubin, conjugated and unconjugated
Alkaline phosphatase
γ-Glutamyltranspeptidase
Glucose
Ammonia
Coagulation studies: PT, PTT, factors V, VII, and XI
Albumin, prealbumin
Urea nitrogen, creatinine, uric acid
Hepatitis A, B, C
Cytomegalovirus, EBV, herpes simplex, toxoplasmosis, HIV
Viral cultures of stool and urine

In infancy
Rubella, parvovirus B19, echovirus, and a variety of enterovirus
  subtypes
Bacterial cultures of blood and urine

Abbreviations: EBV, Epstein-Barr virus; HIV, human immunodeficiency virus;
PT, prothrombin time; PTT, partial thromboplastin time.

hemolytic disorder, such as glucose-6-phosphatase deficiency. In later life mild jaundice aggravated by fasting or intercurrent illness is the only symptom, and the condition is often discovered accidentally. Crigler–Najjar syndrome leads to severe nonhemolytic jaundice, severe neurologic damage, and death despite the use of phototherapy and plasmaphoresis. Kernicterus is a common sequel in survivors. Liver transplant has proven successful in a number of patients, and Crigler–Najjar syndrome is certainly an attractive candidate for gene therapy.

CHOLESTATIC LIVER DISEASE IN EARLY INFANCY

Cholestatic liver disease may aggravate or prolong physiologic neonatal jaundice. The jaundice becomes obviously pathologic when conjugated hyperbilirubinemia is recognized (conjugated bilirubin >15% of total). An important early sign is a change in the color of the urine from colorless or only faintly yellow to distinctly yellow or even brown. The significance of this finding is often missed as this color is similar to adult urine. Of course, by this time, the sclerae are yellow. With chronic direct hyperbilirubinemia, the skin becomes yellow and may have a greenish hue.

Transient conjugated hyperbilirubinemia can be observed in neonates, especially premature infants, after moderate perinatal asphyxia. It is associated with a high hematocrit and a tendency to hypoglycemia; it has an excellent prognosis.

(*text continues on page 196*)

Table 16.2. Differential diagnosis of metabolic disease involving the liver

Leading symptomatology	Age of presentation	Diseases to be considered	Characteristic findings
Cholestatic liver disease (Conjugated hyperbilirubinemia)	< 3 Months	α_1-Antitrypsin deficiency	$\Downarrow\alpha_1$-Globulin, $\Downarrow\alpha_1$-antitrypsin
		Cystic fibrosis	$\Uparrow$Sweat chloride
		Tyrosinemia type I	$\Uparrow$AFP
		Niemann–Pick type C	Foam cells in marrow
		Peroxisomal diseases	Encephalopathy
		Bile acid synthesis defects	Prominent malabsorption
		Progressive familial intrahepatic cholestasis (e.g., Byler disease)	Progressive cirrhosis
	> 3 Months	Rotor syndrome	Normal liver function
		Dubin–Johnson syndrome	Normal liver function
		Neonatal hemochromatosis	$\Uparrow\Uparrow\Uparrow$Ferritin, $\Uparrow\Uparrow\Uparrow\Uparrow$AFP
		Galactosemia	Cataracts, urinary reducing substance
Acute or subacute hepatocellular necrosis	< 3 Months	Tyrosinemia type I	$\Uparrow\Uparrow\Uparrow$AFP
		Urea cycle defects	$\Uparrow\Uparrow\Uparrow\Uparrow$Ammonia
		Respiratory chain defects	$\Uparrow\Uparrow\Uparrow$Lactate
		Long-chain fatty acid oxidation defects	$\Downarrow\Downarrow$Glucose, $\Downarrow$ketones, $\Uparrow$lactate, $\Uparrow$urate, $\Uparrow$CK, $\Uparrow$ammonia, (cardio-myopathy, myoglobinuria
		Niemann–Pick type A, B	Foam cells in marrow
		Phosphomannose isomerase deficiency (CDG Ib)	$\Downarrow\Downarrow$ Transferrin

continued

Table 16.2. *Continued.*

Leading symptomatology	Age of presentation	Diseases to be considered	Characteristic findings
Acute or subacute hepatocellular necrosis (*continued*)	3 Months–2 years	Fructose intolerance	⇓Glucose
		Tyrosinemia type I	⇑⇑⇑AFP
		Fatty acid oxidation defects	⇓⇓Glucose, ⇑uric acid, ⇑⇑CK, ⇓ketones, ⇑lactate, ⇑ammonia
	> 2 Years	Respiratory chain defects	⇑⇑Lactate
		Urea cycle defects	⇑⇑⇑Ammonia
		Wilson disease	Corneal ring, hemolysis, neurologic degeneration, renal tubular abnormalities
		α_1-Antitrypsin deficiency	⇓α_1-Globulin, ⇓α_1-antitrypsin
		Fatty acid oxidation defects	⇓⇓Glucose, ⇑uric acid, ⇑⇑CK, ⇓ketones, ⇑lactate, ⇑ammonia
Cirrhosis	< 1 Year	Glycogenosis type IV	Myopathy
		Galactosemia	Cataracts, urinary reducing substance
		Neonatal hemochromatosis	⇑⇑⇑iron, ⇑⇑⇑ferritin, ⇓AFP, ⇓transferrin
		Tyrosinemia type I	⇑AFP
	> 1 Year	α_1-Antitrypsin deficiency	⇓α_1-Globulin, ⇓α_1-antitrypsin
		Wilson disease	Corneal ring, hemolysis, neurologic degeneration, renal tubular abnormalities

Hepatomegaly			Splenomegaly
	< 3 Months	Lysosomal storage diseases, specifically Wolman disease	+Adrenal calcifications
		CDG type Ia	Lipodystrophy, inverted nipples
		Defects of gluconeogenesis	$\Downarrow$Glucose, $\Uparrow$lactate
		Mevalonic aciduria	Severe failure to thrive, splenomegaly, anemia
		Glycogen storage diseases	$\pm \Downarrow$Glucose, $\Uparrow$lactate, $\Uparrow$lipids, myopathy
		Defects of gluconeogenesis	$\Downarrow$Glucose, $\Uparrow$lactate
		Lysosomal storage diseases	Splenomegaly
		α_1-Antitrypsin deficiency	$\Downarrow\alpha_1$-Globulin, $\Downarrow\alpha_1$-antitrypsin
	3 Months —2 years		
	>2 Years	Hemochromatosis	Diabetes mellitus, hypogonadism
		Cystic fibrosis	Pulmonary involvement, malnutrition, $\Uparrow$sweat chloride
		Lysosomal storage diseases, specifically	Splenomegaly
		Niemann-Pick type B	+ Pulmonary infiltrates
		Cholesterol ester storage disease	+ Hypercholesterolemia

Known infectious diseases should have been ruled out by laboratory tests listed in Table 15.1 and extrahepatic biliary disease by imaging techniques.

Abbreviations: AFP, α-fetoprotein; CK, creatine kinase.

Table 16.3. Second-line investigations in suspected metabolic liver disease

Plasma/serum
Lactate, pyruvate, 3-hydroxybutyrate, acetoacetate
Free fatty acids
Cholesterol, triglycerides
Serum iron and ferritin
Amino acids
Free and total carnitine, acylcarnitine profile
α-Fetoprotein
α_1-Antitrypsin activity and Pi phenotyping
Transferrin isoelectric focusing (for CDG)
Lysosomal enzymes (see Chapter 29)

Urine
Amino acids
Ketones
Reducing substances/sugars (galactose, fructose)
Organic acids (especially orotic acid and succinylacetone)
Individual bile acids (bile acid synthesis defects)

Sweat chloride (cystic fibrosis)

Infancy
Galactose-1-phosphate uridyl transferase (galactosemia)
Chromosomes (especially when liver disease is accompanied by
    malformations suggesting trisomy 13 or 18)
Free T_4 and TSH (hypothyroidism)
Transferrin isoelectric focusing (CDG)
Very-long-chain fatty acids (peroxisomal disorders)

Abbreviations: CDG, congenital disorders of glycosylation; Pi, protease inhibitor; T_4, thyroxine; TSH, thyroid stimulating hormone.

Biliary Obstruction

Infants with cholestatic liver disease often appear well. Early differentiation between extrahepatic biliary atresia or a chole-dochal cyst and a "neonatal hepatitis syndrome" is crucial. Structural cholestasis can also be due to Alagille syndrome in which a dominantly inherited dysplasia of the pulmonary artery occurs with distinctive dysmorphic features and paucity of intrahepatic bile ducts, which result in cholestatic liver disease. Routine clinical chemical investigations seldom differentiate between biliary obstruction and neonatal hepatitis syndrome, although low albumin concentrations and decreased coagulation that is unresponsive to vitamin K point to a longer disease course, such as in prenatal infections or inherited disorders. The differentiation between biliary obstruction and neonatal hepatitis syndrome must be vigorously pursued by ultrasonographic and possibly radioisotopic studies as surgical correction of extrahepatic biliary atresia or a choledochal cyst must be performed before intrahepatic biliary disease begins.

α_1-Antitrypsin Deficiency

Prenatal and active infections must be sought as important causes of the neonatal hepatitis syndrome that results in cholestatic liver disease; this search must occur in parallel with an investigation for the major inherited metabolic disease that presents in this way, α_1-antitrypsin deficiency. Cholestatic liver disease occurs in 10% to 20% of infants with the Pi-ZZ α_1-antitrypsin phenotype, which in turn accounts for between 14% and 29% of the neonatal hepatitis syndrome once infectious and toxic causes have been excluded. Bleeding may occur as a result of deficiency of vitamin K. In the acute stages, liver biopsies of infants with α_1-antitrypsin deficiency may be indistinguishable from idiopathic neonatal hepatitis, except that giant cell transformation is rarely prominent in the former. In dysmorphic infants, very-long-chain fatty acids, as well as chromosomes, should be investigated as well as peroxisomal diseases; and trisomies 13 or 18 are also associated with the neonatal hepatitis syndrome. Cholestatic liver disease in infancy furthermore may be the initial presentation of cystic fibrosis, Niemann–Pick disease type C, or tyrosinemia type I in some patients.

Defects of Bile Acid Biosynthesis

Recently, researchers have described a newly discovered group of inherited metabolic diseases that are characterized by progressive familial intrahepatic cholestasis starting in infancy. These defects in bile acid biosynthesis involve four different enzyme defects for the process of modifying the steroid nucleus of bile acids. Malabsorption of fat-soluble vitamins is pronounced, which results in spontaneous bleeding and rickets. Although the level of alkaline phosphatase is often highly elevated, it is not diagnostic. Determination of total bile acids is not helpful. After exclusion of other diseases, patients with cholestatic liver disease in infancy should be investigated for defects of bile acid biosynthesis by determining individual bile acid metabolites by gas chromatography mass spectrometry (GC-MS) analysis of plasma, urine, or bile. More widespread availability of fast atom bombardment mass spectrometry for rapid analysis of urine samples may lead to a quicker recognition of these disorders in the future. After diagnosis, these disorders have a good clinical and biochemical response to supplementation with bile acids, such as cholic acid, in combination with chenodeoxycholic or ursodeoxycholic acids.

HEPATOCELLULAR NECROSIS IN EARLY INFANCY

The differential diagnosis in early infancy is wide, ranging from toxic or infectious causes to a number of inherited metabolic diseases (Table 16.2). Jaundice is usually present, but more important and characteristic features are elevated liver transaminases and markers of hepatic insufficiency, such as hypoglycemia, hyperammonemia, hypoalbuminemia, and a decrease of vitamin K–dependent and other liver-produced coagulation factors. Failure to thrive is generally present. Deranged liver function may result in spontaneous bleeding or neonatal ascites, indicating end-stage liver disease. Encephalopathy is not necessarily obvious, especially in neonates. Acute disease may progress rapidly to hepatic failure. In severely compromised infants, routine clinical chemical measurements do not help to differentiate acutely presenting inherited metabolic diseases from severe viral hepatitis or septicemia, although disproportionate hypoglycemia, lactic acidosis, and/or hyperammonemia all point to a primary metabolic disease. Furthermore, for septicemia to complicate and aggravate inherited metabolic diseases is common. Help in the differential diagnosis may come from judgment of liver size. Decompensated inherited metabolic diseases are often accompanied by significant hepatomegaly caused by edema, whereas rapid atrophy can develop in viral hepatitis.

Galactosemia

In babies with acute hepatocellular necrosis, rapid diagnosis of the inherited metabolic diseases listed in Table 16.2 is essential, as specific therapy, which must be initiated as soon as possible, is available for most of them. Testing of urine for sugar by using a glucose oxidase method (Clinistix, Tes-tape) detects only glucose, not galactose. This is a strong argument for the continued use of the older methods of screening urine for reducing substances as they also detect galactose (Benedict or Fehling test, Clinitest). Urinary excretion of galactose depends on the dietary intake; it is not detectable 24 to 48 hours after discontinuation of milk feedings. However, babies with severe liver disease from any cause may have impaired galactose metabolism and gross secondary galactosuria. Therefore, for any baby who has received milk and who has subsequently developed liver disease, the investigation should include determination of the enzymatic activity of galactose-1-phosphate uridyl transferase in erythrocytes regardless of the results of neonatal screening. Two to 3 days after discontinuing galactose intake, a baby with galactosemia begins to recover. Cataracts may already have developed; they slowly clear after removal of the toxic sugar.

Tyrosinemia Type I

Determination of amino acids in plasma and urine and analysis of organic acids in urine (particularly succinylacetone, dicarboxylic acids, and orotic acid) should elucidate the presence of urea cycle disorders, fatty acid oxidation defects, and hepatorenal tyrosinemia. Tyrosinemia type I usually presents with pronounced acute or subacute hepatocellular damage and only occasionally with cholestatic liver disease in infancy. Patients who have an acute onset of symptoms very quickly develop hepatic decompensation. They may have jaundice and ascites along with hepatomegaly. Gastrointestinal bleeding may occur. The mothers of several infants have noted a peculiar odor similar to that of sweet cabbage. Generalized renal tubular dysfunction occurs, leading to glucosuria, aminoaciduria, and hyperphosphaturia. Very low levels of phosphate in serum are common findings, as are hypoglycemia and hypokalemia. In some patients the diagnosis of tyrosinemia type I can be difficult, as increases of tyrosine and methionine occur in many forms of liver disease. Although high elevations of α-fetoprotein are very suggestive, they do not constitute proof as neonatal hemochromatosis also involves very high elevations of α-fetoprotein. These two conditions should be differentiated on the basis of gross elevations of iron and ferritin in the latter. The demonstration of succinylacetone in urine and the confirmation of the enzyme defect in fibroblasts or biopsied liver constitute diagnostic proof of tyrosinemia type I. Urinary elevations of succinylacetone may be small in young infants. Repeated analyses with special requests for specific determination by stable isotope dilution analysis may be warranted when clinical suspicion is strong.

Defects of Fatty Acid Oxidation and of Oxidative Phosphorylation

Genetic defects of fatty acid oxidation and of the respiratory electron transport chain have recently become recognized as causes of rapidly progressive hepatocellular necrosis in infancy. Defects of fatty acid oxidation are suggested in prolonged intermittent or subacute presentations with myopathy, cardiomyopathy, hypoketotic hypoglycemia, hyperuricemia, elevation of creatine kinase (CK), moderate lactic acidosis, and dicarboxylic aciduria (see also Chapter 6, "Approach to the Child Suspected of Having a Disorder of Fatty Acid Oxidation"). Defects of the respiratory chain causing hepatocellular necrosis are characterized by additional multiorgan involvement, especially of the bone marrow, pancreas, and brain, that varies; severe lactic acidosis; and ketosis (see also Chapter 6, "Work-up of the Patient with Lactic Acidemia"). During acute hepatocellular necrosis in infancy, these differentiating features may be masked by generalized metabolic derangement. Any baby with progressive hepatocellular necrosis should have repeated determinations of metabolites, such as lactate, pyruvate, 3-hydroxybutyrate, acetoacetate, free and total carnitine, and analysis of acylcarnitines, in addition to determinations of amino acids in the blood and organic acids in the urine. If the clinical and biochemical presentation suggests a defect of fatty acid oxidation or of the respiratory chain, appropriate enzymatic confirmation or molecular studies of nuclear or mitochondrial DNA should be sought (see also Chapter 6). If the results are negative, defects of fatty acid oxidation in patients who were initially thought to have a defect of the respiratory chain should be investigated and vice versa. Small infants with primary defects of fatty acid oxidation may present with overwhelming lactic acidosis, and infants with severe liver disease due to defects of the respiratory chain may present with hypoketotic hypoglycemia and dicarboxylic aciduria. The latter presentation is the rule, rather than the exception, for the recently recognized mitochondrial DNA depletion syndromes. When cardiomyopathy is present, lactic acidosis can also result from heart failure and poor perfusion.

Neonatal Hemochromatosis

Neonatal hemochromatosis should be considered in the differential diagnosis of rapidly progressive hepatocellular necrosis in infancy. As hepatic accumulation of iron occurs in a number of diseases of known origin, such as prenatal infection, tyrosinemia type I, congenital hepatic fibrosis, and Down syndrome, neonatal hemochromatosis is more likely to present as one of these disorders than as an individual disease. However, reports of approximately 100 infants who presented with liver disease from birth exist where no known cause could be defined, and extrahepatic siderosis and occurrence in siblings suggested a primary genetic disorder of fetoplacental iron handling. Diagnosis is by exclusion of other causes and demonstration of increased concentrations of serum iron, ferritin, and α-fetoprotein, as well as from decreased concentrations of transferrin. Complete or near complete saturation of iron-binding capacity is suggestive, and demonstration of extrahepatic siderosis appears to be especially characteristic. The latter can be assessed by salivary gland biopsy or with abdominal magnetic resonance imaging (MRI). Successful treatment depends on early recognition and successful management of hepatic failure, rapid referral to a transplant center, and early liver transplantation.

CHOLESTATIC LIVER DISEASE IN LATER INFANCY AND CHILDHOOD

Dubin–Johnson and Rotor Syndromes

After 3 months of age, the initial clinical and biochemical presentation usually allows a clearer suspicion and differentiation of inherited metabolic liver disease than in neonates. In patients with α_1-antitrypsin deficiency, cholestatic liver disease gradually subsides before 6 months of age. In later infancy, three distinct metabolic diseases present with cholestatic liver disease (Table 16.2). Dubin–Johnson and Rotor syndromes are both autosomal recessively inherited disorders characterized by isolated conjugated hyperbilirubinemia. Patients are usually asymptomatic except for the obvious jaundice. Bilirubin levels can range from 2 to 25 mg/dL (34 to 428 μmol/L). Both conditions are rare; they can be differentiated by differences in urinary porphyrins and by the appearance of the liver, which is deeply pigmented in Dubin–Johnson syndrome and unremarkable in Rotor syndrome. Excretion of conjugated bilirubin is impaired in both disorders; the genes that are involved have not yet been identified.

Progressive Familial Intrahepatic Cholestasis

Progressive familial intrahepatic cholestasis is a heterogeneous group of autosomal recessive liver disorders characterized by early onset of cholestasis that progresses to cirrhosis and liver failure before adulthood. Three types exist. One type appears to be caused by defects in bile acid synthesis and often presents early in infancy (see earlier). A second type, called *Byler disease*, results from defective bile salt secretion. Symptoms start later in infancy with attacks of jaundice, pruritus, and conjugated hyperbilirubinemia that are often provoked by intercurrent illnesses. Although patients initially recover completely between attacks, liver function slowly deteriorates and terminal liver failure usually occurs before 15 years of age. Liver transplantation has become the treatment of choice, but it may be complicated by severe encephalopathic reactions. Two loci for Byler disease have been identified, one on chromosome 18 (PFIC1) and one on chromosome 2 (PFIC2). Patients with bile acid synthesis defects and Byler disease have normal serum levels of γ-glutamyltransferase (GGT1).

High serum GGT activity and liver histology that shows portal inflammation and ductular proliferation in an early stage distinguish a third type of progressive familial intrahepatic cholestasis from those caused by defects of bile acid synthesis or secretion. The histologic and biochemical characteristics of this subtype resemble those of the mdr2 -/- knockout mice very closely. Lack of multidrug resistance gene 3 (MDR3) mRNA negative canalicular staining for MDR3 P-glycoprotein has been demonstrated in the liver of patients. One patient was found to be homozygous for a frameshift deletion; another was homozygous for a nonsense arg957-to-ter mutation. Interestingly, a heterozygous mother of an affected child experienced recurrent episodes of intrahepatic cholestasis during pregnancy.

HEPATOCELLULAR NECROSIS IN LATER INFANCY AND CHILDHOOD

Hepatocellular necrosis in later infancy or early childhood may present in a fashion similar to that in neonates with elevated transaminases, hypoglycemia, hyperammonemia, a decrease of coagulation factors, spontaneous bleeding, hypoalbuminemia, and ascites. Renal tubular dysfunction or rickets indicates an inherited metabolic disease. The association of acute hepatocellular necrosis with a prominent noninflammatory encephalopathy suggests a diagnosis of Reye syndrome; many patients with this syndrome are now found to have inherited metabolic disease.

The most common form of acute hepatocellular necrosis in older children is acute or decompensated chronic viral hepatitis. A small or rapidly decreasing liver size is a strong argument against an inherited metabolic disease. Autoimmune disease must also be taken into consideration. Autoantibodies are present in most affected children, and an increase in immunoglobulin G (IgG) always occurs.

Disorders of fatty acid oxidation and urea cycle defects should be high on the list of differential diagnosis of children presenting with acute hepatocellular necrosis. If disproportionate hyperammonemia or hypoketotic hypoglycemia has been observed, vigorous emergency measures should be initiated promptly and diagnostic confirmation should be sought by specialized metabolic investigations (see Chapter 6). Both are potentially lethal in the acute episode. Tyrosinemia type I and fructose intolerance are usually diagnosed in infancy or early childhood; urea cycle and, more especially, fatty acid oxidation defects continue to be important causes of acute hepatic dysfunction throughout life and may present at any age.

In later childhood Wilson disease and α_1-antitrypsin deficiency are important metabolic causes of severe hepatocellular necrosis.

Courses may be subacute or chronic, and initial presentation varies, ranging from isolated hepatomegaly, jaundice, or ascites to a chronic active hepatitis-like picture or acute liver failure. Hemolysis, when present, may be an important clue to Wilson disease.

Tyrosinemia Type I

If tyrosinemia type I does not become symptomatic until later in infancy, patients usually follow a less rapid course. Vomiting, anorexia, abdominal distension, failure to thrive, rickets, and easy bruising may be the presenting features. Hepatomegaly is also usually present. Although transaminases may be normal or only slightly elevated, prothrombin time and partial thromboplastin time are usually markedly elevated, as is α-fetoprotein, which may range from 100,000 to 400,000 ng/mL. Individual patients may present with different clinical pictures, such as with acute liver disease and hypoglycemia as a Reyelike syndrome. They may also present with isolated bleeding and may undergo an initial investigation for coagulation disorders before the hepatic disease is identified.

Renal tubular disease in tyrosinemia type I is that of a renal Fanconi syndrome with phosphaturia, glucosuria, and aminoaciduria. Proteinuria and excessive carnitine loss may also occur. Renal tubular loss of bicarbonate leads to systemic metabolic acidosis. Affected infants have been observed to develop vitamin D–resistant rickets at less than 4 months of age.

Beyond infancy, neurologic crises very similar to those of acute intermittent porphyria are a more common cause of admission to hospital than is hepatic decompensation. Succinylacetone inhibits porphobilinogen deaminase (the enzyme affected in acute intermittent porphyria); increased urinary excretion of δ-aminolevulinate and porphobilinogen occurs during neurologic crises in tyrosinemia type I. About half of the affected patients experience such crises, starting with pains in the lower extremities, followed by abdominal pains, muscular weakness, or paresis and paresthesias. Head and trunk may be positioned in extreme hyperextension, suggesting opisthotonus or meningismus. Systemic signs include hypertension, tachycardia, and ileus. Symptoms can continue for up to a week, and they slowly resolve. These episodes should be much less frequent now that therapy is available for this disorder. Intellectual function is usually not affected in tyrosinemia type I.

Until recently, most children with tyrosinemia type I died during their early years—most before 1 year of age. Chronic liver disease is that of macronodular cirrhosis. Splenomegaly and esophageal varices that develop are complicated by bleeding. A common complication is hepatocellular carcinoma, which may first be suspected because of a further rise in the level of α-fetoprotein. Liver or combined liver–kidney transplantation was the only promising option of treatment until the advent of 2(2-nitro-4-trifluoro-methyl-benzoyl)-1,3-cyclohexanedione (NTBC). This drug is a potent inhibitor of p-hydroxyphenylpyruvate dioxygenase, which thus prevents the formation of the highly toxic fumarylacetoacetate, and its products succinylacetoacetate and succinylacetone. If treatment is instituted early, hepatic and renal function slowly improve to normal; and neurologic crises are prevented. Concentrations of succinylacetone, α-fetoprotein, and δ-aminolevulinate gradually decrease to near normal values.

The differential diagnosis of the patient with elevated levels of tyrosine in the blood includes tyrosinemias type II and III and transient neonatal tyrosinemia. p-Hydroxyphenylpyruvate dioxygenase is the enzyme defect responsible for tyrosinemia type III. Tyrosinemia type II is caused by deficiency of the enzyme, tyrosine aminotransferase. Tyrosinemia type II, known as the Richner-Hanhart syndrome, results in oculocutaneous lesions, including corneal erosion, opacity, and plaques. Pruritic or hyperkeratotic lesions may develop on the palms and soles. About half of the patients described in the literature have been characterized as having low-normal to subnormal levels of intelligence, but this may reflect the investigator's bias.

The phenotype of tyrosinemia type III is similar. It may include oculocutaneous lesions and neurologic manifestations, such as psychomotor retardation and ataxia. As treatment with NTBC in patients with tyrosinemia type I shifts the metabolic block from fumarylacetoacetate hydrolase to p-hydroxyphenylpyruvate dioxygenase (i.e., from tyrosinemia type I to tyrosinemia type III), treatment with NTBC must be supplemented by dietary treatment with a phenylalanine-reduced and tyrosine-reduced diet, which constitutes the rational approach to treatment in tyrosinemias types II and III.

Metabolic investigations or neonatal screening, particularly in premature infants, sometimes detects tyrosinemia and hyperphenylalaninemia not due to a defined inherited metabolic disease. The protein intake is often excessive, especially when an evaporated milk formula is being used. This form of tyrosinemia is thought to result from physiologic immaturity of p-hydroxyphenylpyruvate dioxygenase; it is a warning that protein intake should be moderate during the first weeks of life. Maternal vitamin C deficiency may play a role. This condition is sometimes associated with prolonged jaundice and feeding problems, and can cause diagnostic confusion. If the clinician is in doubt, molecular analysis of the phenylalanine hydroxylase gene should be performed.

Hereditary Fructose Intolerance

Symptoms develop in hereditary fructose intolerance with the introduction of fructose or sucrose into the diet. The recessively inherited deficiency of fructose-1-phosphate aldolase results in an inability to split fructose-1-phosphate into glyceraldehyde and dihydroxyacetone phosphate. Fructose-1-phosphate accumulates in the liver, kidney, and intestine. Pathophysiologic consequences are hepatocellular necrosis and renal tubular dysfunction, very similar to what occurs in galactosemia. An acute depletion of adenosine 5'-triphosphate (ATP) is caused by the sequestration of phosphate and the direct toxic effects of fructose-1-phosphate.

Depending on the amount of fructose or sucrose ingested, infants may present with isolated asymptomatic jaundice or with rapidly progressive liver failure, jaundice, bleeding tendency, and ascites, suggesting septicemia or fulminant viral hepatitis. Hepatosplenomegaly, if present, argues against the latter diagnosis. Postprandial hypoglycemia develops in 30% to 50% of patients affected with fructose intolerance; it may progress to coma and sudden death. Most patients present subacutely with vomiting, poor feeding, and diarrhea or sometimes with failure to thrive. Pyloric stenosis and gastroesophageal reflux are common initial diagnoses. The clinical picture may be more blurred in later life, and laboratory findings may be unrevealing. Hereditary fructose intolerance deserves consideration as a cause of renal calculi, polyuria, and periodic or progressive weakness or even paralysis. A major clue to diagnosis may be an accurate dietary history that reveals an aversion to fruits and sweets.

Characteristic clinical chemical laboratory features include elevated transaminases, hyperbilirubinemia, hypoalbuminemia, hypocholesterolemia, and a decrease of vitamin K–dependent, liver-produced coagulation factors. An occasional pattern of consumption coagulopathy is seen. In addition, patients may have hypoglycemia, hypophosphatemia, hypomagnesemia, hyperuricemia, and metabolic acidosis in a renal Fanconi syndrome with proteinuria, glucosuria, aminoaciduria, and loss of bicarbonate. A high urine pH despite acidosis may also be seen. In these circumstances fructose in the urine is virtually diagnostic of the disease; however, it may be absent. Elevated plasma levels of tyrosine and methionine, when combined with markedly elevated excretion of tyrosine and its metabolites in urine, may misleadingly suggest a diagnosis of tyrosinosis type I.

The prognosis in hereditary fructose intolerance depends entirely upon the elimination of fructose from the diet. After withdrawing fructose and sucrose, clinical symptoms and laboratory findings quickly reverse. Vomiting disappears immediately, and the bleeding tendency ends within 24 hours. Most clinical and laboratory findings become normal within 2 to 3 weeks, but hepatomegaly may take longer to resolve.

The excellent response to treatment supports a presumptive diagnosis of fructose intolerance. Confirmation of diagnosis should first be attempted by molecular analysis. Several frequent mutations, such as A149P in Caucasians, are known. If the diagnosis remains uncertain, a fructose tolerance test (see Chapter 11) should be performed after the end of clinical symptoms and after ingestion of a diet that has been fructose-free for several weeks. Demonstrating the enzyme defect in liver tissue is necessary only in exceptional constellations.

Wilson Disease

In Wilson disease, or hepatolenticular degeneration, copper accumulates in various organs; and serum levels of ceruloplasmin are low. Clinical manifestations vary greatly, but hepatic disease occurs in approximately 80% of individuals who are affected. This usually manifests at school age and rarely before the age of 4 years. If left untreated, about half of the patients with hepatic disease develop neurologic symptoms in adolescence or adulthood. Neurologic manifestations are the presenting symptoms in other patients with Wilson disease.

One extreme of the clinical spectrum of Wilson disease is a rapid, fulminant course in children past the age of 5 years that progresses within weeks to hepatic insufficiency that is manifested by icterus, ascites, clotting abnormalities, and disseminated intravascular coagulation. This is followed by renal insufficiency, coma, and death, sometimes without diagnosis. The liver disease associated with intravascular hemolysis and renal failure is highly suggestive of Wilson disease.

Wilson disease can also present with a picture of acute hepatitis. Nausea, vomiting, anorexia, and jaundice are common presenting complaints, and the episode may subside spontaneously. In the presence of splenomegaly, the diagnosis may appear to be infectious mononucleosis. Recurrent bouts of hepatitis and a picture of chronic active hepatitis in children more than 6 years of age suggest Wilson disease. These patients experience anorexia and fatigue. Hepatosplenomegaly is prominent. In some patients, isolated hepatosplenomegaly may be discovered accidentally. Any hepatic presentation of Wilson disease leads to cirrhosis; the disease may also present as cirrhosis. The histologic picture is indistinguishable from chronic active hepatitis. Hepatic coma or a hepatorenal syndrome may occur in the terminal stage.

In adolescents and adults, the onset of Wilson disease is classically neurologic, predominantly with extrapyramidal signs. Choreoathetoid movements and dystonia reflect lenticular degeneration and are frequently associated with hepatic disease. This condition has a poor prognosis. Progression tends to be much slower in patients presenting with parkinsonian and pseudosclerotic symptoms, such as drooling, rigidity of the face, and tremor. Speech or behavior disorders, and sometimes frank psychiatric presentations, can occur even in children. The lack of overt liver disease can make diagnosis difficult. Ultimately, dementia develops in untreated patients.

Hemolytic anemia may be a prominent feature of Wilson disease in children, and its presence is very suggestive of the diagnosis. Renal tubular disease is subtle; a generalized aminoaciduria often displays an unusually high excretion of cystine, other sulfur-containing amino acids, and tyrosine. Later, a full-blown Fanconi syndrome may occur, and patients may develop renal stones or diffuse nephrocalcinosis.

The availability of effective treatment for Wilson disease with copper-chelating agents makes early diagnosis crucial. A key finding is the demonstration of Keyser–Fleischer rings as gray-to-green to red-gold pigmented rings around the outer margin of the cornea. Slit lamp examination may be required. The rings are hardest to see in green-brown eyes. They are pathognomonic in neurologic disease, but they take time to develop. They may be absent in about one-third of children who present with hepatic disease.

Biochemical diagnosis of Wilson disease may be difficult. The diagnosis is usually made on the basis of an abnormally low serum ceruloplasmin. In most patients, it is below 10 mg/dL (100 mg/L) (control children display levels of 25 to 45 mg/dL). However, some patients have intermediate and even normal values. Levels of copper in the serum are usually elevated, but measurement of urine copper is more reliable. Urinary excretion of copper increases to more than 100 µg/day (1.6 µmol/day) (control children excrete < 30 µg/day [0.5 µmol/day]). Further increase in urinary copper excretion can be provoked by loading the patient with 10 mg/kg of D-penicillamine. After loading, controls excrete less than 600 µg (9.4 µmol)/ day, whereas in Wilson disease excretion ranges from 1,500 µg (23.6 µmol) to 3,000 µg (47 µmol)/day. The most sensitive test is the measurement of the copper concentration in the liver, so this test may be required for diagnosis. Disposable steel needles or Menghini needles should be used. They are washed with ethylene diamine tetraacetate (EDTA) and are rinsed with demineralized water. Glucose (5%) in water (not saline) is used as the propellant solution. Patients with Wilson disease usually have highly elevated concentrations of copper in the liver (100 to 2,000 µg [1.6 to 31.4 µmol] of copper per gram of dry weight; controls show < 50 µg [0.8 µmol]). Elevated concentrations of copper in the liver may also be found in children with extrahepatic biliary obstruction or cholestatic liver disease.

Primary molecular diagnosis of Wilson disease is not yet clinically available, but mutations of the gene have been found.

Once the diagnosis of Wilson disease is established, all family members (particularly siblings) should be thoroughly investigated. Examination of liver tissue will be necessary in the unusual case of an asymptomatic sibling who has a low ceruloplasmin level, which can be consistent with heterozygosity, as well as with homozygosity. Early diagnosis must be vigorously pursued, as the best prognosis is found with early treatment of asymptomatic patients.

CIRRHOSIS

Cirrhosis is the end stage of chronic hepatocellular disease. The list of diseases that can result in cirrhosis and failure of the liver is extensive; it includes infectious, inflammatory, and vascular diseases; biliary malformations; and toxic and metabolic disorders. Cirrhosis can result from most of the diseases discussed in this chapter. Exceptions are primary defects of bilirubin conjugation or excretion and some of the storage disorders that lead to hepatomegaly.

Glycogenosis type IV, a branching enzyme deficiency, causes primarily cirrhotic destruction of the liver. In Wilson disease and, even more frequently, in α_1-antitrypsin deficiency, a cirrhotic process may be quiescent for a long period with no evidence of liver disease. Patients may be recognized following family investigations or while investigating an unrelated disease, or the disease may remain unrecognized until decompensation leads to full-blown liver failure. Table 16.2 lists specific metabolic diseases leading to cirrhosis.

As cirrhosis progresses, signs and symptoms of decompensation eventually emerge. Regardless of the primary disease, patients develop weight loss, failure to thrive, muscle weakness, fatigue, steatorrhea, ascites, or anasarca, as well as chronic jaundice, digital clubbing, spider angiomatoma, and epistaxis or other bleeding (Table 16.4). Complications of cirrhosis include portal hypertension, bleeding varices, and splenomegaly. In a terminal condition, hepatic coma may occur. Liver transplantation provides the only realistic therapy.

Glycogenosis Type IV

Infants with this rare form of glycogen storage disease present around their first birthday with hepatic cirrhosis, an enlarged nodular liver, and splenomegaly. Hypotonia and muscular atrophy are usually present; they may be severe. Treatment is either symptomatic and palliative, or it involves transplantation of the liver; untransplanted patients usually succumb to complications of cirrhosis before the age of 3 years. Cardiomyopathy may be present.

The disorder is due to a deficiency of the brancher enzyme α-1, 4-glucan:α-1,4-glucan-6-glucosyl transferase, which leads to a decrease in the number of branch points, producing a straight chain of insoluble glycogen-like starch or amylopectin. The content of glycogen in liver is not elevated, but the abnormal structure appears to act like a foreign body and causes cirrhosis. The diagnosis can be established by enzyme assay of leukocytes, cultured fibroblasts, or liver cells.

α_1-Antitrypsin Deficiency

α_1-Antitrypsin deficiency is an important cause of neonatal cholestasis, as well as of chronic active hepatitis (see above). In patients with α_1-antitrypsin deficiency manifesting as cholestatic liver disease in infancy, cholestasis gradually subsides before 6 months of age, and patients become clinically unremarkable. However, 20% to 40% of these children go on to develop hepatic

Table 16.4. Signs and symptoms of hepatic cirrhosis

General	Malnutrition, failure to thrive, muscle wasting, hypogonadism, elevated temperature, increased infections
CNS	Lethargy progressing to coma, behavioral changes, depression, intellectual deterioration, pyramidal tract signs, asterixis
Gastrointestinal tract	Nausea and vomiting, splenomegaly, caput medusa, hemorrhoids, epistaxis hematemesis, abdominal distension, ascites
Kidney	Fluid and electrolyte imbalance, progressive renal insufficiency
Skin	Jaundice, flushing, palmar erythema, spider angiomatoma, digital clubbing

Abbreviation: CNS, central nervous system.

cirrhosis in childhood. As high as 50% of apparently healthy children with the homozygous Pi-ZZ phenotype have subclinical liver disease, as indicated by elevated levels of aminotransferases and γ-glutamyltranspeptidase. Some patients with α_1-antitrypsin deficiency with no history of neonatal cholestasis develop cirrhosis eventually and may present with unexplained liver failure. These patients have possessed the Pi-types ZZ, MZ, and S. In addition, hepatomas and hepatocellular carcinomas have been described with the ZZ and MZ phenotypes. In the presence or absence of a history of neonatal cholestasis or hepatitis, α_1-antitrypsin should be quantified in any child, adolescent, or adult with unexplained cirrhosis (in fact, with every unexplained liver disease). The Pi Z mutation results from a glutamine to lysine exchange at position 342 that alters the charge and tertiary structure of the molecule. The frequency of this particular allele is very high in Caucasians. In Sweden, 5% of the population consists of MZ heterozygotes; in the United States, the proportion is 2%. The frequency of the homozygous Pi-ZZ phenotype is one in 1,600 in Sweden and one in 6,000 in the United States. Normal serum levels of α_1-antitrypsin are from 20 to 50 μmol/L, and in the ZZ phenotype, they fall between 3 to 6 μmol/L. Patients with values below 20 μmol/L should have Pi phenotyping performed.

A major proportion of patients with α_1-antitrypsin deficiency remain free of liver disease throughout life. In adulthood 80% to 90% of patients with the Pi-ZZ phenotype develop destructive pulmonary emphysema. α_1-Antitrypsin protects the lung, because it is an effective inhibitor of elastase and other proteolytic enzymes that are released from neutrophils and macrophages during inflammatory processes. Emphysema results from the imbalance between protease and antiprotease activity in the lung. Children with the rare Pi null variant may have severe emphysema early in life. Intravenous infusions of α_1-antitrypsin have been shown to impede the development of emphysema in affected individuals.

HEPATOMEGALY

Hepatomegaly is often the first clinical sign of liver disease. Two clinical aspects are helpful in the diagnostic evaluation of the patient: (a) the presence or absence of splenomegaly and (b) the consistency and structure of the enlarged liver.

Splenomegaly is the hallmark of storage diseases and is much more prominent than in portal hypertension, infections, or autoimmune disorders. Functional impairment of the liver, such as decreases of coagulation factors and serum albumin or impaired glucose homeostasis, is usually absent in classical lysosomal storage diseases, and aspects of liver cell integrity are unremarkable. Exceptions are Niemann–Pick diseases, both types A and C (Table 16.2). In lysosomal storage diseases, the liver and spleen are firm, but not hard, on palpation. The surfaces are smooth, and the edges are easily palpated. The liver is not tender. A presumptive diagnosis of lysosomal storage disease is strengthened by the involvement of the nervous system and/or mesenchymal structures, resulting in coarsening of the facial appearance and in skeletal abnormalities. In addition, a gradual progression is evident. Chapter 29 details the logistics of the diagnostic work-up of a patient suspected of a lysosomal storage disease.

Any acutely developing liver disease that results from infection, inflammation, or toxic or metabolic processes may cause hepatomegaly as a result of edema and/or inflammation. In these disorders, other manifestations of the disease have usually led to the consultation, and the ensuing physical examination reveals hepatomegaly. On palpation, the liver may feel firm but not hard, and the surface is smooth. The liver may be tender. Clinical or routine chemical studies are likely to reveal abnormalities that direct further diagnostic evaluation. Inherited metabolic diseases in this category have been discussed under acute or subacute hepatocellular necrosis (Table 16.2).

If the enlarged liver feels hard, is not tender, and has sharp or even irregular edges, a detailed evaluation of the causes of cirrhosis should be performed, even if liver function tests are unremarkable. A hard, irregular, or nodular surface is virtually pathognomonic of cirrhosis. Metabolic causes of silent liver disease associated with hepatomegaly that may lead to quiescent cirrhosis are Wilson disease and α_1-antitrypsin deficiency. Another important metabolic disorder is hemochromatosis, in which hepatomegaly may be the only manifestation in adolescence and young adulthood. Although this disease usually does not progress to hepatic failure as does Wilson disease, early recognition and initiation of treatment allow the prevention of irreversible sequelae.

In patients with persistent isolated hepatomegaly, additional findings (Table 16.5) are helpful for the differential diagnosis; they should be specifically sought. Defects of gluconeogenesis result in severe recurrent fasting hypoglycemia and lactic acidosis (see Table 11.5). Of the three enzymatic defects of gluconeogenesis, hepatomegaly is a consistent finding in fructose-1,6-diphosphatase deficiency, whereas patients with deficiency of pyruvate carboxylase or phosphoenolpyruvate carboxykinase usually present with lactic acidemia and multisystem disease without hepatomegaly.

Confronted with an infant or young child with a moderately enlarged smooth, soft liver and an otherwise completely unremarkable history and physical examination, investigations may be postponed until confirmation of persistence of hepatomegaly on repeat clinical examinations a few weeks later. If unexplained hepatomegaly persists or if additional indications of liver disease develop, a liver biopsy should be obtained for histologic and electron microscopic investigation. Additional tissue should be frozen at −80°C for biochemical analyses. Patients with hepatomegalic glycogenoses may present with a moderately enlarged smooth, soft liver and an otherwise completely unremarkable history and physical examination in infancy and early childhood. Similarly, patients with hemochromatosis may present with hepatomegaly without other symptoms in late childhood and adolescence.

**Table 16.5.   Differential diagnosis
of metabolic causes of hepatomegaly**

Additional findings	Suggestive disorder
Cardiomyopathy	Glycogenosis III, hemochromatosis, phosphoenolpyruvate carboxykinase deficiency, disorders of fatty acid oxidation or of oxidative phosphory-lation
Muscular weakness	Glycogenoses III and IV, fructose intolerance, disorders of fatty acid oxidation or of oxidative phosphorylation
Enlarged kidneys	Glycogenosis I, Fanconi-Bickel syndrome
Renal Fanconi syndrome	Glycogenoses I and III, Wilson disease, fructose intolerance, tyrosinemia type I, Fanconi-Bickel syndrome, mitochondrial ox-phos defects
Hemolytic anemia	Wilson disease, fructose intolerance
Fasting intolerance, hypoglycemia	Glycogenoses I and III, fructose-1, 6-diphosphatase deficiency, disor-ders of fatty acid oxidation or of oxidative phosphorylation
Diabetes mellitus, hypogonadism	Hemochromatosis
Neurologic deterioration (Kayser-Fleischer rings)	Wilson disease
Early onset emphysema	α_1-Antitrypsin deficiency
Susceptibility to infections	Glycogenoses IB and IC
Malnutrition	Cystic fibrosis
Lipodystrophy, inverted nipples	CDG type Ia

Abbreviations: CDG, congenital disorders of glycosylation; Ox-phos, oxida-tive phosphorylation.

The Glycogenoses

Several glycogen storage diseases involve isolated hepatomegaly. The frequency of glycogenoses varies considerably according to the ethnic background; it is from one in 20,000 to one in 25,000 in Europe. Von Gierke first described the condition in 1929. Cori and Cori established glycogenosis I as the first inborn error to be defined enzymatically. The current classification of the glyco-genoses has been extended to eight entities. Glycogenosis type 0, also referred to as *aglycogenosis* (both misnomers), is the defi-ciency of glycogen synthase. As the glycogen content in the liver is actually reduced, it is not a storage disorder, but rather, a disorder of gluconeogenesis (see Chapter 6, "Work-up of the Patient with Hypoglycemia"). The symptoms of glycogenoses types II, V, and VII are primarily those of muscle disease.

Advances in techniques of enzymatic and molecular diagnosis may provide definitive diagnosis without requiring a liver biopsy. However, quantitative determination of the glycogen content of the liver is still necessary in the work-up of many patients with suspected glycogen storage disease. Glucagon challenges may help in differentiating between glycogenoses I and III (see Chapter 11, "Monitored Prolonged Fast" and "Glucagon Stimulation").

Glycogen Storage Disease Type I

Glycogen storage disease (GSD) type I results from a deficiency of any of the proteins of the microsomal membrane–bound glucose-6-phosphatase complex. In classic Ia glycogen storage disease (von Gierke disease), glucose-6-phosphatase is deficient. Type Ib is due to defective microsomal transport of glucose-6-phosphate; Ic, to defective transport of phosphate; and Id, to defective transport of glucose. Molecular studies contradict the classification of types Ib and Ic as separate entities. They are both caused by mutations in the glucose-6-phosphate translocase and now are taken together as glycogen storage disease type I non-a. A variant of type Ia results from a deficiency of the regulatory protein. So far, researchers have classified only one patient with this variant.

Type I is the most serious of all hepatic glycogenoses because it leads to a complete blockage of glucose release from liver, so glucose production from glycogen or gluconeogenesis is impaired. The hallmark of the disease is severe fasting hypoglycemia with concomitant lactic acidosis, elevation of free fatty acids, hyperlipemia, elevated transaminases, hyperuricemia, and metabolic acidosis. Lactic acidosis may be further aggravated by ingestion of fructose and galactose as the metabolic block in the liver again traps the converted glucose. Affected patients may be symptomatic in the neonatal period and may have hepatomegaly, hypoglycemic convulsions, and ketonuria. However, the condition often remains undiagnosed until hypoglycemic symptoms reappear in the course of intercurrent illnesses or when the infant begins to sleep longer at night at 3 to 6 months of age. Infants are chubby, and their linear growth usually lags. The liver grows slowly. An immense liver that extends down to the iliac crest is generally found by the end of the first year when the serum triglycerides reach very high levels. Because of the accumulation of lipids, the liver is usually soft and the edges may be difficult to palpate. With increasing activity of the child at around the first birthday, the frequency of manifestation of hypoglycemic symptoms tends to increase. As with any of the diseases that cause severe hypoglycemia, convulsions, permanent brain injury, or even death may occur. However, many children adapt to low glucose levels; and in the untreated state, the brain may be fueled by ketone bodies and lactate. Increased bleeding tendency may result in severe epistaxis and multiple hematomas, and abnormal hemostasis and persistent oozing may complicate traumatic injuries or surgery.

Patients with glycogen storage disease type I non-a (types Ib and Ic) develop progressive neutropenia and impaired neutrophil functions during the first year of life. As a result, they have recurrent bacterial infections, including deep infections and abscesses, ulcerations of oral and intestinal mucosa, and diarrhea. In the second or third decade, they may develop inflammatory bowel disease.

If glycogen storage disease type I is suspected, liver biopsy will provide the diagnosis. Hepatocytes are usually swollen because of extensive storage of glycogen and lipids. The structure of the stored glycogen is normal. Enough liver must be obtained to allow assay of glucose-6-phosphatase and, if necessary, of associated transport proteins. Primary molecular diagnosis of glycogen storage disease type Ia and I non-a is increasingly available. This is helpful because it obviates the need for liver biopsy.

A number of late complications have been observed in patients with type I glycogen storage diseases. Most patients have osteoporosis, and some have spontaneous fractures. Hyperuricemia may result in symptomatic gout after adolescence. Xanthomas may develop. Pancreatitis is another consequence of hypertriglyceridemia. Multiple hepatic adenomas develop, sometimes to sizable tumors. They are usually benign; however, malignant transformation has occurred. Renal complications include a Fanconi syndrome, hypercalciuria, nephrocalcinosis, and calculi. Over time, microalbuminuria may be followed by proteinuria, focal segmental glomerulosclerosis, interstitial fibrosis, and renal failure. Pulmonary hypertension is a rare but very serious complication in adult patients.

Glycogen Storage Disease Type III

Glycogen storage disease type III results from a deficiency of the debranching enzyme, amylo-1,6-glucosidase. The physical and metabolic manifestations of liver disease are usually less severe than those in type I glycogenosis, and fasting intolerance gradually diminishes over the years. The predominant long-term morbidity of this disease is myopathy. In infancy, distinguishing type I from type III on clinical grounds may be impossible. Hypoglycemia and convulsions with fasting, cushinoid appearance, short stature, and nosebleeds characterize both diseases. However, in contrast to type I glycogenosis, concentrations of uric acid and lactate are usually normal. The transaminases and creatine phosphokinase are elevated. This may be the earliest evidence of myopathy.

In glycogen storage disease type III, glycogen accumulates in muscle, as well as in liver. With time the major problem is a slowly progressive, distal myopathy that is characterized by hypotonia, weakness, and muscle atrophy. It is often notable in the interossei and over the thumb. Some patients have muscle fasciculations that are suggestive of motor neuron disease, and storage has been documented in peripheral nerves. Weakness generally is slowly progressive. Ultimately, the patient may be confined to a wheel chair. Rarely, the myocardium may also be involved with left ventricular hypertrophy or even clinical cardiomyopathy.

The liver and muscle of approximately 85% of patients are affected; this is referred to as glycogenosis type IIIa. When the deficiency is only found in the liver, the disorder is referred to as IIIb.

A number of functional tests have been designed to differentiate glycogen storage disease type I from type III. Following a glucose load, the blood lactate, which is initially elevated, will decrease in glycogenosis type I. In type III lactate levels are usually normal. In type I, gluconeogenesis is blocked and the alanine concentration is increased. In type III gluconeogenesis is overactive, resulting in significantly lowered concentrations of alanine. One of the most useful tests is a glucagon challenge 2 to 3 hours after a meal; this yields a good response in GSD type III (no increase in glucose occurs in GSD type I). After a 14-hour fast, glucagon usually does not provoke a rise in blood glucose in GSD type III because all the terminal glycogen branches have been catabolized (see Chapter 11, "Monitored Prolonged Fast" and "Glucagon Stimulation"). Finally, the diagnosis of glycogenosis type III can be proven by demonstrating the deficiency of the debranching enzyme amylo-1, 6-glucosidase in leukocytes, fibroblasts, liver, or muscle. Prenatal diagnosis is possible through enzyme analysis in amniocytes or chorionic villi.

Glycogen Storage Disease Type VI

Defects of the phosphorylase system are sometimes listed as two, or even three, separate groups of glycogen storage diseases. When sorted this way, category type VI is restricted to rare primary defects of hepatic phosphorylase; type VIII, to impaired control of phosphorylase activation; and type IX, to deficient activity of the phosphorylase kinase complex. Deficiencies of the phosphorylase kinase complex can be divided even further into five different subtypes of tissue-specific deficiencies that involve four different subunits. By far, the most common of these defects is an X-linked recessive defect of phosphorylase kinase, which affects approximately 75% of all patients with defects of the phosphorylase system.

The clinical symptoms of type VI glycogenosis are similar to, but milder than, those in types III or I. Hepatomegaly is a prominent finding that may be the only indication of a glycogen storage disease. Muscle hypotonia, tendency to fasting hypoglycemia, elevation of transaminases, and hypercholesterolemia are mild; they may be normal after childhood.

Following a glucose or galactose load in glycogenosis type VI, the blood lactate will show a pathologic increase from normal or only moderately elevated levels. Overactive gluconeogenesis results in lowered concentrations of plasma alanine. In glycogenosis type VI, the response to the administration of glucagon even after a 12- to 14-hour fast is usually normal. Demonstrated enzyme deficiency in the affected tissue, liver, or muscle provides the diagnosis of glycogenosis type Vl. Primary molecular diagnosis is possible for the common X-linked inherited defect of phosphorylase kinase.

Fanconi–Bickel Syndrome

The rare hepatic glycogenosis with renal Fanconi syndrome (Fanconi–Bickel syndrome) has been recently shown to be due to a primary defect of the liver-type facilitated glucose transporter 2. Hepatomegaly and glycogen storage, intolerance to galactose, failure to thrive, and consequences of full-blown Fanconi syndrome are usually obvious in early childhood.

Hemochromatosis

Hepatomegaly is the most frequent early manifestation of hemochromatosis. In most patients, it develops in late childhood or adolescence. Other symptoms that may appear in adolescence include diabetes insipidus, hypogonadism, skin pigmentation, recurrent epigastric pain, cardiac arrhythmias, and congestive heart failure. Recessively inherited hemochromatosis is one of the most common genetic disorders in Caucasians. Prevalence rates are between two and five persons in 1,000.

Hemochromatosis is usually considered an adult disorder; however, early manifestations are increasingly recognizable in adolescents and children. The value of early diagnosis cannot be overemphasized because optimal outcome can be achieved through treatment of presymptomatic or oligosymptomatic patients before the onset of irreversible damage. Laboratory investigations of symptomatic patients reveal increased concentrations of iron and ferritin in the serum, as well as an increased saturation of transferrin that is between 77% to 100%. Determination of the iron content of the liver provides the diagnosis of hemochromatosis. Molecular methods are now available as only two major mutations account for nearly all mutant alleles.

ADDITIONAL READING

Green A, ed. The liver and inherited diseases. *J Inher Metab Dis* 1994;14(Suppl 1).

Suchy FJ, ed. *Liver disease in children.* St. Louis: Mosby-Year Book; 1994.

17 ❧ Approach to the Patient with Gastrointestinal and General Abdominal Symptoms

Gastrointestinal manifestations of metabolic disorders include vomiting, diffuse abdominal pain, pancreatitis, slowed transit time and constipation, maldigestion and malabsorption (which may result in diarrhea), and ascites. These symptoms may occur as part of a systemic disorder of intermediary metabolism in which other symptoms predominate, or they may be the major or exclusive symptoms. Vomiting is typical of the organic acidurias and hyperammonemic syndromes. Pain and constipation occur in the porphyrias and familial fevers. Pancreatitis occurs with many organic acidurias, lipid and fatty acid disorders, and defects of oxidative phosphorylation. Malabsorption and diarrhea can be due to disorders of digestive enzymes, especially disaccharidases, defects of carrier proteins, and mitochondrial dysfunction. Ascites occurs in many lysosomal disorders.

VOMITING

Vomiting is a characteristic feature of many disorders of intermediary metabolism, including those characterized by acidosis (the organic acidurias), hyperammonemia due to disorders of the urea cycle, and fatty acid oxidation defects (Table 17.1). Initial laboratory investigations for vomiting, including acid–base balance, lactate, ammonia, and urinary organic acids, can point the way to a diagnosis.

Chronic or recurrent vomiting in infancy, leading to formula changes before the underlying acidosis is discovered, is a common feature in the organic acidurias due to defects in the metabolism of branched-chain amino acids, such as propionic, methylmalonic, and isovaleric acidurias (see also Chapter 26). The hyperammonemia of disorders of the urea cycle often provokes vomiting. In severe cases, this is rapidly followed by deterioration of the level of consciousness; in milder cases, the vomiting can be intermittent. Hyperammonemia can also be prominent in the fatty acid oxidation disorders, especially medium-chain acyl-CoA dehydrogenase (MCAD) deficiency. Symptoms in these disorders occur intermittently and result from fasting or intercurrent infections. Chapter 6 discusses the appropriate investigations in more detail ("Work-up of the Patient with Hypoglycemia").

Vomiting leads to alkalosis, so the discovery of acidosis when investigating a vomiting infant or child should immediately raise the possibility of an underlying organic aciduria. Hyperammonemia can provoke hyperventilation that leads to respiratory alkalosis, so the discovery of alkalosis when acidosis is expected (e.g., during a work-up for suspected sepsis, especially in an infant) should lead to measurement of the blood ammonia level immediately.

Table 17.1.   Important causes of vomiting in metabolic disorders (neonatal, early infancy, or later)

With or without encephalopathy
  Organic acidurias
  Urea cycle defects/hyperammonemia syndromes
  Fatty acid oxidation disorders

With severe abdominal pain
  Porphyrias (acute intermittent porphyria, coproporphyria,
    variegate porphyria)
  As a symptom of associated pancreatitis

With acidosis/ketoacidosis
  Organic acidurias

With liver dysfunction
  Organic acidurias (chronic or recurrent)
  Urea cycle defects/hyperammonemic syndromes
  Galactosemia
  Fructose intolerance
  Tyrosinemia type I
  Fanconi-Bickel syndrome
  Fatty acid oxidation disorders (acute)

Cyclic Vomiting of Childhood (Ketosis and Vomiting Syndrome)

Vomiting is a prominent feature of a relatively common and poorly understood condition, characterized by ketosis and abdominal pain, that is triggered by fasting, often in the setting of infection (e.g., otitis). In some children strenuous exercise can also provoke episodes. Typically, episodes begin in the second year and end with puberty. The abdominal pain may be intense, similar to that which occurs in diabetic ketoacidosis. Urinary organic acid analysis shows prominent ketosis but no pathologic metabolites, and acylcarnitine analysis shows prominent acetylcarnitine. Treatment with intravenous glucose usually results in rapid resolution of symptoms. Phenothiazine antiemetics are of limited effectiveness in management, but ondansetron can be quite beneficial. Reassurance that this condition is difficult but not dangerous is helpful. Some patients with this pattern of symptoms have been shown to have deficiencies of either β-ketothiolase or succinyl-CoA:3-oxoacid CoA transferase. Abdominal migraine appears to be the explanation in others. However, for a substantial number of children with this syndrome, a coherent explanation has not been found. Impaired uptake of ketones into peripheral tissues is one possibility. This disorder is sometimes confused with ketotic hypoglycemia; but the blood glucose level is not abnormally low, the patients do not have the slight body build of many children with ketotic hypoglycemia, and the treatments for ketotic hypoglycemia (such as avoiding fasting, cornstarch at bedtime) do not seem to be beneficial in cyclic vomiting.

ABDOMINAL PAIN

Crampy abdominal pain occurs with intestinal dysfunction (e.g., malabsorption, infectious diarrhea, or mechanical problems), whereas diffuse pain is often due to an inflammatory response. Metabolic disorders are usually not considered until several episodes of abdominal pain have occurred without an obvious explanation. This section addresses diffuse abdominal pain; pancreatitis is discussed separately. Abdominal pain due to the disorders discussed here is often intense; it may lead to surgical exploration for suspected appendicitis. Recent advances in imaging may help lessen fruitless surgery. However, when the patient has a metabolic disorder associated with recurrent abdominal pain, the physician must be careful in each episode that an actual case of appendicitis or another surgical problem is not being attributed to the metabolic disorder.

The Porphyrias

Diffuse or colicky abdominal pain and constipation occur in three of the hepatic porphyrias—acute intermittent, variegate, and hereditary coproporphyria (see also Fig. 22.1). All three show autosomal dominant inheritance, and enzyme activity is typically about 50% of normal. Symptoms are uncommon in childhood. The dominant porphyrias are among the few dominantly inherited enzymopathies. Although many of the porphyrias intermittently have the characteristic red (or dark) urine, this feature is not always evident, especially in coproporphyria. The porphyrias are disorders of the synthesis of heme, a component of cytochromes, as well as of hemoglobin. Episodes of illness in all three porphyrias with abdominal symptoms appear to be related to increased activity of the first step of porphyrin synthesis, δ-aminolevulinic acid synthase. Most of the porphyrias have prominent photodermatitis, with reddening and easy blistering after sun exposure; hypertrichosis can also occur. In unusual cases an individual (doubly heterozygous) may have more than one form of porphyria and may present with severe symptoms, even in childhood.

Acute intermittent porphyria, which does *not* have skin lesions, is the most common form in most populations. It is caused by deficient activity of porphobilinogen deaminase, also called *hydroxymethylbilane synthase*, previously known as uroporphyrinogen synthase. The incidence of carriers (heterozygote frequency) is generally thought to be between five and ten in 100,000, but it may be as high as one in 1,000 in some areas (northern Sweden). Only about 10% of gene carriers have symptoms. Ethanol, barbiturates, oral contraceptives or other drugs, and hormonal changes may trigger episodes of mental depression, abdominal pain, peripheral neuropathy, or demyelination; but often no precipitating factor is identified.

Hereditary coproporphyria, due to defects in coproporphyrinogen III oxidase (coproporphyrin decarboxylase), is generally milder than acute intermittent porphyria and is less likely to have neurologic symptoms. Onset in childhood is unusual. The rare homozygote may experience the onset of symptoms in infancy with persistent jaundice and hemolytic anemia.

Variegate porphyria is the result of protoporphyrinogen oxidase deficiency. The heterozygote frequency among Afrikaners in South Africa is three persons in 1,000. About half have symptoms that have typically been triggered by medications and have been worsened by iron overload (consider concurrent hemochromatosis). Heterozygotes rarely develop manifestations in childhood, but symptoms can begin as early as infancy in the rare homozygote or compound heterozygote. Photosensitivity is more common in variegate porphyria than in hereditary coproporphyria.

The diagnosis of any of the porphyrias can be difficult. Sometimes a positive family history of porphyria or an illness suggestive of porphyria (e.g., depression, recurrent abdominal pain) is present. Dark or red urine can be a major clue. A positive urine screening test, such as the Watson–Schwartz test or similar reaction, may be present only during acute illness, so it cannot be relied upon for accurate diagnosis. Comprehensive evaluation of blood, urine, and stool for porphyrins is the most reliable diagnostic approach (Table 17.2). In the conditions characterized by abdominal pain, erythrocyte porphyrins are normal. Determination of enzyme activities or molecular analyses should never be the primary diagnostic measures.

The Periodic Fevers

Diffuse abdominal pain also occurs in the periodic fevers. Familial Mediterranean fever (FMF) is an autosomal recessive condition characterized by episodes of noninfective peritonitis, pericarditis, meningitis (Mollaret meningitis), orchitis, arthritis, and erysipelas-like erythroderma. Onset in childhood is common in the severe forms. Amyloidosis leading to renal failure can develop. FMF is so common in some ethnic groups, including Sephardic and Armenian Jews and some Arab communities, that pseudodominant pedigrees are regularly encountered. Defects in marenostrin (pyrin), a protein in the myelomonocytic-specific proinflammatory pathway, have recently been shown to be the underlying cause of FMF. Marenostrin apparently acts to down-regulate the inflammatory response, particularly to the neutrophil chemotactic factor C5a. Diagnosis based on molecular testing of the FMF gene (called MEFV) is replacing the metariminol challenge that was formerly performed.

Autosomal dominant familial periodic fever, sometimes called familial Hibernian fever, is a similar disorder that is much less common than FMF. It was originally reported in an Irish/Scottish family. This condition is caused by mutations in the tumor necrosis factor receptor-1 gene TNFRSF1A.

Abdominal pain and fever also occur in mevalonic aciduria (the form known as hyper-IgD [immunoglobulin D] with periodic fever) (see Chapter 23), and in juvenile hemochromatosis.

PANCREATITIS

Pancreatitis remains one of the most mysterious of the acute life-threatening conditions. Except for mechanical obstruction of

Table 17.2. Characteristic laboratory findings in porphyrias with abdominal symptoms

Disease	McKusick number	Enzyme	Urine	Stool
Acute intermittent porphyria	176000	PBG deaminase	ALA, PBG	
Hereditary coproporphyria	121300	Coproporphyrinogen oxidase	ALA, PBG, coproporphyrin	
Variegate porphyria	176200	Protoporphyrinogen oxidase	ALA, PBG, coproporphyrin	Coproporphyrin, protoporphyrin

Abbreviations: ALA, delta-aminolevulinic acid; PBG, porphobilinogen.

pancreatic secretion due to gallstones, the mechanisms of pancreatitis are not understood, even when a precipitating or proximate cause, such as chronic ethanol use, is known. Gallstones in children are usually associated with hemolytic disorders; in adults, often no obvious cause is found.

The organic acidurias primarily associated with pancreatitis are found in the catabolic pathways for branched-chain amino acids. They include maple syrup urine disease, isovaleric aciduria, 2-methylcrotonyl-CoA carboxylase deficiency, propionic aciduria, methylmalonic aciduria, and β-ketothiolase deficiency. Acidosis, ketosis, vomiting, and abdominal pain are common during episodes of metabolic decompensation in these disorders, so pancreatitis may not be suspected. Conversely, pancreatitis may be the presenting illness in mild forms of these conditions, especially in isovaleric acidemia. A search for an underlying organic aciduria (urine organic acids, plasma or blood acylcarnitines, and plasma amino acids) should therefore be part of the initial investigation in pancreatitis (Table 17.3).

Pancreatitis occurs in disorders of oxidative phosphorylation, especially cytochrome oxidase deficiency, and with mitochondrial encephalomyopathy, lactic acidemia, and strokelike episodes (MELAS) syndrome due to mutations in the tRNA leucine gene, and carnitine-palmitoyl-CoA transferase (CPT) I deficiency. Lipid disorders, especially hyperlipidemia due to lipoprotein lipase deficiency and hypo/abetalipoproteinemia, are also often associated with pancreatitis. Homocystinuria due to cystathionine β-synthase deficiency is the aminoacidopathy that is most commonly associated with pancreatitis. Depletion of antioxidants (vitamin E, glutathione, selenium, and so on) or oxidative stress may play a role in the pathogenesis of pancreatitis.

CONSTIPATION/SLOWED TRANSIT/PSEUDOOBSTRUCTION

Constipation and pseudoobstruction occasionally are manifestations of systemic metabolic disease, although in most cases they are due to diet, habit, or intestinal motility abnormalities that are

Table 17.3. First-line investigations for pancreatitis

Urinary organic acid analysis
Plasma amino acids
Plasma total homocysteine
Blood spot or plasma acylcarnitine analysis
Blood lipid profile (lipoprotein electrophoresis)
Selenium
Total glutathione
Zinc
Vitamins A, C, and E
Calcium

associated with neuronal dysfunction. The porphyrias are noted for constipation, especially during times of crisis. The syndrome of hyper-IgD with fever may include constipation (compared to familial Mediterranean fever in which diarrhea is more likely). Constipation may also be prominent in the Fanconi–Bickel syndrome of glycogen storage and renal tubular dysfunction and in malonyl-CoA decarboxylase deficiency.

In the organic acidurias and hyperammonemias, constipation can be troublesome, as altered bowel function may lead to decompensation of the primary metabolic disorder because of the accumulation of intermediate compounds (e.g., propionate or ammonia) produced by gut flora. Treatment of the constipation can lead to significant improvement in metabolic control. Metronidazole is often used to alter bowel flora to diminish the intestinal production of propionate in patients with disorders of propionate metabolism.

ASCITES

Ascites is rarely the sole presenting symptom of metabolic disease, but it does accompany several of them. In severe or early-onset disorders, the ascites may occur before birth as nonimmune hydrops fetalis. Ascites or hydrops occurs in many lysosomal diseases, including sialidosis (mucolipidosis I), galactosialidosis, sialic acid storage disease, Farber lipogranulomatosis, Gaucher disease, Niemann–Pick disease, mannosidosis, and mucopolysaccharidoses IV-A and VI. Hydrops is especially common in mucopolysaccharidosis (MPS) VII (Sly disease, β-glucuronidase deficiency) (see Chapter 29).

DIARRHEA

Mitochondrial neurogastrointestinal encephalopathy syndrome (MNGIE) (myoneurogastrointestinal disorder and encephalopathy) is a generalized disorder of mitochondrial dysfunction. The onset of intestinal symptoms occurs in childhood or early to middle adult life and includes chronic diarrhea, stasis, nausea, and vomiting, resulting in impaired growth. Wasting and cachexia may occur. Skeletal growth may be retarded. Eventual loss of longitudinal muscle, diverticuli (which may rupture), intestinal scleroderma, and pseudoobstruction are seen. Electrophysiologic studies have shown visceral neuropathy with conduction failure. Prokinetic drugs have been generally ineffective. Lactic acidosis is often present. The extraintestinal symptoms vary but are typical of a mitochondrial disorder (Table 17.4).

In vitro analysis of mitochondrial function reveals a variety of impairments, especially deficiency of complex I or complex IV, or combined deficits. Mitochondrial DNA analysis (liver, muscle) shows depletion and multiple DNA deletions. Recurrences in siblings, a high frequency of parental consanguinity, and lack of vertical transmission are consistent with autosomal recessive inheritance. Mapping of MNGIE to distal 22q has been followed by identification of pathologic mutations in the gene ECGF1,

Table 17.4.   Extraintestinal manifestations in mitochondrial neurogastrointestinal disorder and encephalopathy syndrome

Organ	Findings
Growth	Slow; cachexia and wasting
Brain	Leukodystrophy, increased CSF protein, ataxia
Eye	Ophthalmoplegia, ptosis
Ear	Sensorineural deafness
Cranial nerves	Dysarthria, dysphonia, facial palsy
Heart	Heart block
Skeletal muscle	Ragged-red fibers, weakness
Peripheral nerves	Demyelinating neuropathy, axonal degeneration

Abbreviation: CSF, cerebrospinal fluid.

which codes for thymidine phosphorylase. Impaired function of this gene leads to impaired mitochondrial DNA synthesis.

A similar autosomal recessive condition whose cause is unknown has been called either oculogastrointestinal myopathy or familial visceral myopathy with external ophthalmoplegia. A destruction of the gastrointestinal smooth muscle is seen, whereas the myenteric plexus appears normal. Abdominal pain, diarrhea, diverticuli, and dilatation of the bowel occur. Patients also suffer from a demyelinating and axonal neuropathy, focal spongiform degeneration of the posterior columns, ptosis, and external ophthalmoplegia. The onset is in childhood or adolescence with death by the age of 30 years in many patients. Most reports of this condition were made in the 1980s, so a considerable overlap may exist with MNGIE, which was generally not excluded enzymatically or molecularly.

Chronic diarrhea also occurs in Menkes disease, perhaps because of autonomic dysfunction.

MALDIGESTION

Generalized impairment of digestion resulting from pancreatic problems (e.g., cystic fibrosis) or liver disease is well known. The Pearson marrow–pancreas syndrome, usually caused by sporadic heteroplasmic deletion of mitochondrial DNA, has exocrine pancreatic failure in infancy or childhood that is usually recognized by steatorrhea. Sideroblastic anemia and progressive failure of blood cell lines may occur, along with chronic lactic acidosis. The same deletion (and pancreas failure) can be found in Kearns–Sayre syndrome (KSS); Pearson syndrome occasionally evolves into KSS.

Failure of the exocrine and/or endocrine pancreas and other endocrine organs may also occur in other mitochondrial disorders (see Chapter 6).

Several disorders of digestion involve primary enzymes of carbohydrate metabolism (Table 17.5). A deficiency typically results in severe watery (osmotic) diarrhea when the affected substrate or its precursors is ingested. Excessive gas production and bloating may also occur. All are autosomal recessive.

Disaccharide Intolerance I: Sucrase/Isomaltase Deficiency

Sucrase/isomaltase deficiency is a rare cause of infantile diarrhea, which becomes evident with the introduction of sucrose in the diet. Several different mechanisms exist for enzyme deficiency, including impaired secretion, abnormal folding, deficient catalytic activity, and enhanced destruction.

Glucose–Galactose Malabsorption

Glucose–galactose malabsorption is clinically similar to sucrase/isomaltase deficiency with severe, life-threatening watery diarrhea from early infancy. Elimination of glucose and galactose from the diet is necessary. Fortunately, fructose is well tolerated, so a fructose-based formula is effective. This condition is most often recognized in Middle Eastern Arab populations. The defect in the

Table 17.5.   Disorders of carbohydrate digestion

Disorder	McKusick number	Enzyme	Major substrate
Disaccharide intolerance I	222900	Sucrase/ isomaltase	Sucrose
Disaccharide intolerance II— congenital alactasia	223000	β-Glycosidase complex— lactase, glycosyl-ceramidase	Lactose
Disaccharide intolerance III— adult lactase deficiency	223100	β-Glycosidase complex— lactase, glycosyl-ceramidase	Lactose
Trehalase deficiency	275360	Trehalase	Trehalose (mush-rooms)
Not recognized	154360	Glucoamylase (maltase) I and II	

sodium–glucose cotransporter SGLT1 is due to mutations in the solute carrier gene SLC5A1.

Disaccharide Intolerance II: Infantile Lactase Deficiency and Congenital Lactose Intolerance

Congenital lactase deficiency is extremely rare. In nearly all cases, lactase deficiency in infants and young children is due to infection and the loss of the mature brush border.

Congenital lactose intolerance appears to be distinct from congenital lactase deficiency. In the former, excessive gastric absorption of lactose (leading to lactosemia and lactosuria), vomiting, failure to thrive, liver dysfunction, and renal Fanconi syndrome are found. Congenital lactase deficiency may be fatal if not recognized and treated by the elimination of lactose from the diet. Interestingly, lactose is well tolerated after 6 months of age. The basis for this condition is not known.

Disaccharide Intolerance III: Adult Lactase Deficiency

Adult lactase "deficiency" is a common polymorphism. In fact, declining expression of intestinal lactase during childhood is the usual state, mirroring the declining importance of milk in mammalian nutrition after infancy. In a few regions, including northern Europe, unfermented milk remains an important dietary component after infancy. The ability to digest milk is clearly an advantage, so among individuals from those regions a minority is lactose intolerant. The custom of drinking unfermented milk may have arisen because of a chance mutation that interrupts the usual decline in lactase activity with age. Intestinal lactase activity depends on the summed expression from both alleles. Recent studies indicate that differences in lactase expression do not reside in the coding sequence itself but are probably found in a cis-acting regulatory element.

MALABSORPTION

Malabsorption in metabolic disorders can be due to abnormalities in ion channels, transport molecules, carrier proteins for lipids, or cotransport molecules. Symptoms are attributable to the deficiency of the substance that is not being properly absorbed (e.g., essential fatty acids, fat-soluble vitamins) and to the effects caused by abnormally high amounts of the substance within the gut. Ion-channel defects distort the balance of water and electrolytes, leading to diarrhea; abnormalities of transport molecules lead to diarrhea; and the deficiency of a cotransport molecule (e.g., intrinsic factor) can have major consequences because of the resulting deficiency of an essential nutrient. First-line investigations for metabolic causes of malabsorption should include stool pH and an analysis of reducing substances in stool. Characterization of stool sugars may confirm what has been suggested by the history. A breath hydrogen test after dietary challenge can confirm malabsorption.

Electrolytes

Chloride Diarrhea

In chloride diarrhea, a recessively inherited disorder, voluminous watery diarrhea with high chloride content (greater than the sum of sodium and potassium) occurs from an early age. Polyhydramnios is common, perhaps universal. The defect is in the brush border chloride–bicarbonate exchange mechanism. Treatment with potassium chloride was the initial therapy, but inhibitors of prostaglandin synthase (Ketoprofen) and the gastric proton pump (Omeprazole) have been found to be effective. Mutations have been discovered in the gene DRA.

Defects of the Na^+/H^+ exchange mechanism result in sodium diarrhea and metabolic acidosis. The presentation is similar to congenital chloride diarrhea, but the stool electrolyte composition shows high sodium and an alkaline pH. Treatment with oral Na-K-citrate normalizes the electrolyte status of the patient.

Microvillus inclusion disease is another recessive cause of intractable diarrhea in infancy, perhaps the most common noninfectious one. Jejunal biopsy shows intracytoplasmic inclusions consisting of brush-border microvilli that suggest that this is a disorder of intracellular transport that impairs their assembly.

Protein-Losing Enteropathy

Protein-losing enteropathy, often due to infection or impaired function of intestinal lymphatics, is a cardinal feature of the congenital disorder of glycosylation CDG 1B, which is caused by phosphomannose isomerase deficiency. Liver disease and a bleeding diathesis may also occur. Unlike the other CDG syndromes, mental retardation and severe neurologic problems are not seen. Diagnosis is based on isoelectric focusing of transferrin and enzyme assay. Treatment with oral mannose is effective. The CDG syndromes are discussed in greater detail in Chapter 23.

Amino Acids

The two main disorders of intestinal amino acid transport are those involving tryptophan and methionine. Tryptophan malabsorption (Hartnup disease) occurs as an autosomal recessive disorder that may be clinically silent. The transport of several neutral amino acids in the intestine and kidney is involved, but tryptophan is the one most likely to be limiting. If niacin in the diet is also inadequate, a deficiency of nicotinic acid and nicotinamide causes a rash (pellagra), light sensitivity, emotional instability, and ataxia. In severe cases, this progresses to an encephalopathy with delirium and seizures. An increase in stool indoles and urinary indican may occur, reflecting the action of intestinal bacteria on the unabsorbed tryptophan. The diagnosis is suggested by finding high urinary levels of the neutral amino acids alanine, serine, threonine, asparagine, glutamine, valine, leucine, isoleucine, phenylalanine, tyrosine, tryptophan, histidine, and citrulline. Plasma levels of these amino acids are normal or slightly low.

A few infants with methionine malabsorption have been reported. Clinical manifestations included white hair, tachypnea, mental retardation, seizures, diarrhea, and a peculiar odor similar to that of hops drying in an oasthouse. The urine may show increased α-hydroxybutyric acid after a methionine load. The condition appears to be autosomal recessive.

Vitamin B$_{12}$

The intricate story of vitamin B$_{12}$ illustrates the interaction of diet, digestion, absorption, and intermediary metabolism. Vitamin B$_{12}$ is the precursor of substances known as cobalamins. Two forms are essential for human metabolism: methylcobalamin, which is a cofactor for the remethylation of homocysteine to methionine, and adenosylcobalamin, which is used by methylmalonyl-CoA mutase. Defects of the cobalamin pathway can therefore cause problems with either or both of these reactions.

Vitamin B$_{12}$ in food (primarily meat and dairy products) is first released by digestion that occurs in the stomach. It binds to specific glycoproteins (r-proteins), especially transcobalamin I (TC I). In the duodenum the pancreatic proteases act to release the B$_{12}$ again, which then binds to intrinsic factor (IF) produced by gastric parietal cells. The intrinsic factor–B$_{12}$ complex (B$_{12}$-IF) binds to a specific receptor (cubilin) on ileal enterocytes. The receptors internalize the B$_{12}$-IF, which then dissociates. The absorbed B$_{12}$ is transported to the bloodstream coupled to transcobalamin II (TC II); this B$_{12}$–TC II complex is the main way of distributing newly absorbed B$_{12}$ to the tissues. However, most of the B$_{12}$ in the bloodstream is bound to TC I as methylcobalamin.

Autosomal recessive genetic defects in intrinsic factor or the ileal receptor system typically lead to megaloblastic anemia with neurologic changes (developmental delay, hypotonia, hyporeflexia, coma). Onset usually occurs after the first year. Infants in the first year of life apparently do not depend on the ileal receptor system for B$_{12}$ uptake, which explains the lack of symptoms in young infants with problems in this system. The receptor defect is called the Imerslünd–Grasbeck syndrome (megaloblastic anemia I, common in Finland), which may be characterized by proteinuria, as well as anemia. Defects in TC II, on the other hand, become apparent in the first few months of life with symptoms of megaloblastic anemia, failure to thrive, and neurologic delay. Congenital B$_{12}$ deficiency can occur in the offspring of vegan–vegetarian mothers who have not had adequate intake of B$_{12}$. Deficiency of B$_{12}$ leads to mild methylmalonic aciduria and hyperhomocysteinemia. Infants with congenital B$_{12}$ deficiency may be recognized by increased propionylcarnitine on newborn screening. Late-onset B$_{12}$ deficiency is usually caused by a lack of intrinsic factor due to atrophic gastritis, another disease of the stomach, or an unexplained mechanism. The defects of B$_{12}$ metabolism after uptake from the bloodstream lead to variant forms of homocystinuria (cblE and cblG defects), methylmalonic aciduria (cblA and cblB defects), or both (cblC, cblD, and cblF defects).

Investigation of suspected B_{12} disorders includes determining erythrocyte indices, plasma homocysteine, acylcarnitine analysis for propionylcarnitine, and urine methylmalonic acid. Serum cobalamin levels are low in defects involving intrinsic factor and gut uptake but may be normal in TC II deficiency.

ADDITIONAL READING

Gross U, Hoffmann GF, Doss MO. Erythropoietic and hepatic por-phyrias. *J Inher Metab Dis* 2000;23:641–661.

Kahler SG, Sherwood WG, Woolf D, et al. Pancreatitis in patients with organic acidemias. *J Pediatr* 1994;124:239–243.

Pfau BT, Li BU, Murray RD, et al. Differentiating cyclic from chronic vomiting patterns in children: quantitative criteria and diagnostic implications. *Pediatrics* 1996;97:364–368.

18 ♣ Renal and Electrolyte Disturbances

GENERAL REMARKS: DEHYDRATION

Renal and electrolyte abnormalities present frequently with acidosis and dehydration, which may indicate a metabolic disease. More commonly, this picture of abnormal clinical chemistry results from infectious diarrhea. Rarely, an inherited disorder of intestinal absorption causes chronic diarrhea (see Chapter 17). Patients with clinical manifestations of dehydration, decreased skin turgor, depressed fontanel, sunken eyes, decreased urine output, or documented acute loss of weight fortunately have measurements of electrolyte concentrations, urea nitrogen, and creatinine in the blood regularly included in the assessment. One of the clinical signs of dehydration is poor skin turgor. However, the fact that turgor is measured by the relative rate that a pinched-up piece of skin returns to its resting state is not so widely known. In fact, in rats, measured weight loss in experimentally induced dehydration had a straight-line correlation with the length of time (measured with a stop-watch) that the skin took to flatten.

Electrolyte analysis in the dehydrated patient usually reveals hyperchloremic dehydration. The anion gap is not increased. Most commonly, this results from acute diarrhea, although chronic diarrhea can lead to chronic acidosis and chronic dehydration. Hyperchloremic acidosis also results from renal tubular acidosis (see later). Metabolic acidosis developing from the classic inborn errors of metabolism is hypochloremic, with an increased anion gap (see Chapter 6). Acute infectious diarrhea can, of course, precipitate an attack of metabolic imbalance in most inborn errors of metabolism. Recurrent or episodic attacks of dehydration characterize dehydration resulting from inherited disease (Table 18.1). A combination of the electrolyte pattern and the clinical manifestations clearly permits a ready dissection of the heritable causes of recurrent dehydration. In actuality, many of the chronic diarrheas, such as the disaccharidase deficiencies, often do not lead to dehydration because patients are so accustomed to their problem that they compensate with ample fluid intake. The water intake of infants and children with nephrogenic diabetes insipidus is enormous. These patients often get into trouble when exogenous forces, such as intercurrent illness, interfere with their ability to compensate. Admission to the hospital and a requirement for parenteral fluids, even with fairly trivial surgery, can lead to major morbidity and mortality if physicians do not recognize and supply the very large quantities of water necessary for maintaining these patients.

Intestinal losses deplete intracellular potassium, resulting in hypochloremic alkalosis. In small infants hypochloremic alkalosis is the hallmark of pyloric stenosis. Infants with congenital chloride diarrhea and those with cystic fibrosis (CF) both have diarrhea, but those with CF are edematous from hypoproteinemia and pale from anemia. Those with Bartter syndrome and Gitelman syndrome do not have diarrhea. A teenager or adult with bulimia can mimic Bartter syndrome, as can one with chronic laxative abuse.

Table 18.1. Recurrent or episodic dehydration

Hyperchloremic acidosis	
Diarrhea	Lactase deficiency
	Sucrase, isomaltase deficiency
	Glucose, galactose malabsorption
	Acrodermatitis enteropathica
Failure to thrive, rickets,	Renal tubular acidosis
polyuria	Cystinosis
Hypochloremic alkalosis	
Diarrhea	Congenital chloride diarrhea
Diarrhea, hypoproteinemia,	Cystic fibrosis
anemia	Bartter and Gitelman syndromes
Polyuria	Pyloric stenosis
Vomiting	Bulimia
Hypernatremia	Nephrogenic diabetes insipidus
	Diabetes insipidus
Hyponatremia, hyperkalemia	Congenital adrenal hyperplasias
	Adrenal aplasia, hypoplasia
	Pseudohypoaldosteronism
Hypochloremic acidosis	Propionic acidemia
Increased anion gap	Methylmalonic aciduria
Ketoacidosis	Diabetic ketoacidosis
	Isovaleric acidemia
	3-Oxothiolase deficiency

The adrenal hormone deficiency diseases are readily recognized in females with ambiguous genitalia. However, they are frequently missed in those without ambiguous genitalia, such as male infants with adrenal hyperplasia or infants with absent or hypoplastic adrenals or pseudohypoaldosteronism. The hyponatremia, renal salt wasting, and hyperkalemia should be giveaways for the diagnosis.

Manifestations of renal disease other than dehydration or renal tubular dysfunction include urinary tract calculi and crystalluria (see later). They also include failure to thrive, myoglobinuria (see Chapter 6), unusual odor (see Table 4.1), and abnormal color (see Table 4.2). Renal cystic disease occurs in Zellweger syndrome (see Chapter 27), carnitine palmitoyltransferase II deficiency, and multiple acyl-CoA dehydrogenase deficiency (glutaric aciduria type II) due to deficiency of electron transfer flavoprotein (ETF) and ETF dehydrogenase (see Chapter 6).

Methylmalonic aciduria is a classic organic aciduria. It may be complicated by a variety of renal manifestations. Isolated renal tubular dysfunction may lead to acidosis and hyperchloremia along with proximal renal tubular bicarbonate wasting. It may also be complicated by interstitial nephritis and renal glomerular failure. Patients with cobalamin C disease have displayed a hemolytic uremic syndrome with combined methylmalonic aciduria and homocystinuria.

Renal disease is also a late complication of glycogenosis type I, glucose-6-phosphatase deficiency (von Gierke disease). These patients may have proteinuria, increased blood pressure, urinary tract calculi, or nephrocalcinosis that have been attributed to hyperuricemia. However, glomerulosclerosis and interstitial fibrosis also occur, leading to glomerular dysfunction and possibly to renal failure.

URINARY TRACT CALCULI

Kidney stones or calculi anywhere in the urinary tract represent a common affliction among adults but are rarely found in children. In adults the composition of the stone is usually a salt or a mixture of salts of calcium, calcium oxalate, and calcium phosphate. The calculi found in pediatric populations are largely the products of inborn errors of metabolism (Table 18.2).

Lithiasis in the urinary tract may present with pain, which is referred to as renal colic. This sudden-onset pain is of such extreme intensity that it may lead to nausea and vomiting. The pain reflects the movement of a stone along the ureter and may be well localized by the patient to this curvilinear distribution. Pain may vanish on entry of the calculus into the bladder, only to reappear once the calculus enters the urethra. Associated frequency or dysuria may occur. Some patients may have these symptoms as a result of crys-

Table 18.2.   Urinary tract calculi

Stone	Disorder	Enzyme
Cystine	Cystinuria	—
Uric acid	Lesch–Nyhan	HPRT
	PRPP synthetase superactivity	PRPP synthetase
	Glycogenosis I	Glucose-6-phosphatase
2,8-Dihydroxyadenine	APRT deficiency	APRT
Xanthine	Xanthinuria	Xanthine oxidase
Oxalate	Oxaluria, glycolic aciduria	Alanine:glyoxylate aminotransferase
	Oxaluria, glyceric aciduria	D-Glycerate-dehydrogenase
Calcium salts	Hypercalciuria + uricosuria	Multifactorial
	Wilson disease	P-type ATPase transporter

Abbreviations: APRT, adenine-phosphoribosyl transferase; ATPase, adenine triphosphatase, HPRT, hypoxanthine guanine phosphoribosyl transferase; PRPP, phosphoribosylpyrophosphate.

talluria, as well as with discrete stones. Hematuria also can result from crystalluria or calculi.

Urinary tract infection is a common complication of urinary tract calculi. It may present with pyuria, dysuria, and fever. Infection usually does not disappear until the stone is removed by passage, lithotripsy, or surgery. Repeated episodes of pyelonephritis and obstruction may lead to renal failure.

Patients with symptoms should be investigated for the possibility of stones, but those with diseases in which calculi are common should also be monitored. Stones containing calcium are radiopaque, but urate stones are not; cystine stones are difficult to visualize roentgenographically. Ultrasonography is useful in detecting hydronephrosis or hydroureter, but it may miss small stones. Intravenous urography is useful for delineating calculi and defining their presence or absence and the degree of obstruction. Retrograde pyelography permits visualization without intravenous injection of dye, but it does require cystoscopy. Computed tomography (CT) scan may permit detection of radiolucent stones that are not evident with other methods.

Cystinuria results from mutation in the gene for the cystine transporter of the kidney and intestine. It leads to increased urinary excretion of lysine, ornithine, and arginine, as well as of cystine. Only the cystinuria causes symptoms, all of which result from lack of solubility and formation of calculi. Treatment involves ensuring ample fluid throughout the day and at night to keep the cystine soluble. Cystine crystallizes above 1,250 μmol/L at pH 7.5.

Uric acid stone disease occurs commonly in Lesch–Nyhan disease, as well as in the other variant hypoxanthine–guanine phosphoribosyltransferase deficiencies. Patients with phosphoribosylpyrophosphate (PRPP) synthetase superactivity and glucose-6-phosphatase deficiency also overproduce purine and excrete it as uric acid in large quantities. Deafness is common in patients with PRPP synthetase mutations. Other patients with uric acid calculi have uricosuria as a result of increased urate clearance by the kidney. Some well-defined kindreds have been reported. Most have normal blood concentrations of uric acid; some are hypouricemic, and some, like the Dalmatian dog, are hyperuricemic.

Adenine phosphoribosyltransferase mutations, common in those of Japanese descent, leads to deficiency of enzyme activity and to increased excretion of the very insoluble dioxygenated derivative of adenine. Xanthine oxidase deficiency is associated with stones composed of the highly insoluble xanthine, as well as with hypouricemia. Xanthine stones also occur in patients with hyperuricemia who are treated with allopurinol; however, in many finding a dosage regimen that minimizes or avoids the propensity for stone formation is possible because hypoxanthine is very soluble. The two forms of oxaluria, known as types I and II, are characterized by very-early-onset renal stone disease and early renal failure. Successful treatment has included combined transplantation of both the liver and kidney.

RENAL TUBULAR DYSFUNCTION

Fanconi Syndrome

The Fanconi syndrome is a generalized disruption of renal tubular function in which the proximal tubular reabsorption of amino acids, glucose, phosphate, bicarbonate, and urate is impaired, leading to a generalized amino aciduria, glycosuria, phosphaturia, uricosuria, and increased urinary pH. As a consequence, vitamin D–resistant rickets and osteomalacia are found.

Obligatory polyuria in this syndrome can lead to clinically important dehydration, especially when fluid intake is restricted. Chronic hyperchloremic acidosis may worsen in acute situations. Losses of ions and metabolites in the urine may lead to symptomatic depletion. Thus, hypokalemia may lead to muscle weakness or even paralysis, constipation, and ileus, as well as to disturbances of cardiac rhythm and function. Excretion of carnitine may deplete the body stores and may lead to disturbed fatty acid oxidation and hypoketotic hypoglycemia (see Chapter 6), muscle weakness, or congestive cardiac failure. Losses of calcium may lead to tetany or convulsions. Hypomagnesemia may also develop. Shortness of stature or failure to thrive occurs regularly.

A number of genetically determined diseases lead to the Fanconi syndrome (Table 18.3). The most common of these is cystinosis (see later). With these disorders, associated syndromic features lead to the diagnosis and the appropriate confirmatory test. Hepatic dysfunction occurs in hepatorenal tyrosinemia, usually as the major clinical feature; and urinary organic acid analysis for succinylacetone provides the diagnosis. Hepatic dysfunction also occurs with cataracts in galactosemia and with hypoglycemia in hereditary fructose intolerance. Confirmation of each is by enzyme assay; in the latter, enzyme assay of the liver is necessary. Mutational analysis reveals the common Caucasian mutations. Fanconi syndrome has been reported in glycogenosis types I, III, and XI. Type I can be diagnosed clinically by glucagon testing (see Chapter 11, "Glucagon Stimulation"), by enzyme assay of the liver, or by mutation analysis. The clinical chemistry is characterized by hypoglycemia, lactic acidemia, hyperalaninemia, hyperlipidemia, and hypercholesterolemia. Other renal complications are common in glycogenosis type I, including distal renal tubular disease, amyloidosis, nephrocalcinosis, and calculi (see earlier). Renal failure, with proteinuria, focal glomerulosclerosis, and interstitial fibrosis, may be a late complication. In Lowe syndrome and Wilson disease, the full Fanconi picture is often absent from the urine; but a generalized amino aciduria is the rule. In Wilson disease the pattern also includes increased cystine and methionine, indices of the liver dysfunction. In electron transport defects, various patterns of renal tubular acidosis occur, including the complete Fanconi syndrome. A molecular defect has not been found in some clearly genetic kindreds, and these are classified as idiopathic Fanconi syndrome. In addition, an acquired Fanconi syndrome has been observed with a variety of renal insults, including the ingestion of outdated tetracycline, 6-mercaptopurine, and heavy metal poisoning. Deficiency

Table 18.3. **Heritable causes of the Fanconi syndrome**

Disorder	Molecular defect	Distinguishing characteristics
Cystinosis	Lysosomal cystine transporter	Corneal deposits, shortness of stature
Hepatorenal tyrosinemia	Fumarylacetoacetate hydrolase	Hepatic dysfunction
Galactosemia	Galactose-1-phosphate uridyltransferase	Hepatic dysfunction, cataracts, mental retardation
Hereditary fructose intolerance	Fructose-1-phosphate aldolase	Hepatic dysfunction, hypoglycemia
Glycogenosis	Glucose-6-phosphatase Amylo-1,6-glucosidase Phosphorylase-b-kinase	Hepatomegaly, hypo-glycemia, hyperlipi-demia, hypercholes-terolemia, lactic acidemia
Lowe syndrome	OCRL-1 gene on Xq25–26	Cataracts, glaucoma, hypotonia, develop-mental retardation
Wilson disease	P-type ATPase transporter	Hepatic dysfunction, Kayser–Fleischer ring, neurologic dysfunction
Electron transport defects	mtDNA deletions mtDNA depletion Cytochrome C oxidase Complex III or IV	Lactic acidemia, encephalomyopathy
Idiopathic	—	

of vitamin D leads to a moderate generalized aminoaciduria but not usually to the rest of the Fanconi syndrome.

Cystinosis

Cystinosis is one of the most important causes of the Fanconi syndrome; as such, it manifests all of the features of the syndrome (see earlier). In addition, some clinical manifestations are unique to this disease. Patients generally have fair skin, hair, and irises. Ophthalmic abnormalities include photophobia caused by deposits of cystine in the cornea. The slit lamp may reveal these refractile crystalline bodies early. They may lead ultimately to thickened, hazy corneas and may be complicated by corneal ulcers. Crystalline cystine may also be identified in conjunctiva. In addition, a charac-teristic peripheral retinopathy is visible as pigmentation and depigmentation. Some adults with the disease are legally blind.

Hypothyroidism results late from deposition of cystine in the gland. Myopathy may follow cystine deposition in muscle or carnitine depletion caused by losses in the urine. Some patients have developed diabetes mellitus. Late neurologic abnormalities include tremor, seizures, or mental retardation. Hydrocephalus and cerebral atrophy have also been documented.

The diagnosis is usually made by assay of cystine content in leukocytes or cultured fibroblasts. The molecular defect is in the transporter for cystine from lysosomes.

Renal Tubular Acidosis

Renal tubular acidosis (RTA) includes the Fanconi syndrome and cystinosis (see earlier). A few patients have renal tubular acidosis without any of the features of the Fanconi syndrome. These patients are characterized by failure to thrive as infants and shortness of stature later. Vomiting is frequently encountered in infants, and many are anorexic. Infants are often described as irritable or apathetic. Metabolic bone disease manifests itself as rickets and osteomalacia, particularly in proximal RTA. The diagnosis is often first suggested by roentgenographic examination of a patient with failure to thrive. Older patients with distal RTA sometimes have urolithiasis.

A low serum bicarbonate, hyperchloremia, and a normal anion gap are characteristic. Patients seldom have a HCO_3 of more than 19 mEq/L, but its values are usually higher than 10 mEq/L. The serum bicarbonate is the most reliable indicator, as the pH and pCO_2 may change in a crying infant. Relative alkalinity of the urine is often the key to the diagnosis. In distal RTA the urine pH remains high and the net excretion of acid is low even when the serum bicarbonate is low. That a urinary pH of 6 may be relatively alkaline may not be readily evident in some acidotic patients. Moreover, modern clinical chemistry laboratories have largely dispensed with pH meters to determine urinary pH, yet dipsticks may not be precise.

Defective acidification of the urine leads to renal losses of sodium and potassium and to polyuria. Bone resorption leads to hypercalciuria. The serum calcium is normal. Phosphaturia may lead to hypophosphatemia, and alkaline phosphatase may be increased. The excretion of citrate may be low. Hypercalciuria may lead to nephrocalcinosis and nephrolithiasis. Renal ultrasonography is useful for early detection.

The distinction between the two major types of RTA, proximal RTA (sometimes called type II) and distal RTA (sometimes called type I), is best made by assessing urinary loss of bicarbonate and serum concentration during intravenous or oral loading with $NaHCO_3$ that causes a progressive increase in the serum level. Doing so requires collecting urine under oil and maintaining it in oil until it is analyzed. The fractional excretion of bicarbonate ($FEHCO_3\%$) is calculated as the [$UHCO_3/U$ creatinine (Cr)] $\times$ [$SCr/ SHCO_3$] $\times$ 100, where U and S indicate urine and serum, respectively. The percentage in patients with distal RTA is less than 10, whereas in proximal RTA values of 10% to 15% occur when the serum level is 20 mEq/L. A massive bicarbonaturia may occur with values of more than 15%. Patients with distal RTA and hyperkalemia may have values from 5% to 10%, whereas those with classic hypokalemia usually have values of less than 5%. The hyperkalemia in patients may represent a generalized tubular dysfunction, which is sometimes referred to as type IV. These patients may have hypoaldosteronism, pseudohypoaldosteronism, or hyporeninemic hypoaldosteronism.

Some discrete syndromes are associated with RTA. Pyruvate carboxylase deficiency and methylmalonic aciduria are associated with proximal RTA. A mixed proximal and distal RTA occurs in patients with carbonic anhydrase deficiency in which a genetically determined syndrome of RTA, osteopetrosis, and cerebral calcifications is found. A mixed RTA also occurs in carnitine palmitoyltransferase I (CPT I) deficiency.

Bartter Syndrome

Bartter syndrome is an uncommon cause of hypokalemic alkalosis in which calcium excretion is normal or increased. In this way, it is distinguished from Gitelman syndrome, in which hypocalciuria and hypomagnesemia accompany hypokalemic alkalosis.

Bartter syndrome results from mutation in the Na–K–Cl cotransporter gene SLC 12A, previously called NKCC2, on chromosome 15q15–21, which codes for a protein that mediates electrolyte transport in the loop of Henle at the site of action of diuretics, furosemide, and butanide. Mutations in this gene have also been found in antenatal Bartter syndrome, in which ultrasonography has revealed fetal nephrocalcinosis *in utero*. Bartter syndrome may also be caused by mutations in the inwardly rectifying potassium channel, ROMK, which recycles reabsorbed K^+ back into the tubule.

In Bartter syndrome presentation usually occurs before 5 years of age. The initial presentation may be with dehydration and hypovolemia. Some patients present with cramps or weakness in the muscles resulting from the hypokalemia. Some have had convulsions or tetany. Chvostek and Trousseau signs may be positive. Polyuria, nocturia, or enuresis may occur. A craving for salt is common. Some patients display vomiting, and constipation is common.

Shortness of stature or failure to thrive is the rule. About two-thirds of children suffering from this syndrome are mentally retarded. Some have abnormal electroencephalograms. Ileus and attacks of hypoventilation, both concomitants of hypokalemic alkalosis, sometimes occur. Rickets has been reported rarely. Many have nephrocalcinosis, especially those with so-called antenatal or infantile forms of Bartter syndrome.

Hypokalemia, alkalosis, hyperaldosteronism, and hyperreninemia are regular laboratory findings. Bartter and colleagues noted unresponsiveness of the blood pressure to intravenous angiotensin II and hypothesized that increased production of renin was a compensatory response to maintain blood pressure and that aldosterone production was also stimulated. Volume expansion can reduce levels of renin and aldosterone. Histologically, hyperplasia of the renal juxtaglomerular apparatus also exists. Renal prostaglandin production increases. Large urinary losses of sodium and potassium lead to contraction of volume. Hypokalemia is usually profound at less than 2.5 mEq/L. Patients cannot form concentrated urine, and this isosthenuria does not respond to the administration of antidiuretic hormone.

Less common laboratory findings include hypomagnesemia, hypocalcemia, and glucose intolerance without fasting hyperglycemia. Some patients have hyperuricemia or clinical gout.

The differential diagnosis of Bartter syndrome includes Gitelman syndrome (see later). It also includes primary hyperaldosteronism, a renin-producing tumor, and renal artery stenosis, all of which are differentiated by the presence of hypertension. Chronic diarrhea, especially laxative abuse, and bulimia may mimic Bartter syndrome, as may chronic or surreptitious diuretic use.

Gitelman Syndrome

Gitelman syndrome is a disorder in which depletion of magnesium and potassium leads to hypokalemic alkalosis, which was once thought to be a variant of Bartter syndrome but which is caused by mutations in the thiazide-sensitive Na–Cl cotransporter gene on chromosome 16q13. This gene, referred to as SLC12A3, codes for a transporter that mediates sodium and chloride reabsorption in the distal convoluted tubule. This transporter is the target of the thiazide diuretics used to treat hypertension. At least 17 different nonconservative mutations have been found.

Patients with this disorder present later, often in adulthood, than those with Bartter syndrome without hypovolemia; some patients overlap both syndromes.

Episodic muscle weakness has been one presentation. Tetany has been another, often precipitated by intercurrent infectious illness. Paresthesias or carpopedal spasm may occur. Patients have been described with a chronic dermatosis, in which the skin was thickened and had a purple-red hue. Erythema of the skin has been observed in experimental magnesium depletion in rats.

In Gitelman syndrome hypokalemic metabolic alkalosis is accompanied by hypomagnesemia and hypocalciuria. Renal wasting of potassium and magnesium is characteristic. Administration of furosemide intravenously leads to excretion of sodium, chloride, and magnesium and a cessation of hypocalciuria, which is consistent with a defect in transport in the distal tubule as opposed to the loop of Henle.

Investigation for Renal Tubular Dysfunction

Initial clinical chemistry carries out determinations of Na, K, Cl, HCO_3, and pH. This establishes the presence or absence of acidosis, and whether the acidosis is hyperchloremic. Other useful blood chemistry values include those for Ca, PO_4, Mg, alkaline phosphatase, urea, and creatinine.

The urine is studied to assess the presence of a Fanconi syndrome by analyzing glucose, amino acids, Ca, PO_4, and creatinine. Proteinuria or an increased amount of retinol-binding protein or N-acetylglucosaminidase indicates tubular damage and proximal tubular leak. Decreased urinary concentrating ability may also indicate generalized tubular dysfunction.

If acidosis is present, urine pH is measured. In a patient suspected of having RTA in whom acidosis is not present, an ammonium chloride load may be useful.

19 ♣ Metabolic Myopathies

The metabolic disorders that affect muscle cells cause weakness and hypotonia, rhabdomyolysis, or both. Rhabdomyolysis disorders can be conveniently separated according to the patient's tolerance of short, intense exercise as compared to that of longer, milder efforts. Most metabolic disorders that affect skeletal muscle do so by altering energy metabolism. Muscle at rest uses fatty acids as its main energy source. During intense exercise anaerobic glycolysis and utilization of muscle glycogen occur. During sustained exercise fatty acids become an important source of fuel. Exercise, fasting, cold, infections, and medications may elicit symptoms of metabolic disorders that affect muscle. Important causes of metabolic myopathy include adenosine monophosphate (myoadenylate) deaminase deficiency and disorders of glycolysis, glycogenolysis, fatty acid oxidation, and oxidative phosphorylation. In many cases other organs are involved. Diagnosis requires careful attention to dietary and exercise history, as well as appropriate laboratory investigations. Exercise testing, electromyogram, and muscle biopsy can provide essential information. Treatment depends on avoiding precipitating factors and on optimizing muscle energetics. Malignant hyperthermia can occur with anesthesia in patients with metabolic myopathies.

Many metabolic disorders cause muscle dysfunction or damage (Table 19.1). The pathophysiologic basis in many disorders is impairment of energy production under stress, especially that induced by exercise, cold, fasting, or infection (especially of viral origin). In some situations the problem is confined to skeletal muscle; but in many cardiac involvement also is found. The liver, brain, retinas, and kidneys, all of which have significant energy requirements, may also be involved. More extensive or patchy involvement (e.g., pancreas and bone marrow) is characteristic of the mitochondrial disorders, where heteroplasmy may occur (see Chapter 6, "Mitochondrial DNA and Oxidative Phosphorylation," under "Work-up of the Patient with Lactic Acidemia").

SPECIAL ASPECTS OF SKELETAL MUSCLE METABOLISM

Skeletal muscle relies on different fuel sources at different times and circumstances. Impairment of muscle energy metabolism will lead to clinical symptoms. The history of the events that elicit the symptoms is a guide to the likely area of the biochemical defect.

Resting muscle in the fed state uses fatty acids as the primary fuel; glucose is stored as muscle glycogen (in the cytoplasm). Preformed high-energy phosphate compounds and muscle glycogen, in addition to glucose and fatty acids in the bloodstream, are the energy source for short-term, intense activity. Lactate is the end product of anaerobic glycolysis. Impaired ability to utilize muscle glycogen (e.g., glycogen storage diseases III—debrancher deficiency, V—muscle phosphorylase deficiency, and muscle phosphorylase kinase deficiency) results in a significant limitation when the patient attempts short, intense exercise. Production of pyruvate and, hence, of lactate diminishes. The situation is magnified if a tourniquet deprives the muscle being tested of oxygen and continuous fuel. This constitutes the basis for the ischemic exercise test (see Chapter 11, "Forearm Ischemia Test").

Defects of glycolysis in muscle (e.g., deficiencies of muscle phosphofructokinase [PFK], phosphoglycerate kinase [PGK], phosphoglycerate mutase [PGM], and lactate dehydrogenase [LDH]) can cause symptoms similar to muscle phosphorylase deficiency. Figure 19.1 shows the pathways of glycogenolysis and glycolysis.

When sustained muscle activity is initiated, the initial reliance is on glucose and glycogen as a fuel source. Metabolic disorders affecting their use typically cause symptoms at this time. After a few minutes glycogen stores are depleted, and fatty acids become more important as a fuel. The carnitine cycle and the β-oxidation spiral of fatty acid oxidation are essential at this point, so defects in these pathways result in easy fatigability and impaired tolerance of sustained exercise.

BASIC PATTERNS OF METABOLIC MYOPATHIES

The two major distinct syndromes of muscle metabolic disorders are rhabdomyolysis (with or without myoglobinuria), and weakness (with or without hypotonia). Rhabdomyolysis can be divided further into syndromes in which it occurs during strenuous exercise and those in which it occurs afterward.

Rhabdomyolysis, the destruction of skeletal muscle cells, often results from failure in energy production that leads to an inability to maintain muscle membranes. The hallmark of rhabdomyolysis is elevation of muscle enzymes in the blood, particularly of creatine kinase (CK or CPK). This elevation can persist for several days after an acute event. Chronic elevation of CK indicates ongoing damage.

Rhabdomyolysis during short-term intensive exercise is a primary feature of the disorders of carbohydrate metabolism, including muscle phosphorylase, phosphofructokinase, and phosphoglycerate kinase deficiencies. After a period of intense pain either with or without cramping, considerable relief and an ability to continue to exercise, called the "second wind" phenomenon, may occur as the muscle switches to the increased use of fatty acids for fuel. Postexercise cramps and rhabdomyolysis are more common in fatty acid disorders, especially with deficiencies of carnitine palmitoyltransferase (CPT) II, very-long-chain acyl-CoA dehydrogenase (VLCAD), long-chain hydroxyacyl-CoA dehydrogenase (LCHAD), and short-chain hydroxyacyl-CoA dehydrogenase (SCHAD) (see also Chapter 6, "Approach to the Child Suspected of Having a Disorder of Fatty Acid Oxidation"), and in mitochondrial oxidative phosphorylation disorders. Rhabdomyolysis may also be a chronic feature of the various muscular dystrophies, which are disorders of the structural proteins of muscle (e.g., dystrophin, actin, tropomyosin).

(*text continues on page 249*)

Table 19.1. Summary table of major presentations of metabolic myopathies

	Enzyme (position in pathway— Fig. 19.1)	Rhabdomyolysis	Hypotonia, weakness	Cramps	Worsened by fasting?	Worsened by exercise?	Worsened by cold?	Worsened by infection?
A. Rhabdomyolysis and myoglobinuria presentation								
1. Intense exercise not tolerated; second-wind phenomenon		++	+	++		++		
GSD type V	Muscle phosphorylase (II)	++	+	++		++		
GSD type VIII	Muscle phosphorylase kinase (II)	+	+	+		+		
GSD type VII	Muscle phosphofructokinase (8)*	+	+	+		+	++	
PGK deficiency	Muscle phosphoglycerate kinase (III)*	++		++		++		
PGM deficiency	Phosphoglycerate mutase (III)*	++		++		++		
LDH deficiency	Lactic dehydrogenase, M subunit (12)*	++				++		

Incr. baseline CK	Abnormal EMG	Muscle biopsy	Organic acids	Carnitine level	Acylcarnitine profile	Cardiomyopathy	Hepatic dysfunction[†]	Encephalopathy[†]	Diagnostic tissues	Comments
+	+	+								*Disorders of glycogenolysis and glycolysis; AMP deficiency*
+		+							M	Occ. severe inf. form. Proximal > distal
+		+				1 form			M	Four syndromes, two involving skeletal muscle
++	+	++				+			M, E	Hemolytic anemia. Rare. Hyperuricemia. Muscle cannot utilize glucose—worse after glucose, high-CHO meal. Severe infantile form with cardiomyopathy.
++		++	–				+	+	M	Hemolytic anemia, X-linked, neurologic abnormalities.
++	–	++	–						M	Very rare.
		–	–						M	Very rare. Ischemic exercise: lactate does not rise when pyruvate is elevated.

continued

Table 19.1.   *Continued.*

	Enzyme (position in pathway— Fig. 19.1)	Rhabdomyolysis	Hypotonia, weakness	Cramps	Worsened by fasting?	Worsened by exercise?	Worsened by cold?	Worsened by infection?
Myoadenylate deaminase deficiency	Muscle AMP deaminase	+	+	+		+		
2. Short, intense exercise tolerated; prolonged exercise not tolerated.		+	+	++	++	++	++	++
Translocase deficiency	Carnitine-acylcarnitine translocase (22)*							
CPT II deficiency	Carnitine palmitoyl-transferase II (23)*	++			++	++	++	++
VLCAD deficiency	Very-long-chain acyl-CoA dehydro-genase (24)*	++	+		++	+		+
LCAD deficiency	Long-chain acyl-CoA dehydrogenase (24)*							
LCHAD/trifunctional enzyme deficiency	Long-chain 3-hydroxy-acyl-CoA dehydro-genase (26)*	++						

Incr. baseline CK	Abnormal EMG	Muscle biopsy	Organic acids	Carnitine level	Acylcarnitine profile	Cardiomyopathy	Hepatic dysfunction[+]	Encephalopathy[+]	Diagnostic tissues	Comments
−	+	++							L	Impaired ammonia production with ischemic exercise.
+	+	++	++	+	++	++	++	++		*Disorders of fatty acid oxidation and carnitine-assisted transport into mitochondria.*
			+	+	++	++	++	+	F	
		++	+	↓	++	++	++	+	F, M, L, W	Heterozygote may have symptoms; vulnerable to malignant hyperthermia. Lactic acidosis. Sensorimotor neuropathy.
+	++		++	++	++	++	++	+	F, W, L	
									F, W, L	Uncommon; see text.
			++	++	++	++	++	++	F, M, L, D	HELLP syndrome in pregnant heterozygote.

continued

Table 19.1.   *Continued.*

	Enzyme (position in pathway— Fig. 19.1)	Rhabdomyolysis	Hypotonia, weakness	Cramps	Worsened by fasting?	Worsened by exercise?	Worsened by cold?	Worsened by infection?
MCAD deficiency	Medium-chain acyl-CoA dehydrogenase (24)*	–	(+)		++	+	–	++
SCAD deficiency	Short-chain acyl-CoA dehydrogenase (24)*		++					
SCHAD deficiency	Probably a form of MAD (see below).	++						+
B. Hypotonia and weakness presentation		+	++		+	+		
Carnitine transporter deficiency	Plasma membrane carnitine transporter (20)*	–	++		++			
Secondary carnitine depletion			++			+	+	+
MAD deficiency	Electron-transfer flavoprotein (ETF) or ETF dehydrogenase (ETF-QO)		+					

Incr. baseline CK	Abnormal EMG	Muscle biopsy	Organic acids	Carnitine level	Acylcarnitine profile	Cardiomyopathy	Hepatic dysfunction[†]	Encephalopathy[†]	Diagnostic tissues	Comments
			+	++	++	+	++	++	F, L, W, D	Myopathy is minimal; this is the most common disorder of fatty acid oxidation. Most early cases called systemic carnitine deficiency.
	+		++				++	++	F, M, L	Rare. Extremely variable.
						++	++		F, M, L	Very rare.
+	+	+		+		+	+			*Carnitine deficiency or depletion; Pompe disease; glycogen brancher and debrancher deficiencies.*
+	+	++	+	↓↓		++	++	+	F, M, L, K	
	+	+	+	↓↓		+	++	+		Occurs in many settings
	+	+	++	+	++	++	++	++	F, M, L	Mild forms exist—may respond to riboflavin.

continued

Table 19.1.   *Continued.*

	Enzyme (position in pathway— Fig. 19.1)	Rhabdomyolysis	Hypotonia, weakness	Cramps	Worsened by fasting?	Worsened by exercise?	Worsened by cold?	Worsened by infection?
Lysosomal glycogen storage disease (Pompe)	Acid maltase		++					
GSD type III	Glycogen debrancher (II)*	+	++	+				
GSD type IV	Glycogen brancher enzyme (I)*		+					
C. Mitochondrial myopathies	Many disorders and mechanisms. (See Chapter 6, "Work-up of the Patient with Lactic Acidemia".)	+	++	+		+	+	+

Abbreviations for diagnostic tissues: D, DNA (predominant or common mutation); E, erythrocytes; F, fibroblasts; H, heart; K, kidney, L, liver; M, muscle; W, leukocytes. This list is only a guide. Which tissue is required and which test is to be done depend on the laboratory performing the test and, in some cases, on the organs affected.

Incr. baseline CK	Abnormal EMG	Muscle biopsy	Organic acids	Carnitine level	Acylcarnitine profile	Cardiomyopathy	Hepatic dysfunction[†]	Encephalopathy[†]	Diagnostic tissues	Comments
++	+	++				++			W, M, F	Variable. Macroglossia, severe cardiomyopathy in infantile Pompe form.
++		++				Most, but symptoms rare	++		E, F, H, L, M, W	Liver ± muscle. Distal > proximal.
		++				+	++		L, M, W, E, F, D	Severe liver disease. Neuropathy, dementia in adult form.
+	+	++	+	+	+	++	+	++	M, W, L, H, F	Several syndromes. See "Mitochondrial DNA and Oxidative Phosphorylation," Chapter 6. Lactate/pyruvate ratio usually increased.

Abbreviations: AMP, adenosine monophosphate; CHO, carbohydrate; CK, creatine kinase; CPT, carnitine palmitoyltransferase; EMG, electromyogram; GSD, glycogen storage disease; HELLP, hemolysis, elevated liver function, and low platelets; incr., increased; inf., infantile; LCAD, long-chain acyl-CoA dehydrogenase; LCHAD, long-chain hydroxyacyl-CoA dehydrogenase; LDH, lactic dehydrogenase; MAD, multiple acyl-CoA dehydrogenase; MCAD, medium-chain acyl-CoA dehydrogenase; occ., occasional; PGK, phosphoglycerate kinase; PGM, phosphoglycerate mutase; SCAD, short-chain acyl-CoA dehydrogenase; SCHAD, short-chain hydroxyacyl-CoA dehydrogenase; VLCAD, very-long-chain acyl-CoA dehydrogenase.

++ Often present or abnormal. + Occasionally present or abnormal. See text for details about specific disorders.

* The numbers in parentheses refer to Fig. 19.1 and to their place in the pathways, which is given in the legend.

[†] Hepatic dysfunction together with encephalopathy is a "Reyelike syndrome."

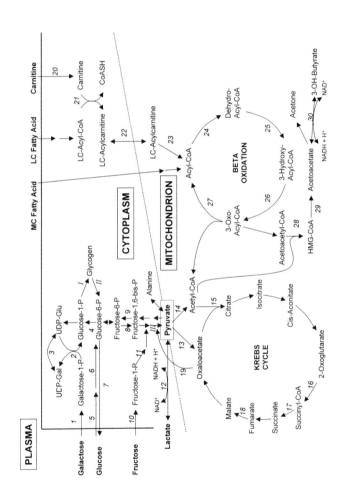

Myoglobinuria is an extreme result of rhabdomyolysis. When muscle cells lyse, they release myoglobin. When myoglobin appears in the urine in visible amounts, extensive damage can result. Typically, no myoglobin is found in the urine if the CK is less than 10,000 IU, so the absence of myoglobinuria provides no reassurance regarding the absence of rhabdomyolysis.

Myoglobinuria is an emergency situation, as the pigment may precipitate in the renal tubules, leading to possibly irreversible renal failure. Severe rhabdomyolysis can raise the serum potassium level dangerously high, leading to disturbances of cardiac

←

Figure 19.1.   Major aspects of carbohydrate metabolism illustrating the different steps and interrelations of glycogenolysis, glycolysis, and mitochondrial energy metabolism.
Single arrows and *Arabic numerals* represent single steps; *sequential arrows* and *Roman numerals* represent multiple steps.

I.   Glycogen synthesis—glycogen synthase, brancher enzyme.
II. Glycogenolysis—phosphorylase kinase, phosphorylase, debrancher enzyme.
III. Glycolysis—the individual enzymes, such as phosphoglycerate kinase and phosphoglyceromutase, are listed below.

1. Galactose kinase
2. Galactose-1-phosphate uridyl transferase
3. Epimerase
4. Phosphoglucomutase
5. Glucose transporter
6. Hexokinase
7. Glucose-6-phosphatase
8. Phosphofructokinase
9. Fructose-1,6-diphosphatase
10. Fructokinase
11. Fructose aldolase
12. Lactate dehydrogenase
13. Pyruvate carboxylase
14. Pyruvate dehydrogenase complex
15. Citrate synthase
16. 2-Oxoglutarate dehydrogenase complex
17. Succinyl-CoA synthetase
18. Fumarase
19. Phosphoenolpyruvate carboxykinase
20. Carnitine transporter
21. Carnitine palmitoyltransferase I (CPT I)
22. Carnitine-acylcarnitine translocase
23. Carnitine palmitoyltransferase II (CPT II)
24. Acyl-CoA dehydrogenases (very-long-chain [VLCAD], long-chain [LCAD], medium-chain [MCAD], short-chain [SCAD])
25. 2-Enoyl-CoA hydratase (trifunctional enzyme, crotonase)
26. 3-Hydroxyacyl-CoA dehydrogenase (long-chain [trifunctional enzyme/LCHAD], short-chain [SCHAD])
27. 3-Oxoacyl-CoA thiolase (long-chain [trifunctional enzyme], short-chain) Acetoacetyl-CoA is the 4-carbon 3-ketoacyl-CoA.
28. Hydroxymethylglutaryl-CoA (HMG-CoA) synthase
29. Hydroxymethylglutaryl-CoA (HMG-CoA) lyase
30. 3-OH-butyrate (β-hydroxybutyrate) dehydrogenase

rhythm. Accordingly, dark urine in a patient suffering from muscle symptoms (pain, weakness, cramping) must be tested for myoglobin using a specific test that distinguishes the pigment from hemoglobin. Hemoglobinuria most often accompanies hematuria, which is readily detectable by finding erythrocytes on microscopic analysis of the urine. Intravascular hemolysis occasionally results in hemoglobinuria without hematuria.

Myoglobinuria is treated with diuresis and careful monitoring of electrolyte, fluid status, and urine output until the myoglobinuria resolves. Investigation for the underlying cause of myoglobinuria begins at the same time as treatment.

Chronic weakness and hypotonia are typical features of disorders of glycogen breakdown, carnitine availability, fatty acid oxidation, and oxidative phosphorylation. Important causes include lysosomal glycogen storage disease (acid maltase deficiency—Pompe disease); glycogen debrancher deficiency; carnitine transporter defect and secondary carnitine deficiencies; VLCAD, LCHAD, and SCHAD deficiencies; and the mitochondrial myopathies. Chronic weakness may certainly result from the repeated destruction of muscle, which occurs with recurrent rhabdomyolysis.

APPROACH TO METABOLIC MYOPATHIES

The most urgent issues in assessing myopathy involve determining if the weakness is so severe that it impairs respiration, if damage is sufficient enough to lead to myoglobinuria, and if cardiac involvement is seen. Hepatic involvement, often manifesting itself as hypoglycemia and fasting intolerance, occurs in many metabolic disorders, particularly in those that involve glycogen or fatty acid metabolism. Encephalopathy may also be present.

The history of muscle dysfunction may be easy to elicit from either an adult or a child, but determining it in infants can be more difficult. Hypotonia and weakness may first become evident as a developmental delay. Careful assessment may then reveal that social, fine-motor, and language skills are appropriate for the child's age and that the only area of delay is in gross motor skills.

As a young child grows older, problems with exercise intolerance and easy fatigability become easier to detect, particularly if an unaffected older sibling serves as a reference point for the parents. Occasionally, a child with a muscle disorder is thought to be seeking attention or malingering, but careful history and observation can usually eliminate this possibility. Laboratory tests that demonstrate ongoing muscle injury (elevated CK, for example) are most persuasive.

Disorders made worse by fasting may not be evident in infancy as most infants are fed frequently. An inability to tolerate intense or prolonged exercise will not be evident in infancy and may not be seen until adulthood. Rhabdomyolysis in response to cold also may not become apparent until adolescence or adulthood. Rhabdomyolysis triggered by infection (usually of viral origin) or fasting may occur in infancy as sudden weakness accompanied by dark urine. Rhabdomyolysis is often, but not always, quite painful.

Some conditions can cause severe and potentially fatal rhabdomyolysis in children, particularly in the setting of viral infection. Children with such conditions, like those with disorders of fatty acid oxidation and mitochondrial dysfunction, need to be monitored carefully during infections.

The history of exercise can provide helpful preliminary guidance in determining the most likely causes of a myopathy. An inability to perform sudden intense exercise suggests a problem with glycogenolysis or glycolysis, whereas inability to sustain performance hints at a problem with fatty acid oxidation.

Many mitochondrial disorders of oxidative phosphorylation first become apparent because of skeletal muscle weakness. Rhabdomyolysis is uncommon. Mitochondrial disorders may have prominent muscle involvement, and they can involve any organ at any age. Other organs commonly affected include the brain, retina, extraocular muscles, heart, liver, kidney, pancreas, gut, and bone marrow. Systemic growth may be impaired. Mild hypertrichosis often accompanies systemic lactic acidosis. Despite the diversity of mitochondrial dysfunctions, many patients can be conveniently grouped into several common syndromes. These include myoclonic epilepsy with ragged red fibers (MERRF); mitochondrial encephalomyopathy, lactic acidemia, and stroke-like episodes (MELAS); and infantile myopathy.

Genetics

Most metabolic myopathies, like other metabolic disorders, are inherited in an autosomal recessive manner. All disorders of fatty acid oxidation and most disorders of glycogen and glucose metabolism are inherited this way. However, X-linked recessive (one form of phosphorylase b kinase deficiency, as well as phosphoglycerate kinase deficiency), autosomal dominant (heterozygous carnitine palmitoyltransferase II [CPT II] deficiency), mitochondrially transmitted, and sporadic mitochondrial disorders occur.

Because of the highly variable nature of most metabolic disorders of muscle, all siblings of the patients should be checked for the condition. If the disorder may be dominant, X-linked, or mitochondrially inherited, other relatives should also be examined carefully.

Physical Examination

The general physical examination of a patient suspected of myopathy includes assessment of growth and development. The muscles should be examined for bulk, regional (proximal, distal) or local evidence of wasting, texture, consistency, and tenderness. Deep tendon reflexes, which are generally preserved in myopathies but lost in peripheral neuropathies, should be tested carefully. Attention should also be directed to extraocular movements and the retina, the appearance of the tongue, the heart, and the size and character of the liver.

Laboratory Investigations

Laboratory investigation of suspected myopathies should be undertaken during the acute episode, if possible, and should be completed later, as indicated. Useful information can be obtained from serum electrolytes; the routine measurement of glucose, urea, creatinine, "muscle enzymes" including creatine kinase, lactate dehydrogenase (LDH) (including isoforms), aldolase, serum glutamic-oxaloacetic transaminase (SGOT) or aspartate aminotransferase (AST), serum glutamic-pyruvic aminotransferase (SGPT) or alanine aminotransferase (ALT), and total and free carnitine; a plasma or blood spot acylcarnitine profile; and levels of plasma lactate and pyruvate, phosphate, calcium, thyroid hormone, plasma and urine amino acids, and urine organic acids.

Following the assessment of the first-order laboratory tests, further tests may be warranted. Functional testing using ischemic exercise (for suspected glycogen storage and glycolytic disorders and adenosine monophosphate deaminase deficiency) can be helpful (see Chapter 11, "Forearm Ischemia Test"). Graded exercise or bicycle ergometry (for fatty acid oxidation disorders, mitochondrial disorders) may help pinpoint the metabolic error or may define the general area of impairment if history and blood tests have not done so. A "diagnostic fast" to evoke abnormal metabolites or to provoke symptoms has become a second-line investigation; challenges to fibroblasts or tissue samples can prove more beneficial. However, a fast under controlled circumstances can provide valuable information regarding the length of time that a particular child can safely fast when healthy (see Chapter 11, "Monitored Prolonged Fast").

Third-order tests include the electromyogram (EMG) (often coupled with nerve conduction studies), chest X-ray, electrocardiogram, echocardiogram, and muscle biopsy (perhaps with nerve biopsy). Light and electron microscopic examination and special stains for glycogen, lipids, and various enzymes may all be essential. Many enzymes can be studied in fibroblasts or lymphocytes, and DNA, for certain mutations, can be obtained from the blood or a buccal brush instead of from tissue biopsy. Mitochondria for functional and molecular studies can be prepared from muscle, liver, leukocytes, and other samples. Chapter 12 gives details of these tests. Table 19.1 provides a guide to the principal features of the major metabolic myopathies and to the usefulness of the various diagnostic tests.

SPECIFIC DISORDERS OF MUSCLE METABOLISM
Rhabdomyolysis and Myoglobinuria Presentation

Intense exercise is not tolerated, although mild prolonged exercise is. Fasting is tolerated. Diet modification is helpful.

Muscle Glycogen Phosphorylase (Myophosphorylase) Deficiency: McArdle Disease (Glycogen Storage Disease Type V)

McArdle disease, a dramatic disorder of muscle glycogen metabolism, is a relatively common cause of rhabdomyolysis and myoglobinuria. Although it is inherited in an autosomal recessive manner, most symptomatic patients are men. Symptoms usually begin between late childhood and late middle age. Strenuous exercise leads rapidly to cramping and fatigue, but after a period of rest (adaptation), exercise is tolerated. Some patients with McArdle disease have chronic progressive weakness and wasting without pain or cramping.

Exceptional cases include a rapidly fatal form in infants or young children that includes hypotonia and generalized weakness, late-onset cases with chronic weakness, and late-onset cases with severe symptoms (pain, cramping, weakness, and muscle swelling) after decades of normal activity. Inadvertent discovery of elevated CK in a child without symptoms has also been reported.

The symptoms and response to ischemic exercise suggest the diagnosis. The enzyme is expressed mainly in muscle. Muscle biopsy may show myopathic changes and increased glycogen content.

Specific treatment is generally not needed as avoiding strenuous exercise prevents symptoms in most patients. Some have suggested a high-protein, low-carbohydrate diet to help improve endurance. Others have found increased carbohydrate intake (glucose, fructose) immediately before exercise helpful.

Muscle Glycogen Phosphorylase Kinase Deficiency (Formerly Phosphorylase B Kinase Deficiency, GSD VIII)

A few instances of a few men with deficiency of muscle phosphorylase kinase have been reported. Some patients have weakness without cramps; others report cramps without weakness. Increased muscle glycogen content, elevation of CK, and rhabdomyolysis have been observed. Enzyme deficiency in the muscle was demonstrated. The gene encoding the alpha subunit of phosphorylase kinase in muscle is found on the X chromosome, but it is distinct from the liver isoform (which is also on the X). Three autosomal components of the glycogen phosphorylase kinase system are also found. Autosomal recessive defects have been found in the beta and gamma peptides. No defects in the three delta subunit isoforms, which are calmodulins, have been reported.

Muscle Glycolytic Disorders

Deficiencies of the three glycolytic enzymes in muscle are rare causes of myopathy that are similar to muscle phosphorylase deficiency. They are phosphofructokinase, phosphoglycerate kinase, and phosphoglycerate mutase (Fig. 19.1). Hemolytic anemia occurs in all. Phosphoglycerate kinase deficiency is X-linked recessive. Patients may have neurologic problems (e.g., mental retardation, behavioral abnormalities, seizures, strokes). The other disorders are autosomal recessive.

Lactate Dehydrogenase (LDH-A) Deficiency

Lactate dehydrogenase catalyzes the conversion of pyruvate and NADH to lactate and NAD^+. The enzyme is a tetramer of H and M peptides, produced respectively from LDH-B and LCH-A genes. Homozygous deficiency of the M protein results in impaired muscle LDH activity. The result is impaired regeneration of NAD+ for anaerobic glycolysis and diminished production of lactate (with resulting high levels of pyruvate) with exercise, detectable by the ischemic exercise test. Cramps, weakness, and myoglobinuria can occur with strenuous exercise. Deficiency of LDH can result in failure of LDH to increase after tissue damage, producing a "false-negative" result. No syndrome is attributable to LDH-B deficiency.

Adenosine Monophosphate (Myoadenylate) Deaminase Deficiency

Adenosine monophosphate (AMP) (myoadenylate) deaminase deficiency, an autosomal recessive disorder of purine metabolism, is probably the most common metabolic myopathy; it causes impaired exercise tolerance, postexercise cramps, and myalgias (see also Chapter 28). Myoglobinuria is uncommon, but CK is often elevated after exercise. The onset of symptoms (usually consisting of pain after exercise) ranges from childhood to later adult life. In the U.S. population, perhaps 2% are homozygous for the deficiency, but most have no symptoms. Because AMP deaminase (AMPDA) deficiency is so common, it has sometimes been found by coincidence with a less common muscle disorder that by itself would account for the symptoms (e.g., muscle phosphorylase or phosphofructokinase deficiency). As only ischemic exercise testing or a specific assay or molecular test will reveal the enzyme deficiency, a selection bias for patients with muscle problems exists.

AMP deaminase catalyzes the deamination of AMP to IMP (inosine monophosphate) in the purine nucleotide cycle (see Fig. 28.1). During exercise an increased production of IMP and ammonia will occur; maintenance of the adenylate energy charge is accomplished by preventing AMP accumulation. A decrease in ATP and an increase in ammonia will also stimulate glycolysis by increasing the activity of phosphofructokinase. The increase in IMP may enhance glycogen phosphorylase as well. Finally, during intense exercise, AMP deaminase moves from the cytosol and binds to myosin, which suggests its importance in muscle metabolism during such times.

The diagnosis of AMP deaminase deficiency is approached by ischemic exercise, which ordinarily provokes a rise in blood ammonia level (see Chapter 11, "Forearm Ischemia Test"). If AMP is deficient, ammonia production will be diminished. Although this test is very sensitive, it does not distinguish between inherited and acquired AMP deficiency. Muscle biopsy may be normal, or it may show some myopathic changes. Specific staining for AMP deaminase is a generally reliable diagnostic test. Enzyme activity in deficient muscle ranges up to 15% of normal; some authorities regard activity of more than 2% as adequate enough to prevent symptoms. A common mutation accounts for most cases of inherited AMP deaminase deficiency. This nonsense mutation in exon 2, Q12X, can result in a severely truncated protein. However, an alternative splicing mechanism allows for phenotypic rescue by producing a shortened, but functional, protein. This may account for the great variability in symptoms among homozygotes with this mutation. The allele frequency was 0.13 (Caucasians) and 0.19 (African-Americans) in one study, which accounts for the observed homozygote frequency of about 0.02.

Many patients discovered to have AMP deaminase deficiency have other symptoms as well, especially neuromuscular disease. Diminished synthesis of AMP deaminase occurs in a variety of situations. This is called *acquired deficiency* and does not seem to have a direct genetic basis; the common mutation is not present at a frequency above the background rate in the general population.

Short, intense exercise is tolerated; prolonged exercise is not. Fasting is detrimental; diet effects are less pronounced. Symptoms may be triggered by infection. Restriction of long-chain fats, with increased medium-chain lipids, may be helpful, especially for cardiomyopathy.

Carnitine-Acylcarnitine Translocase Deficiency

An inability to import long-chain acylcarnitines into the mitochondrial matrix would be expected to cause serious difficulties, especially in cardiac and skeletal muscle and in the liver. The severe infantile form of translocase deficiency typically demonstrates this, beginning a day or two after birth. Cardiac (cardiomyopathy, usually hypertrophic) and hepatic (hypoglycemia, vomiting, hyperammonemia) dysfunction are more prominent than are hypotonia and weakness. Urinary organic acids show dicarboxylic aciduria, and the plasma–blood spot acylcarnitine profile is dominated by long-chain species (C16:1, C18:1, C18:2), which can be formed but not used, as well as dicarboxylic acylcarnitines.

CPT II Deficiency

Carnitine palmitoyltransferase II (CPT II) deficiency is the most common disorder of fatty acid oxidation to cause episodic rhabdomyolysis. CPT II is needed to synthesize long-chain acylcarnitines once they have been translocated into the mitochondria, so the clinical features are similar to translocase deficiency. Prolonged exercise, cold, infection, and emotional stress (which will increase catecholamines and fatty acid metabolism) may precipitate episodes, which usually do not occur in children. Cardiac involvement is uncommon in this form of CPT II deficiency.

Although this is an autosomal recessive disorder, heterozygosity for a mutation may be associated with subtle myopathy and the risk of malignant hyperthermia in response to anesthetics or muscle relaxants.

Plasma or blood spot acylcarnitine analysis shows prominent long-chain species, especially saturated and unsaturated C16 and C18 forms; and dicarboxylic aciduria, similar to translocase deficiency, may be found.

A severe form of infantile CPT II deficiency also exists. Hepatic encephalopathy with hypoketotic hypoglycemia, severe cardiac involvement, renal malformations, and low plasma and tissue carnitine levels may be present. This form is usually fatal because of cardiac complications. It is discussed in more detail in Chapter 15.

Treatment includes the avoidance of fasting and the provision of adequate fuel for the muscles. Medium-chain fatty acids do not need the carnitine system to enter the mitochondria, so they can be used in place of long-chain fats as a source of energy. There is a form of CPT I that is expressed solely in muscle. No clinical deficiency has been recognized so far.

Very-Long-Chain Acyl-CoA Dehydrogenase Deficiency

Very-long-chain acyl-CoA dehydrogenase (VLCAD) is the first enzyme of the beta-oxidation spiral. It is bound to the inner mitochondrial membrane. Deficiency of VLCAD is a common cause of metabolic myopathy and cardiomyopathy. For several years, the enzyme now known as VLCAD was called LCAD. Reports from before 1993 regarding LCAD deficiency almost always involve what is now called the true VLCAD. VLCAD utilizes fatty acids of 14 to 20 carbons. The fatty acids called very-long-chain fatty acids (VLCFA), with a chain length of more than 20 carbons, are metabolized in the peroxisomes by a different system altogether.

Impairment of VLCAD leads to variable dysfunction of skeletal and cardiac muscle, liver, and brain. Recurrent Reye syndrome with coma and hypoketotic hypoglycemia may occur. Muscle soreness and episodic rhabdomyolysis may be provoked by infection, cold, fasting, or emotional stress (perhaps mediated by catecholamines). Usually, dicarboxylic aciduria is found, although during severe metabolic derangement, it may be completely masked by excessive lactic aciduria so that it is indistinguishable from a primary defect of the respiratory chain. Carnitine depletion with low plasma and tissue levels is common, and acylcarnitine analysis shows prominence of the $C14:1$ (tetradecenoyl) species, which is derived from oleic acid ($C18:1$). Hepatic dysfunction may result in hyperammonemia and lipid accumulation. Muscle biopsy may show lipid storage, and the electromyogram (EMG) is often myopathic.

VLCAD deficiency, like other disorders of fatty acid oxidation, must be promptly treated during the acute episode with enough glucose to maintain the blood glucose level at 6 to 8 mM (see also Chapter 6, "Emergency Treatment of Inherited Metabolic Diseases"). The use of carnitine supplementation has been controversial on theoretical and experimental grounds, particularly because of the fear that long-chain acylcarnitines would accumulate and would provoke arrhythmias. However, few convincing reports have been published. Long-term management emphasizes the intake of adequate calories from carbohydrates, the avoidance of fasting, and supplementation with medium-chain triglycerides, which provides a source of fuel that can be metabolized without requiring VLCAD.

The enzyme now known as the long-chain acyl-CoA dehydrogenase (LCAD) is in the mitochondrial matrix. Its major substrates are unsaturated long-chain fatty acids that are 12 to 18 carbons long. True deficiencies are very uncommon, but, when present, they display clinical symptoms typical of disorders of fatty acid oxidation.

Long-Chain Hydroxyacyl-CoA Dehydrogenase (Including Trifunctional Protein) Deficiency

Long-chain hydroxyacyl-CoA dehydrogenase (LCHAD) deficiency often results in chronic myopathy, with rhabdomyolysis that may be extensive, particularly during viral infections. As in other disorders of long-chain fatty acids, cardiomyopathy and significant liver dysfunction, both of which may be fulminant, are often seen. The extent of chronic liver dysfunction can be greater than in other disorders, and fibrosis often occurs. Reyelike episodes of hepatic encephalopathy may ensue. In addition, peripheral neuropathy and retinopathy exist. The basis for these complications is not yet known.

The enzyme activity called long-chain hydroxyacyl-CoA dehydrogenase resides in an octameric protein ($\alpha 4\beta 4$), which is called the *trifunctional protein* for its ability to catalyze the 3-hydroxyacyl-CoA dehydrogenation, 2-enoyl-CoA hydration, and 3-oxoacyl-CoA thiolysis of long-chain acyl CoAs and which is located in the mitochondrial inner membrane. The first two activities reside in the alpha subunit; thiolase activity is located in the beta subunit. The two subunits depend on each other for stability.

Some relationship between the mutation and the symptoms is found. The most common mutation, 1528G>C (E510Q) in the alpha subunit (87% in one study), usually causes liver dysfunction with hypoketotic hypoglycemia in infancy.

LCHAD deficiency is an autosomal recessive disorder, and carriers are generally symptom-free. A particular complication of heterozygous (carrier) status for LCHAD deficiency, especially the E510Q mutation, causes serious liver disease during pregnancy when the mother is carrying an affected infant. The mother may suffer from acute fatty liver of pregnancy (AFLP) with nausea and anorexia, vomiting, and jaundice or from the HELLP syndrome of hypertension or hemolysis, elevated liver enzymes, and low platelets. This may result from the production of abnormal fatty acid metabolites by the fetus, which may overload the mother's ability to deal with them on top of the increased fatty acid mobilization that occurs during pregnancy. Prospective studies of women with AFLP or HELLP syndrome, however, have not found an increased number of carriers of LCHAD deficiency, indicating that other causes for these conditions exist. Women heterozygous for hepatic CPT I deficiency, which may cause a Reyelike syndrome in homozygotes, may also suffer from AFLP when carrying an affected fetus.

In untreated patients the urine organic acids reveal increased saturated and unsaturated dicarboxylic and hydroxy species. The plasma acylcarnitine profile typically shows elevation of hydroxy-C18:1 species, which, in combination with an elevation of two of the three long-chain species C14, C14:1, and hydroxy-C16, identifies more than 85% of patients with high specificity (less than 0.1% false-positive rate). Blood spot acylcarnitine analysis is not quite as sensitive as plasma because of higher levels of long-chain species in blood samples. Dietary treatment (restricted long-chain fats with supplementation of medium-chain triglycerides) will lower the concentration of the long-chain species, often to a normal level. Carnitine levels are usually low, especially during an acute illness, so it is often given at such times. Its usefulness as a chronic medication for myopathy (and whether it might provoke arrhythmias in certain situations—see "Carnitine Palmitoyl-CoA Transferase Deficiency" in Chapter 15) is a subject of current investigation.

Short-Chain Acyl-CoA Dehydrogenase Deficiency

Short-chain acyl-CoA dehydrogenase (SCAD) deficiency is extremely variable; it has been reported in both infants and adults. Muscle symptoms have ranged from a mild lipid myopathy with low muscle carnitine to a more severe condition with weakness, poor exercise tolerance, and myopathic EMG. Systemic symptoms of hepatic encephalopathy can occur. The impaired metabolism of short-chain acyl-CoAs leads to short-chain dicarboxylic aciduria (ethylmalonic and adipic, similar to multiple acyl CoA-dehydrogenase [MAD] deficiency) and increased butyrate. Acylcarnitine analysis may show increased C4 species.

Short-Chain Hydroxyacyl-CoA Dehydrogenase Deficiency

Short-chain hydroxyacyl-CoA dehydrogenase (SCHAD) deficiency is a very rare condition that is characterized by recurrent rhabdomyolysis, hypertrophic cardiomyopathy, and hypoketotic hypoglycemia. Mild dicarboxylic and hydroxydicarboxylic aciduria has been reported. The enzyme can be assayed in muscle or in mitochondria from skin fibroblasts.

Weakness and Hypotonia Presentation

Carnitine Transporter Deficiency

The carnitine transport defect is the result of a problem with the high-affinity carnitine transporter, which is active in the kidneys, muscle, heart, fibroblasts, and lymphocytes. Renal fractional excretion of carnitine, when calculated in relation to creatinine clearance, approaches 100% (normal < 5%). The severe plasma carnitine depletion that results (levels can be < 5 μmol/L; normal is approximately 45 μmol/L) will lead to tissue carnitine depletion as well. Hepatic carnitine depletion leads to hypoketotic hypoglycemia. Onset of myopathy and cardiomyopathy can occur in the first few months, or it can be delayed for several years. Urine organic acids are typically normal. Muscle biopsy reveals lipid accumulation, and the muscle carnitine level is extremely low. The patient's response to carnitine supplementation is dramatic, but because of the ongoing renal leak of carnitine, maintaining normal plasma carnitine levels or tissue levels is extremely difficult; exercise tolerance may be limited. Oral carnitine supplementation to an amount just short of provoking a fish odor (a trimethylamine) by exceeding the conjugating capacity is the usual approach. Inheritance is autosomal recessive; mutations have been found in the SLC22A5 gene.

Secondary Carnitine Depletion

Adults can synthesize all the carnitine they need. The major dietary source of carnitine is meat. The carnitine content of human breast milk is similar to that of plasma. Carnitine deficiency has occurred in several infants receiving total parenteral nutrition (TPN) (without added carnitine) and has resulted in myopathy and cardiomyopathy, impaired ketogenesis, and hepatic steatosis. Carnitine supplementation (intravenous or oral) in these patients has been rapidly beneficial. This experience suggests that carnitine may be an essential nutrient for the very young and that routine carnitine supplementation of TPN solutions for all infants should be considered.

Severe carnitine depletion can result from a generalized Fanconi syndrome as occurs in cystinosis, Lowe syndrome, and mitochondrial disorders (especially cytochrome C oxidase deficiency). See also Chapter 18, "Fanconi Syndrome." Recognition of the carnitine depletion usually occurs after the discovery of Fanconi syndrome. Plasma carnitine measurement and the determination of the fractional excretion should be part of the investigation of all patients with Fanconi syndrome. Restoration of tissue carnitine levels may take a very long time, even after correction of the renal leak, as occurs after transplantation for cystinosis.

Some medications, such as valproic acid and pivampicillin, are essentially organic acids, which may be excreted as carnitine esters, causing significant urinary losses of carnitine as valproylcarnitine or pivaloylcarnitine; these losses consequently induce secondary systemic carnitine deficiency. The use of pivampicillin has been linked to a life-threatening crisis, especially in patients with an underlying metabolic disorder (e.g., MCAD deficiency).

MCAD deficiency is unusual among fatty acid oxidation disorders because it has only minimal skeletal muscle symptoms. Hepatic and cerebral symptoms (e.g., Reyelike syndrome, hypoketotic hypoglycemia, sudden unexplained death) are the usual features. However, carnitine depletion can occur. MCAD deficiency accounted for nearly all the original patients described as suffering from "systemic carnitine deficiency," before the enzyme deficiency was discovered. It may be the mechanism for chronic weakness and impaired exercise tolerance in some older patients with MCAD deficiency. Long-term carnitine supplementation, whose use in MCAD deficiency is not universally accepted, may ameliorate this situation. Longitudinal studies have not yet been reported.

2,4-Dienoyl-CoA Reductase Deficiency

2,4-Dienoyl-CoA reductase deficiency, an extremely rare disorder, has been described in one infant with hypotonia, normal deep tendon reflexes, poor feeding, and failure to thrive. In this patient plasma carnitine was deficient; a unique unsaturated acylcarnitine (C10:2), which occurred in the plasma, was shown to be derived from long-chain unsaturated fatty acids.

Multiple Acyl-CoA Dehydrogenase Deficiency

Multiple acyl-CoA dehydrogenase deficiency (MAD), also known as glutaric aciduria type II (due to deficiency of electron-transfer flavoprotein [ETF] or ETF dehydrogenase), in its severe form causes overwhelming acidosis shortly after birth. Impairment of the ETF system blocks many different dehydrogenation systems for the degradation of fatty acids and amino acids. Milder deficiency of the same system can cause a lipid-storage myopathy that may not become apparent for years or decades. The gradual onset of weakness and easy fatigability may allow it to be overlooked initially, and the history may first suggest an inflammatory myopathy. Liver dysfunction may occur. Urine organic acids can show dicarboxylic aciduria, including ethylmalonic, adipic, and glutaric acids. Plasma acylcarnitine analysis demonstrates the elevation of short- and medium-chain species. Mitochondrial studies may show deficient activity of complex I and II. Response to supplemental riboflavin (50 to 100 mg/d), the precursor of the cofactor flavin adenine dinucleotide (FAD), is sometimes dramatic in the milder forms. A postulated disorder of riboflavin transport may be the cause of another similar disorder.

Lysosomal Glycogen Storage Disease Type II (Pompe Disease)

Pompe disease is the severe infantile form of acid maltase (lysosomal α-glucosidase) deficiency. It is one of the most common storage diseases presenting in infancy, and it was the first one to be identified. The infant typically presents in the first few months with weakness and profound hypotonia. Feeding and respiratory difficulties are common. Macroglossia with minimal hepatomegaly is found. At least 80% of infants with acid maltase deficiency have significant cardiac involvement. Progressive weakness and cardiomyopathy usually lead to death within a year. Despite the hypotonia the muscles feel firm or even woody.

A spectrum of deficiency of α-glucosidase occurs, with the onset of symptoms reported as late as the eighth decade of life. Various terms, including *juvenile* and *adult onset*, have been used to describe later onset patients. However, the age of onset bears no relation to the rapidity of the course. The older that the patient is, the more likely that symptomatic muscle involvement will be patchy clinically and morphologically. However, enzyme activity is deficient, regardless of the appearance of the cells. The function of lysosomal glycogen is not known. α-Glucosidase activity can be measured in leukocytes, as well as in muscle or liver biopsy or with cultured skin fibroblasts. Muscle biopsy, which is unnecessary for diagnosis if performance of an enzyme assay is possible, shows enlarged lysosomes that are engorged with glycogen, thus altering the ultrastructure of the cell.

No satisfactory treatment of Pompe disease was available until the development of enzyme replacement therapy. Two enzyme products are currently undergoing clinical trials.

Glycogen Debrancher Deficiency: Glycogen Storage Disease Type III (Cori or Forbes Disease)

Glycogen debrancher deficiency, a relatively common disorder of glycogen metabolism, results from varying deficiencies of the amylo-1,6-glucosidase, the debrancher enzyme, a remarkable peptide that has two separate catalytic activities (transferase and glucosidase). Liver involvement is always seen, but muscle involvement varies; it does not occur at all in about 15% of patients (GSD IIIb). In infancy and childhood, the liver symptoms dominate, with hepatomegaly, hyperlipidemia, and fasting hypoglycemia similar to GSD I. Muscle weakness may not be apparent. After puberty the liver symptoms subside, but the myopathy may persist as weakness and may worsen with time. CK concentrations in the blood may be elevated, or they may be normal, even with muscle involvement. Distal wasting, myopathic EMG, and peripheral neuropathy can occur. Mild cardiac involvement may be found as well.

The history suggests the diagnosis. Western blot analysis of fibroblasts or lymphocytes can demonstrate low levels of enzymatic activity. Enzyme assay can be done using fibroblasts, lymphocytes, or muscle or liver tissue. Analysis of glycogen structure in the muscle or liver can demonstrate abnormalities due to the lack of normal glycogen breakdown. Differences in phenotype can be correlated with different mutations. The differences in tissue expression may be traceable to alternate splicing of exon 1 of the amylo-1,6-glucosidase gene. Molecular techniques may eventually replace direct enzyme analysis, but currently, direct evaluation of muscle must be used to be sure about muscle involvement.

High-protein meals and high-protein enteral overnight feeds have been used to treat the myopathy. Alanine supplementation, which lowers levels of CK and transaminases, may be of clinical benefit.

Glycogen Brancher Deficiency: Glycogen Storage Disease Type IV (Anderson Disease)

Type IV glycogen storage disease, a glycogen brancher deficiency, can cause hypotonia and weakness, but the clinical picture is dominated by hepatic fibrosis and dysfunction. Cardiomyopathy may be significant in the severe infantile form.

Mitochondrial Myopathies

The mitochondrial myopathies are an extremely heterogeneous group of disorders. Symptoms may be confined to muscle tissue, or they may involve other organs, particularly the brain, heart, liver, and kidneys. In addition, symptoms may be present at birth, or they may not appear for decades. Myopathy is particularly evident in the syndromes of chronic progressive external ophthalmoplegia (CPEO), including the Kearns–Sayre syndrome (KSS) or ophthalmoplegia-plus; MELAS; MERRF; fatal infantile mitochondrial myopathy; depletion of the mitochondrial DNA; and autosomal dominant and recessive mitochondrial myopathies. Molecular defects can be in the mitochondrially encoded tRNAs, in mitochondrial and nuclear-encoded subunits of the oxidative phosphorylation complexes, and in many other proteins. Table 6.7 shows some of the most relevant disorders and etiologies.

Muscle symptoms are generally those of chronic weakness and impaired exercise tolerance. Cramps are unusual. Rhabdomyolysis can occur, particularly in the setting of sustained exercise or febrile illness. Malignant hyperthermia may occur with anesthesia or muscle relaxants.

Systemic lactic acidosis may be present at rest, or it may be elicited by exercise. CK may be elevated, and plasma amino acids may show increased alanine. Urinary organic acids may show increased lactate, citric acid cycle intermediates, and dicarboxylic fatty acids. The plasma carnitine level may be either normal or low. Plasma acylcarnitine analysis may show a generalized increase in short- and medium-chain species, especially in acetylcarnitine.

EMG may be normal, or it may suggest myopathy; nerve conduction studies may reveal a peripheral neuropathy (usually axonal).

Muscle tissue can be analyzed for carnitine content, acylcarnitine species, and coenzyme Q level. Muscle biopsy may show dense clusters of abnormal mitochondria, especially near the surface of the cell membrane ("ragged-red fibers"), as well as an increase in lipids; however, they may also be normal (see Chapter 12). Cells may stain strongly for succinate dehydrogenase (complex II) yet may not stain for cytochrome oxidase (COX), particularly in CPEO, KSS, and MERRF. Maternally inherited Leigh syndrome patients may have deficient COX staining but no ragged-red fibers. Electron microscopy may show abnormal mitochondrial morphology, including paracrystalline inclusions.

Studies of oxidative phosphorylation are best carried out in fresh muscle biopsy tissue. Some laboratories are able to work with frozen muscle tissue or freshly isolated platelets. Mitochondrial DNA studies are optimally performed from muscle biopsy as well. If a heteroplasmic disorder occurs in the mtDNA, tissues that are more easily obtained (e.g., leukocytes and fibroblasts) sometimes give a misleading normal result. Mitochondrial myopathies are a subset of the mitochondrial cytopathies (see "General Considerations" in Chapter 6).

Mitochondrial disorders of oxidative phosphorylation are generally treated with a high-fat, low carbohydrate diet and supplemental vitamins and antioxidants, especially coenzyme Q (CoQ) (ubiquinone) and riboflavin (which may be quite helpful for complex I deficiency myopathy). Vitamin C, thiamine, vitamin E, vitamin K_3 (used as an artificial electron acceptor-donor), dichloroacetate, carnitine, and succinate have been used in various situations. Responses generally are subtle, but occasionally, a patient responds dramatically to CoQ or other therapies.

Myopathies with Major Cardiac Involvement

Chapter 15 discusses the cardiac manifestations of several disorders discussed in this chapter, including glycogen storage diseases types II and IV, fatty acid oxidation disorders (such as carnitine transport defect, deficiencies of carnitine-acylcarnitine translocase, CPT II, VLCAD, and LCHAD/trifunctional enzyme), and mitochondrial disorders.

Malignant Hyperthermia

Malignant hyperthermia (MH) occurs in response to anesthetics in many different situations and myopathies. MH is most commonly due to the failure to regulate calcium concentration in the sarcoplasmic reticulum. Excess calcium permits continuous muscle contraction, leading to heat generation and a rise in body temperature. Severe myoglobinuria, irreversible kidney damage, and death from hyperthermia or arrhythmia due to hyperkalemia may occur. For these reasons all patients with a myopathy must be carefully monitored during surgery or any other procedure where anesthesia is used; the most risky anesthetics (e.g., halothane) and muscle relaxants (e.g., suxamethonium) should not be used. Premedication with dantrolene can lessen the risk of problematic reactions. MH is often due to mutations in the ryanodine receptor RYR1 (with or without central core disease) or the alpha subunit of the gated sodium channel IV, SCN4A, which is altered in hypokalemic periodic paralysis and paramyotonia congenita. Patients with muscular dystrophies are also vulnerable. Even for these high-risk conditions, MH does not occur with each exposure to a triggering agent. Of the disorders of intermediary metabolism, which are the primary topic of this book, the greatest risk is for patients with CPT II deficiency (perhaps even for those in the heterozygous state) and with mitochondrial disorders; but all patients with metabolic myopathy should be regarded as at potential risk for malignant hyperthermia.

ADDITIONAL READING

Bonnefont J-P, Taroni F, Cavadini P, et al. Molecular analysis of carnitine palmitoyltransferase II deficiency with hepatocardiomuscular expression. *Am J Hum Genet* 1996;58:971–978.

Leonard JV, Schapira AH. Mitochondrial respiratory chain disorders I: mitochondrial DNA defects. *Lancet* 2000;355:299–304.

Leonard JV, Schapira AH. Mitochondrial respiratory chain disorders II: neurodegenerative disorders and nuclear gene defects. *Lancet* 2000;355:389–394.

Vladutiu GD, Bennett MJ, Smail D, et al. A variable myopathy associated with heterozygosity for the R503C mutation in the carnitine palmitoyltransferase II gene. *Mol Genet Metab*,2000;70:134–141.

20 ♣ Approach to the Patient with Psychiatric Problems

A number of inherited metabolic diseases display psychiatric symptoms that are compatible with various psychiatric diagnoses. With improvement in the treatment and prognosis of patients with inherited metabolic diseases, manifestations, such as psychiatric problems, that affect long-term quality of life become increasingly important in an older patient population. Psychiatric features may be the leading clinical correlate of certain inherited metabolic diseases, as well as a phenomenon observed in long-term care. Recognition of inherited metabolic diseases in the differential diagnosis of psychiatric manifestations is important since some metabolic diseases may be mistaken for a diagnosis such as schizophrenia. In acute intermittent porphyria (AIP), for example, psychiatric symptoms may be at the forefront of clinical manifestations. Careful examination of mental and neurologic status and psychiatric history and the recognition of psychotropic drugs or metabolic treatment regimens that exacerbate metabolic crises (e.g., in porphyrias or in Wilson disease) are mandatory.

Inherited metabolic diseases can manifest as acute attacks of delirium or psychosis, as well as intellectual disintegration, mental regression, or chronic psychosis.

ACUTE ATTACKS OF DELIRIUM, HALLUCINATIONS, MENTAL CONFUSIONS, HYSTERIA, OR PSYCHOSIS

Psychiatric features may be the first clinical link to the underlying metabolic defect. They may include hallucinations, delirium, dizziness, aggressiveness, anxiety, agitation, agony, or schizophrenic-like behavior. These presentations may be observed in acute attacks of metabolic diseases characterized by hyperammonemia, such as occur in urea cycle disorders (ornithine transcarbamylase [OTC] deficiency, lysinuric protein intolerance, or others), organic acidurias, or maple syrup urine disease (MSUD). Psychiatric manifestations classically are found in acute intermittent porphyria (AIP) or hereditary coproporphyria. In AIP, a disorder of heme biosynthesis that leads to intermittent elevations in porphobilinogen and related porphyrins, psychiatric manifestations of acute attacks consist of anxiety, depression, psychosis, or altered mental status. AIP is often mistaken for schizophrenia or hysteria. Before the initial attack, a high frequency of histrionic personality traits also occurs in many patients with AIP. An even higher incidence of anxiety disorder has also been found in otherwise asymptomatic carriers. For many patients with AIP, getting the correct diagnosis early is essential because many psychotropic drugs may induce or exacerbate an acute attack of porphyria. The metabolic crisis may induce or aggravate psychiatric symptoms, leading to a long-term psychiatric career that results from misinterpretation as treatment resistance. A correct diagnosis of porphyria requires the demonstration of pathologic metabolites in the urine and/or feces. A diagnostic approach that is primarily enzymatic or even molecular can be misleading. Patients suffering from methylene tetrahydrofolate reductase (MTHFR) deficiency are also sometimes identified as suffering from schizophrenia or psychosis. In these patients further symptoms often include stroke, seizures, and a progressive myelopathy.

PROGRESSIVE NEUROLOGIC AND MENTAL DETERIORATION

In general, psychiatric symptoms associated with inherited metabolic diseases are predominantly recognized in older children, adolescents, or adults (Table 20.1). However, considering the relationship of psychiatric manifestations to the age of the patient can be of interest.

Infancy (1 to 12 Months)

In infancy autistic features may be the leading clinical feature of metabolic disease. They have been observed in untreated phenylketonuria and inborn errors of biopterin metabolism. Autistic features may be present in infants affected by late-onset subacute forms of disorders associated with hyperammonemia, as in urea cycle disorders, as well as in infants with 4-hydroxybutyric aciduria, mevalonic aciduria, Smith–Lemli–Opitz syndrome, adenylosuccinase deficiency, dihydropyrimidine dehydrogenase deficiency, homocystinuria, Salla disease, nonketotic hyperglycinemia, or sulfite oxidase deficiency. In addition, patients with Smith–Lemli–Opitz syndrome often present with severe sleeping problems, as

Table 20.1.   Collection of routine and specific investigations for differential diagnosis of psychiatric symptoms in inherited metabolic diseases

Urine
  Amino acids
  Organic acids
  Porphyrins (urine and feces)
  Purines and pyrimidines
  N-acetylneuraminic acid
  Sulfite test (fresh urine)
  Oligosaccharides
  Copper

Plasma/serum
  Amino acids
  Lactate
  Very-long-chain fatty acids
  Copper

Histology including electron microscopy (skin biopsy, bone marrow, lymphocytes)

Enzyme studies (lysosomal enzymes, respiratory chain enzymes)

Mitochondrial DNA

well as with excessive screaming in early childhood. Children with the treatable pyrimidine nucleotide depletion disease in which cytosolic 5'-nucleotidase superactivity occurs develop a disorder similar to autism.

Childhood (1 to 5 Years)

Psychotic behavior is a typical clinical symptom of the late infantile form of G_{M2} gangliosidosis (Tay–Sachs, Sandhoff). These diseases are characterized mainly by developmental regression, spinocerebellar degeneration, ataxia, and spastic fright reaction. In this age group, awareness of diseases with arrest or regression of cognitive function is especially important. The most significant disorders are Rett syndrome and mucopolysaccharidosis (MPS) type III (Sanfilippo). In Rett syndrome girls are affected; they present with characteristic behavior, regression of developmental achievements, and stereotyped movements of fingers and hands. In MPS type III major clinical manifestations include regression of high-level achievements, as well as the loss of speech. Affected children often show agitation and aggressive behavior.

Childhood and Adolescence (5 to 15 Years)

Progressive neurologic and mental deterioration along with psychiatric manifestations can be found in a number of neurometabolic diseases, including juvenile neuronal ceroid lipofuscinosis (Spielmeyer–Vogt). Intellectual deterioration occurs in addition to loss of sight and retinitis. In patients with this disease, alteration in behavior, which may be seen years before other symptoms become evident, may be the presenting complaint. Dementia and deterioration also occur in metabolic diseases with predominant cerebellar ataxia, such as disorders of mitochondrial DNA like mitochondrial encephalomyopathy, lactic acidemia, and stroke-like episodes (MELAS), and in cerebrotendinous xanthomatosis, G_{M1} gangliosidosis, Gaucher disease, Niemann–Pick type C, the juvenile form of Krabbe disease, Lafora disease, and metachromatic leukodystrophy (MLD).

MLD is a lysosomal storage disease characterized by the accumulation of cerebroside sulfate in the central nervous system myelin, as well as in the kidney, gall bladder, and other visceral organs. Psychiatric manifestations are most often found in the late juvenile and adult age group and are characterized by psychosis with disorganized thoughts, delusions, and auditory hallucinations. In adult patients these findings may lead to a diagnosis of schizophrenia. The subsequent rapid intellectual deterioration to dementia should clue the clinician to suspect an underlying metabolic disease. The discovery of unrelated patients with similar psychiatric symptoms and the same arylsulfatase A mutation suggests that a single gene defect corresponds to a psychiatric presentation of MLD.

In childhood and adolescence a number of metabolic diseases can display psychiatric features as the only presenting symptoms before the recognition of any significant neurologic or extraneurologic signs. These manifestations include behavioral disturbances, personality and character changes, mental regression, dementia, or schizophrenia. In addition to the inherited metabolic diseases discussed earlier, these features may be at the forefront of the presentation in X-linked adrenoleukodystrophy, Hallervorden–Spatz disease, Huntington chorea, urea cycle disorders (especially hemizygous ornithine transcarbamylase deficiency), or Wilson disease.

In Wilson disease toxic tissue levels of copper cause damage primarily to the liver and the basal ganglia. Psychiatric manifestations may vary; they include personality changes, depressive episodes, cognitive dysfunction, and psychosis. The overall prevalence of psychiatric symptoms in Wilson disease is greater than 20%. Ten percent of the cases may present with psychiatric symptoms alone. A positive correlation is found between the presence of psychiatric and neurologic symptoms. Effective chelation treatment does improve most psychiatric symptoms. However, initiation of chelation treatment in Wilson disease may precipitate an acute psychiatric crisis.

Adulthood (> 15 Years)

In adulthood progressive neurologic and mental deterioration with preponderant psychosis and dementia may be found in a variety of the inherited diseases discussed in the preceding section, including MLD, Niemann–Pick type C, ceroid lipofuscinosis, cerebrotendinous xanthomatosis, Huntington chorea, Lafora, and Wilson diseases. In addition, psychiatric abnormalities have been reported in patients with homocystinuria due to cystathionine β-synthase (CBS) deficiency. Major diagnostic categories in patients with CBS deficiency include, in order of decreasing incidence, personality disorders, chronic disorders of behavior, episodic depression, and chronic obsessive-compulsive disorder. Schizophrenia is uncommon in CBS-deficient patients.

Phenylketonuria (PKU) in untreated patients results not only in mental retardation but in varying degrees of psychiatric pathology. Some adult patients with PKU that was treated early have exhibited an atypical pattern of psychopathology with a variety of symptoms, including anxiety and depression. PKU patients no longer observing their dietary restrictions have an increased risk of psychosocial difficulties. Agoraphobia has been recognized as a common symptom. That psychiatric disease, as a common occurrence, simply coexists in some of these patients is also possible. Interestingly, psychiatric symptoms observed in PKU are not clearly related to phenylalanine levels.

ADDITIONAL READING

Estrov Y, Scaglia F, Bodamer OAF. Psychiatric symptoms of inherited metabolic diseases. *J Inher Metab Dis* 2000;23:2–6.

21 ♣ Approach to the Patient with Ophthalmologic Problems

Ocular manifestations are frequent in inherited metabolic diseases. In some, ocular abnormalities are a leading finding, whereas in others these abnormalities are part of a multiple-organ spectrum of disease. The most important ophthalmologic anomalies associated with inherited metabolic diseases include cataracts, corneal opacity, and retinitis pigmentosa (RP). A helpful criterion for the differential diagnosis is the age of onset of cataracts or corneal opacities. The spectrum of diseases associated with cataracts includes defects of peroxisome biogenesis, galactosemia, Wilson disease, Sjögren–Larsson syndrome, and cerebrotendinous xanthomatosis. Corneal opacity is most commonly found in lysosomal disorders, defects of high-density lipoprotein (HDL) metabolism, and Fabry disease. The differential diagnosis of retinal abnormalities includes inborn errors of lipid metabolism, as well as peroxisomal and mitochondrial diseases.

CATARACT

Lens opacities at birth, if not diagnosed or removed, are a major cause of blindness or amblyopia. When cataracts are bilateral, they lead to irreversible nystagmus by 3 months of age. Thus, these cataracts must be quickly removed by surgery, preferably within the first few days or weeks of life. Screening for the orange or red retinal reflex with a dilute dilating eyedrop should be done soon after birth. Often, the retinal reflex can be visualized with an ophthalmoscope alone. The etiologic classification of congenital cataract is diverse, and more than 90% of congenital cataracts remain unexplained. The differential diagnosis includes a wide pathologic spectrum, including metabolic, chromosomal, infectious, traumatic, and toxic causes. They occur in syndromes with deafness, mental retardation, or dwarfism. Isolated cataracts, which may have early or later childhood onset, may be familial and are usually autosomal dominant.

The cataract that occurs after 8 to 9 years of age does not, after treatment, lead to amblyopia. However, the pediatrician must make establishing the child's overall good health a priority. If the clinician discovers cataracts, he or she should do a work-up for an underlying cause.

A number of inherited metabolic diseases must be included in the differential diagnosis of cataracts. Their etiology is usually determined by the constellations of symptoms with which the child presents. The age of onset is a helpful criterion for differential diagnosis of underlying inherited metabolic disease.

At Birth (Congenital)

At birth, cataracts are a constant finding in the X-linked inherited oculocerebrorenal syndrome of Lowe. A hallmark of this condition is the presence of congenital cataracts that develop prenatally and that are always present before birth. Affected neonates usually present with a multisystem disorder in which the nervous system and the kidneys are affected in addition to the major abnormalities found in the eyes. Other ocular abnormalities, such as glaucoma, microphthalmos, decreased visual acuity, and corneal keloid formation, may be present. Additionally, these patients have muscular hypotonia, areflexia, and profound retardation of mental development. Other major features include renal tubulopathy, Fanconi syndrome, and facial dysmorphia. Congenital cataracts in association with dysmorphic features are also frequently present in disorders of peroxisome biogenesis, such as the classic Zellweger syndrome and its variants (see Chapter 27). These neonates often have seizures and muscular hypotonia. When combined with chondrodysplasia punctata and rhizomelic dwarfism, congenital cataracts lead to the diagnosis of rhizomelic chondrodysplasia punctata. Cataracts at birth are also often seen in Cockayne syndrome, which is characterized by encephalopathy, retinitis, deafness, facial dysmorphia, and intracranial calcifications. Sorbitol dehydrogenase deficiency involves isolated cataracts at birth as the only presenting sign.

Newborn (First Week to First Month of Life)

During the first month of life, cataracts associated with liver failure, jaundice, and tubulopathy in a severely ill newborn comprise the phenotype of classical galactosemia due to galactose-1-phosphate uridyltransferase deficiency. In any newborn with cataracts who has received milk, the galactose-1-phosphate uridyl transferase activity should be measured in erythrocytes regardless of the results of neonatal screening. Cataracts are usually reversible after the introduction of a galactose-free diet. They can also occur very early in patients with galactokinase deficiency; these may not be recognized until later because no other signs of illness are present.

Some newborns with galactose-1-phosphate epimerase deficiency and newborns of mothers with the so-called marginal galactokinase deficiency have had cataracts. This occurrence supports the hypothesis that galactitol accumulation in the lens is the major cause of cataracts in these metabolic diseases. Detection of all three defects requires the determination of reducing substances in the urine, blood galactose, and erythrocyte galactose-1-phosphate.

Infancy (First Month to First Year)

In infancy, cataracts are the only clinical symptom for the different variants of galactokinase deficiency (total, partial, marginal maternal), as well as for galactitol or sorbitol accumulation of unknown origin. Cataracts can be part of a multiorgan system complex in lysosomal storage disorders, such as sialidosis or α-mannosidosis, which are also characterized by hepatosplenomegaly, coarse facies, and vacuolated lymphocytes. They can be found in infants with mitochondrial disease that presents with muscular hypotonia, encephalopathy, and lactic acidosis. Rarely, cataracts have been reported in infants with a severe form of mevalonic aciduria, hypobetalipoproteinemia, vitamin E or D deficiencies, or lactose intolerance. Some patients with diseases in which hypoglycemic episodes of various origins occur have also developed cataracts.

Childhood/Adolescence (1 to 15 Years)

Sunflower cataracts occur in 20% to 25% of patients with Wilson disease. At this age most patients present primarily with hepatic signs rather than with neurologic manifestations. In patients with hypocalcemia and bone changes caused by hypoparathyroidism and pseudohypoparathyroidism, cataracts may be a clinical finding. Minute opacities in the anterior fetal Y suture of both lenses that are often surrounded by minute satellites are frequent observations in lysinuric protein intolerance. These opacities are not large enough to cause visual impairment; they may remain stable for several years. In addition to hyperammonemia, hepatosplenomegaly, chronic diarrhea, osteoporosis, and growth retardation identify these patients.

Patients with the Sjögren–Larsson syndrome have cataracts; other features of the syndrome include spastic paraplegia, mental retardation, retinal degeneration, and ichthyosis. The last is usually one of the original clinical signs in this syndrome, which is caused by deficiency of fatty alcohol oxidoreductase. Cataracts may also be present in another syndrome characterized by ichthyosis, the so-called neutral lipid storage disorder. This syndrome whose origin is yet unknown includes ataxia, myopathy, and hepatomegaly as further clinical features. Vacuolated lymphocytes are a frequent finding in the peripheral blood.

Corneal verticillata is the most common ocular finding in Fabry disease, an inborn error of glycosphingolipid catabolism that results from deficient activity of the lysosomal hydrolase α-galactosidase (see later). Cataracts are also common in Fabry disease; they consist of two characteristic types—anterior and posterior subcapsular cataracts. Anterior subcapsular cataracts, which only occur in hemizygous males, appear as granular, radially arranged wedges. Posterior subcapsular cataracts have the appearance of nearly translucent spokelike or dendritic projections; they may also occur in heterozygous female carriers. Posterior subcapsular cataracts may be the initial ophthalmologic manifestation of Fabry disease. Patients with homocystinuria due to cystathionine β-synthetase (CBS) deficiency may also present with cataracts. However, the most common eye finding in CBS deficiency is ectopia lentis (dislocation of the ocular lens), preceded by progressive myopia. In contrast to patients with Marfan syndrome, the dislocation is usually downward, although it may occur in any direction. The dislocation is usually not discovered before 2 years of age.

Adulthood (> 15 Years)

Adults with cerebrotendinous xanthomatosis commonly have cataracts. These patients can be easily diagnosed because of the association of cataracts with xanthomata and because of the neuro-degenerative course in which mental regression, ataxia, and psychotic behavior are seen. Patients with ornithine aminotransferase deficiency (gyrate atrophy of the choroid and retina) frequently have a posterior subcapsular cataract in their second decade. These patients often come to an ophthalmologist in late childhood or puberty for evaluation of myopia or decreased night vision. Affected patients are at high risk for blindness, usually between the ages of 40 to 55 years. Except for the progressive visual impairment, patients with gyrate atrophy are asymptomatic. Hyperornithinemia is the characteristic laboratory finding.

Patients with glucose-6-phosphate dehydrogenase deficiency, who come first to the clinician's attention because of hemolytic anemia, also have developed cataracts. Some with the dominantly inherited X-linked Alport syndrome of hemorrhagic nephritis, progressive sensorineural deafness, and pathognomonic ocular abnormalities, such as anterior lenticonus, also develop cataracts. Isolated cataracts in otherwise healthy adults may suggest heterozygous status for some inherited metabolic diseases, such as galactose-1-phosphate uridyl transferase, galactokinase deficiency, or Lowe syndrome (Table 21.1).

CORNEAL OPACITIES

Corneal clarity is maintained by a crystalline array of stromal fibers and the multiple translucent endothelial layers. The cornea is optically sensitive to abnormal storage products, which may accumulate as a result of a systemic disorder. Inherited lysosomal disorders resulting from a deficiency of a lysosomal hydrolytic enzyme may lead to corneal manifestations as the earliest indication of a metabolic disease. The age of visible corneal opacity is a helpful criterion for the identification of the metabolic causative disease.

Infancy (3 to 12 Months)

Oculocutaneous tyrosinemia (type II, Richner–Hanhart syndrome) is a distinct syndrome that appears during the first months of life, usually with corneal erosions and associated pseudodendrites, or plaques, as well as with systemic symptoms, including painful hyperkeratotic palm and sole lesions. Some patients have mild mental retardation. The disease results from a deficiency of cytosolic tyrosine aminotransferase and causes elevated levels of tyrosine in the blood and urine. Symptoms often worsen in winter when levels of tyrosine are often higher.

Cystinosis is an autosomal recessive disorder characterized by a lysosomal transport defect that results in the accumulation of cystine within lysosomes. Cystine accumulates intracellularly in many tissues, including conjunctiva, the cornea, iris, choroid, and retinal pigment epithelium, as well as in the kidney. Whereas the corneal findings are similar in all age groups, the systemic symptoms may be fatal in infants. In the cornea, the crystals are located in the anterior stroma; they are iridescent and polychromatic, presenting first in the periphery and extending centrally. The corneal

Table 21.1.   Collection of routine and specific investigations for the differential diagnosis of cataracts and corneal opacities in inherited metabolic diseases

Urine
  Amino acids
  Organic acids
  Oligosaccharides
  Copper

Plasma/serum
  Amino acids
  Very-long-chain fatty acids
  Phytanic acid
  Lactate
  3-Hydroxybutyrate
  Triglycerides
  Cholesterol
  Lipoproteins
  Copper
  Cholestanol
  Bile alcohols

Enzyme studies (galactose-1-phosphate-uridyl transferase, galactokinase, UDP-galactose-4-epimerase, glucose-6-phosphate dehydrogenase, lysosomal enzymes, fatty alcohol oxidoreductase, respiratory chain enzymes)

Peripheral blood (vacuolated lymphocytes, cystine content in leukocytes)

Erythrocytes (plasmalogen)

Mitochondrial DNA

Abbreviation: UDP, uridine diphosphate.

changes and associated photophobia are due to the anterior location of the crystal deposition. They may be present before nephropathy is severe; thus, they can be the first indicator of the disease. The anterior location of the crystals can also predispose the patient to recurrent erosions. Cysteamine eyedrops are effective in reducing the deposits of crystals in the cornea and in improving the extreme photophobia that often accompanies this condition. Corneal transplantation may be indicated for visual rehabilitation, as well as for recurrent erosions.

Mucopolysaccharidoses (MPS) are lysosomal storage diseases that result from a deficiency of enzymes involved in the degradation of the glycosaminoglycans, dermatan sulfate, heparan sulfate, and keratan sulfate (see Chapter 29). The incompletely degraded mucopolysaccharides accumulate in the tissues and are excreted in the urine. Because the cornea consists of approximately 4% glycosaminoglycans, the enzyme deficiencies become clinically apparent as stromal clouding. Other systemic features that may also be found include skeletal dysplasia, coarse facies, mental retardation, hepatosplenomegaly, cardiac disease, and inguinal hernias. Relevant metabolic diseases in this group are Hurler (MPS type IH), Scheie (MPS type IS), Maroteaux–Lamy (MPS type VI), and Sly (MPS type VII) syndromes. In addition, I-cell disease (mucolipidosis type II) resembles Hurler syndrome, as does the infantile form of α-mannosidosis that presents with corneal clouding clinically.

Mild corneal opacities, which do not affect vision, occur in about 25% of patients with steroid sulfatase deficiency. Patients have increased levels of cholesterol sulfate in plasma and stratum corneum. The increase of cholesterol sulfate levels in the stratum corneum appears to be responsible for the ichthyotic changes of the skin. The phenotype of affected patients is primarily characterized by the presence of dark, scaly skin that starts between birth and 4 months of age. This disorder is inherited as a X-linked trait.

Early Childhood (1 to 6 Years)

In the age group from 1 to 6 years, corneal opacities became apparent in another MPS, Morquio disease (MPS type IV). Patients exhibit marked dwarfism, a barrel chest, a short neck, kyphoscoliosis, aortic valvular disease, and odontoid hypoplasia; intelligence is usually normal. Corneal clouding with major visual impairment is a prominent feature in patients with mucolipidosis type IV (sialolipidosis). Corneal clouding is one of the early symptoms; later, retinal degeneration and blindness may develop. Cytoplasmic membranous bodies are found in diverse tissues, including the conjunctiva, fibroblasts, liver, and spleen. Affected patients are usually mentally retarded, and progressive neurologic and mental deterioration may occur. The late-onset form of α-mannosidosis also involves corneal clouding, in addition to cataracts, changes in bone, and hearing loss.

Some disorders of high-density lipoproteins (HDL) metabolism, namely, Tangier disease and fish-eye disease, both of which are caused by lecithin:cholesterol acyltransferase (LCAT) deficiency, must be included in the differential diagnosis of corneal opacity that is visible in early childhood. Patients with these diseases have hypoalphalipoproteinemia with low HDL, low Apo A-I, and elevated triglycerides. Those with Tangier disease have striking large yellow tonsils or pharyngeal plaques. They also have peripheral neuropathy manifested by weakness, paresthesias, vegetative dysregulation, and ptosis. In addition, abnormal rectal mucosa, anemia, renal failure, and hepatosplenomegaly may occur. Corneal clouding is the only clinical manifestation in patients with fish-eye disease. Deficiency of LCAT in both syndromes leads to the accumulation of lipoprotein cholesteryl esters. Different mutations in the LCAT gene cause LCAT deficiency, called fish-eye disease. In fish-eye disease, LCAT activity is absent against HDL but not against low-density lipoproteins (LDL).

Late Childhood, Adolescence, and Adulthood

Fabry disease is an X-linked recessive deficiency of the enzyme ceramide trihexosidase. It is characterized by crises in the abdomen or extremities that are sometimes accompanied by fever. Pain may be the only manifestation for many years, followed eventually by the development of the angiokeratomata, which greatly facilitates the diagnosis. Later complications include renal failure, cardiovascular disease, recurrent enteritis, anemia, and neurodegeneration. The corneal changes, occurring in the first decade of life in 90% of cases, are the earliest and the most consistent ocular abnormality. The whorllike supepithelial lines seen on the cornea produce a characteristic pattern. Cornea verticillata may also occur in heterozygotes.

In the juvenile/adult type of galactosialidosis, corneal clouding with loss of visual acuity presents in the second decade of life. Additional ophthalmologic abnormalities include bilateral cherry-red spots, punctate lens opacities, and color blindness. Other clinical symptoms include coarse facies, growth disturbance, cardiac involvement, hernias, angiokeratomata, hearing loss, joint stiffness, vertebral changes, and a progressive neurologic course with mental retardation, seizures, myoclonus, and ataxia (see Chapter 29).

The Kayser–Fleischer ring is the most important ocular sign of Wilson disease. It is a yellow-brown granular deposit on Descemet membrane at the limbus of the cornea; it is usually seen earliest and most densely at the upper and lower poles. In early stages the ring is visible only with a slit lamp. It occurs in nearly all patients with neurologic presentation. However, Kayser–Fleischer rings are absent in more than 30% of children who present with acute liver disease. The rings improve with effective penicillamine chelation, as do cataracts.

Alkaptonuria is a rare autosomal recessive condition caused by deficient homogentisic acid oxidase. Homogentisic acid is excreted in excess in the urine, but its oxidized pigment derivatives (alkapton) also bind collagen, leading to pigment accumulation in connective tissue of the nose, sclera, and ear lobes. Affected patients also develop a degenerative arthropathy. The ocular changes occur in 70% of patients. Just inside the limbus the cornea develops a black "oil-droplet" pigmentation that appears similar to spheroidal degeneration. Pigmentation gradually increases throughout adulthood.

RETINITIS PIGMENTOSA (RP)

RP is a clinically and genetically heterogeneous group of hereditary disorders in which a progressive loss of photoreceptor and pigment epithelial function occurs. The prevalence of RP is between one in 3,000 and one in 5,000, making it the most frequent tapetoretinal degeneration and one of the most common causes of hereditary visual impairment in all age groups. Diagnostic criteria include bilateral involvement, loss of peripheral vision, rod dysfunction, and progressive loss of photoreception function. In the course of evaluation, the anamnestic history of visual symptoms should include information regarding the nature of the earliest symptoms, the age at onset, and progression. The age at onset of RP varies but often begins in early childhood or infancy. The initial symptom is usually defective adaptation to the dark, or night blindness. In adults, careful questioning often elicits a history starting in childhood or adolescence when patients are asked to recall difficulties with outdoor activities at dusk or with indoor activities at night in minimal lighting. Patients rarely note a loss in peripheral vision as an early symptom, although they may be considered clumsy before constricted visual fields are detected. Other symptoms include pendular eye movements and nystagmus. Patients who present with initial symptoms of photophobia, sensations of flashing lights, abnormal central vision, abnormal color vision, or marked asymmetry in ocular involvement may not have RP, but rather, another retinal disease. The ocular examination should include measurements of the patient's best-corrected visual acuity, refraction, examination of the anterior segment, and measurement of intraocular pressure. Attention should also be given to the lens, vitreous, optic disc, retinal vessels, macula, and retinal periphery. The earliest ophthalmoscopic findings are a dull retinal reflex and a threadlike aspect of the retinal arteries. The electroretinogram is abnormal before gross fundoscopic evidence of RP is found.

The pigmented retinopathies can be divided into two groups: primary RP, in which the disease process is confined to the eyes, and secondary RP, in which retinal degeneration is associated with single or multiorgan involvement. Primary RP may segregate as an autosomal dominant, autosomal recessive, or X-linked recessive trait. Linkage studies with X-linked RP revealed at least two distinct genetic loci on the X-chromosome. The rhodopsin gene, the pigment of the rod photoreceptors, has been directly implicated as the cause of the severe type of the autosomal dominant form of RP. The other group, secondary RP, is most often associated with nervous system involvement, dysmorphic features, myopathy, nephropathy, deafness, and skin abnormalities. Some of these conditions accompany well-known and defined nonmetabolic genetic syndromes, whereas others occur in relation to inherited metabolic diseases.

Retinal degeneration occurs in a number of metabolic diseases. The differential diagnosis of retinal abnormalities includes inborn errors of lipid, peroxisomal, and mitochondrial metabolism. Table 21.2 lists screening procedures for diagnosing patients with RP and suspicion of a metabolic disorder.

Sometimes, sophisticated techniques are necessary to establishing a specific diagnosis. However, a detailed clinical investigation and routine metabolic screening usually provide a presumptive diagnosis. An appropriate diagnosis is essential for potential treatment options that prevent progression of the disease, as well as for genetic counseling.

Classifying these diseases according to the presence or absence of neurologic, gastrointestinal, or cutaneous involvement may provide clues to the differential diagnosis of pigmentary degeneration. Retinal degeneration occurs as a unique clinical manifestation in ornithine aminotransferase deficiency.

Retinitis Pigmentosa with Neurologic Involvement

Several inborn errors of lipid metabolism, including abetalipoproteinemia, vitamin E malabsorption, Refsum disease, long-

Table 21.2. Collection of routine and specific investigations for differential diagnosis of retinitis pigmentosa in inborn metabolic diseases

Urine
  Organic acids

Plasma/serum
  Amino acids
  Very-long-chain fatty acids
  Phytanic acid
  Lactate
  3-Hydroxybutyrate
  Free fatty acids
  Triglycerides
  Cholesterol
  Lipoproteins
  Vitamins A, E
  Free and total carnitine, acylcarnitine profile
  Transferrin isoelectric focusing

Peripheral blood (acanthocytes, vacuolated lymphocytes, inclusion bodies in lymphocytes)

Erythrocytes (plasmalogen)

Enyzme studies (lysosomal enzymes, long-chain hydroxyacyl-CoA dehydrogenase, fatty alcohol oxidoreductase, respiratory chain enzymes)

(Electron) microscopy (skin biopsy, fibroblasts, lymphocytes)

Cystine content in leukocytes

Mitochondrial DNA

chain hydroxyacyl-CoA dehydrogenase (LCHAD) deficiency, and Sjögren–Larsson syndrome, involve pigmentary retinopathy. Abetalipoproteinemia involves the absence of apoprotein B and the malabsorption of fat and fat-soluble vitamins, especially vitamins A and E. The most common clinical manifestations are diarrhea and failure to thrive from early infancy, followed by signs of peripheral neuropathy, spinocerebellar ataxia, and muscle weakness. The retinal and neurologic complications may be prevented or stabilized by early supplementation with vitamin E. Nearly every patient with Refsum disease has an inborn error of phytanic acid metabolism that is caused by phytanic acid oxidase deficiency. The clinical triad includes RP, peripheral polyneuropathy, and elevated cerebrospinal fluid protein. Other symptoms include cerebellar ataxia, deafness, anosmia, ichthyosis, and skeletal and cardiac manifestations. Night blindness may be the first clinical symptom at school age or later.

Disorders of mitochondrial fatty acid oxidation, such as LCHAD deficiency, involve life-threatening hypoglycemic coma, liver failure, muscle weakness, cardiomyopathy, myoglobinuria, neuropathy, and RP. Clinical manifestation of Sjögren–Larsson syndrome includes congenital ichthyosis, spastic di- or tetraplegia, mental retardation, and glistening dots in the macular region of the retina. In some patients with a defect of intracellular cobalamin metabolism (Cbl C), RP may be present from the neonatal period or infancy.

Another group of inborn errors of metabolism associated with RP is that of the neuronal ceroid lipofuscinoses (CLN). This is a group of progressive encephalopathies, which are characterized by neural and extraneural accumulation of ceroid and lipofuscin storage material. CLN are among the most common neurodegenerative disorders. Three main types that include RP have been distinguished on clinical and neurophysiologic criteria: the infantile Santavuori–Hagberg form, with onset between 6 and 18 months of age, regression of psychomotor development, myoclonic epilepsy, visual failure, microcephaly, and "vanishing electroencephalogram (EEG)"; the late infantile Jansky–Bielschowsky form, with onset between 2 and 4 years of age, epilepsy, regression of mental skills, ataxia, myoclonic jerks, pathologic EEG, electroretinogram (ERG), and visual evoked potentials (VEP); and the juvenile Spielmeyer–Vogt form, with onset of visual impairment between the ages of 4 and 10 years, psychologic disturbances, motor dysfunction and epilepsy, retinal degeneration, and vacuolated lymphocytes.

Peroxisomal disorders in which pigmentary retinopathy may be observed are associated with defective beta-oxidation of very-long-chain fatty acids (see Chapter 27). Assessment of plasma concentrations of very-long-chain fatty acids in these disorders usually yields the diagnosis. Peroxisomal disorders with retinal degeneration include Zellweger syndrome, neonatal adrenoleukodystrophy, and isolated defects, such as acyl-CoA oxidase deficiency and peroxisomal thiolase deficiency

Patients with disorders of protein glycosylation, which make up a heterogenous group called *congenital disorders of glycosylation* (CDG) syndromes, also develop RP in childhood. This is seen predominantly in CDG type Ia (phosphomannomutase deficiency). Defects in the mitochondrial electron transport chain cause a variety of manifestations, among them retinal degeneration. Among these disorders, retinal degeneration has been consistently reported only in the Kearns–Sayre syndrome, a progressive multisystem disorder, with onset usually before the age of 20 years. Clinical features include chronic progressive external ophthalmoplegia, ptosis, retinopathy, cardiac conduction disturbances, and deafness. The Kearns–Sayre syndrome is caused by deletion-duplications of mtDNA. RP is also seen in patients with the neurodegeneration, ataxia, retinitis pigmentosa (NARP) mutation in mitochondrial DNA, although not as regularly as the name would suggest.

In addition, several well-known autosomal recessive syndromes without known etiology involve RP; these include Hallervorden–Spatz (severe neurologic regression, dystonia, acanthocytosis), Laurence–Moon–Biedl (obesity, polydactyly, mental retardation), Usher type II (deafness, severe mental retardation), Joubert (mental retardation, vermis atrophy, attacks of hyperventilation), and Cockayne (dysmorphia, hypotonia, intracranial calcifications, deafness) syndromes.

RP with Gastrointestinal Symptoms (Failure to Thrive, Chronic Diarrhea, Hypolipidemia)

Metabolic diseases with RP and predominant associated gastrointestinal symptoms include abetalipoproteinemia, vitamin E malabsorption, and infantile Refsum disease.

Retinitis Pigmentosa with Cutaneous Symptoms

Cutaneous symptoms, such as juvenile or congenital ichthyosis, are found in classic Refsum disease or the Sjögren–Larsson syndrome.

Isolated Retinitis Pigmentosa

Isolated RP is a typical finding in patients with the X-linked, autosomal recessive, or dominant types of primary RP and in patients with ornithine aminotransferase deficiency (gyrate atrophy of the choroid and retina). (For details see "Cataract" in this chapter.)

ADDITIONAL READING

Endres W, Shin YS. Cataract and metabolic disease. *J Inher Metab Dis* 1990;13:509–516.

Poll-The BT, Billette de Villemeur T, Abitbol M, et al. Metabolic pigmentary retinopathies: diagnosis and therapeutic attempts. *Eur J Pediatr* 1992;151:2–11.

Vinals A, Kenyon KR. Corneal manifestations of metabolic diseases. *Int Ophthalmol Clin* 1998;38:141–153.

22 ♣ Skin and Hair

Recognizing the significance of skin lesions in inborn errors of metabolism can prove useful for diagnosis. Finding even one characteristic lesion often provides the clue to the identification and to the appropriate test to prove it.

DERMATOSES

Angiokeratomata

Angiokeratomata occurring in substantial number almost always indicates Fabry disease. It can occur in some other lysosomal storage disorders, but in those diseases angiokeratomata are exceedingly sparse (Table 22.1). One or two angiokeratomata may be seen in a patient with G_{M1} gangliosidosis, but usually this patient has already been diagnosed because the hepatosplenomegaly, developmental delay, coarse features, and dysostosis multiplex occur very early in infancy and the skin lesions rarely appear before the first year. Similarly, a patch of angiokeratomata may be seen in fucosidosis, but again it is not among the earliest features, although it may appear between 6 months to 4 years of age. Organomegaly, bone changes, and developmental delay are evident earlier. Similar lesions may be seen in childhood in aspartylglucosaminuria, but they appear long after the patient is known to have coarse features, cataracts, joint laxity, and neurodegeneration. They may also be seen in the juvenile form of galactosialidosis. These patients have corneal opacities, bone findings, and neurologic degeneration that bring the patient to attention usually before the skin lesions appear. Researchers have reported two brothers with β-mannosidosis who had both angiokeratomata and mental retardation.

In Fabry disease the skin lesions are a dominant feature of the disease. They may be the first manifestations of the disease; in some heterozygous females they may represent the only sign of disease. However, males with this X-linked disorder usually have a number of years of often excruciating and unexplained pain. Pain most commonly occurs in the extremities, particularly the lower ones, but may strike in the abdomen or elsewhere. Affected boys may be referred to a psychiatrist because finding out why they are complaining so vehemently is so difficult. The appearance of the skin lesions creates an entirely different scenario.

They are dark red and do not blanch with pressure. They seek out pressure points like the buttocks or knees, but they are often distributed profusely over the scrotum and penis. They may also be seen on the oral mucosa or the conjunctiva. They increase in number and in size with time. Initially, they are usually flat, but they may eventually become slightly palpable.

Pigment Problems

Hypopigmentation

The classic abnormality in pigment deposition is oculocutaneous albinism. In its most extreme form, the patient's skin and hair are milk white and the irides are translucent with a visible red reflex. However, many variations are seen. The abnormalities in tyrosine

Table 22.1. Angiokeratomata

Disease	Diagnostic test
Fabry	Lysosomal enzymes (LE): ceramide trihexosidase, α-galactosidase
Aspartylglucosaminuria	Amino acid analysis— aspartylglucosamine
Fucosidosis	LE; α-fucosidase
Galactosialidosis	LE; β-galactosidase; neuraminidase
G_{m1}, gangliosidosis	LE; β-galactosidase
β-Mannosidosis	LE; β-mannosidase

metabolism are confined to the melanosomes of the melanocytes, which are found in the skin, iris, choroid, and retina. Considerable progress has been made in elucidating the molecular biology. Patients with oculocutaneous albinism have major ocular abnormalities, hearing loss, and a high risk of developing skin cancers.

Most patients with phenylketonuria (PKU) before the development of screening diagnosis and early treatment had fair hair and skin and were blue-eyed. Early treatment has made it clear that the abnormal chemical environment in the untreated state is what interferes with normal pigmentation, not the state itself. PKU actually occurs with all varieties of ethnic pigmentation. The rule is that the affected patient has less pigment than the unaffected members of his or her family do. This is true also for patients with cystinosis and for some with homocystinuria (Table 22.2).

Hyperpigmentation

In alkaptonuria defective activity of homogentisic acid oxidase leads to accumulation of homogentisic acid, which is then oxidized to form black insoluble pigment (Table 22.3). Pigment deposition is greatest in cartilage, so it appears prominently in the ears. It may also be seen early in the sclerae and in the nose, initially as salt and pepper spots; however, these spots may later become confluent. In an older patient it may be widely distributed, especially distally on the fingers. Deposition in joint cartilage leads to early debilitating osteoarthritis. The skin may alert the physician to the diagnosis. Earlier clues can be seen; however, the dark stain

Table 22.2. Fair skin and hair—hypopigmentation

Albinism
Cystinosis
Phenylketonuria
Homocystinuria

Table 22.3. Hyperpigmentation

Alkaptonuria
Adrenoleukodystrophy/adrenomyeloneuropathy
Glycerol kinase deficiency/adrenal insufficiency
Addison disease

that used to occur with diapers disappeared with cloth diapers, and the red staining of plastic diapers is often missed. Later, voided urine is flushed before oxygen produces the coloration. Tests for reducing substance are positive, but these have been largely replaced by tests for glucose in routine urinalyses. Once effective treatment is developed, screening for homogentisic acid may become practical.

Increase in the deposition of melanin that occurs early in childhood without much exposure to sun is characteristic of adrenal insufficiency. Pigment in the oral mucous membranes may also be seen and may be the first substantial clue to the presence of adrenoleukodystrophy or adrenomyeloneuropathy (see Chapter 27). Confirmation is achieved by analysis for very-long-chain fatty acids (VLCFA) in blood or fibroblasts. Adrenal insufficiency also occurs in those patients with glycokinase deficiency who have a contiguous gene deletion syndrome. Dependent on the size of the deletion, some also have Duchenne muscular dystrophy and/or ornithine transcarbamylase (OTC) deficiency (see Chapter 6, "Work-up of the Patient with Hyperammonemia"). Finally, in isolated Addison disease, hyperpigmentation is again an important clue that needs to be recognized, if at all possible, before an endocrine crisis occurs.

Ichthyosis

Ichthyosis is a very striking scaling dermatosis that results from overactive proliferation of skin cells. Extra skin piles up in scales, reminiscent of the skin of fish, and falls off. Depending on the rate of the process, the scales may appear old and black; or they may have the pronounced erythroderma of new skin. Most ichthyosis is not part of an inborn error of metabolism, but in a surprising list of metabolic diseases, ichthyosis can be very prominent in its presentation (Table 22.4).

The purest form is X-linked ichthyosis, which results from defective activity of steroid sulfatase, leading to the deposition of cholesterol sulfate. Patients with this condition may have no manifestations of the disease other than dark, scaly skin. Mild corneal opacities, which do not interfere with vision, are found in about 25% of patients. Mental retardation, hypogonadism, shortness of stature, and chondrodysplasia punctata have been observed.

Patients with multiple sulfatase deficiency are most debilitated by manifestations of metachromatic leukodystrophy and of mucopolysaccharidosis. A patient with features of both who also has

Table 22.4. Ichthyosis

Disease	Diagnostic test
X-linked ichthyosis	Lysosomal enzymes (LE); steroid sulfatase
Multiple sulfatase deficiency	LE; battery of sulfatases (e.g., arylsulfatase A, iduronate sulfatase)
Refsum disease	Phytanic acid (phytanoyl-CoA hydroxylase)
Sjögren–Larsson syndrome	Fatty alcohol oxidoreductase
Neutral lipid storage disorder	Vacuolated lymphocytes
Gaucher disease	LE; glucocerebrosidase, β-glucosidase
Chondrodysplasia punctata	Plasmalogen synthesis
Conradi–Hünermann syndrome	Sterol analysis in plasma/serum (sterol-8-isomerase)
CHILD syndrome	Sterol analysis in plasma/serum (sterol-4-demethylase)
Carbohydrate-deficient glycoprotein (CDG-1f) disease	Sialotransferrin electrofocusing
Serine synthesis defect	CSF amino acids (low serine)

Abbreviations: CHILD, congenital hemidysplasia, ichthyosis, and limb defects; CSF, cerebrospinal fluid.

ichthyosis undoubtedly has multiple sulfatase deficiency, which is sometimes known as Austin disease. This condition results in a failure of posttranslational modification of these sulfatase enzymes from an intrinsic cysteine moiety to a formylglycine.

In patients with Refsum disease, the skin may be the key to diagnosing this multisystem disease. Ataxia is an early manifestation. Deafness, peripheral neuropathy, and retinitis pigmentosa complete the syndrome. The cerebrospinal fluid (CSF) protein is elevated, and no pleocytosis is seen. The diagnosis is made by assay of the blood for phytanic acid.

Patients with Sjögren–Larsson syndrome in which the fatty alcohol oxidoreductase is defective have cataracts and ichthyosis. In addition, they are mentally retarded and have spastic paraplegia. Retinitis pigmentosa may be evident on ophthalmoscopy; glistening dots may appear in the area of the macula.

Cataracts and ichthyosis also occur in neutral lipid storage disorder. The origin of this disease is not yet known. Vacuolated lymphocytes are seen; hepatomegaly distinguishes it from Sjögren–Larsson disease. Patients also have ataxia and myopathy.

Ichthyosis is seen as an early congenital syndrome in neuro-nopathic Gaucher disease. The patient may even have a collodion baby appearance. With time the skin may appear normal, but neurodegeneration is progressive.

Ichthyosis may also be seen in the Conradi–Hünermann or X-linked dominant chondrodysplasia punctata (see Chapter 23). In addition, ichthyotic lesions are prominent in infants with congenital hemidysplasia, ichthyosis and limb defects (CHILD) syndrome, another X-linked disorder considered lethal in males, but studies of skin cell kinetics have indicated that the lesions in this disease are actually psoriasis. Besides ichthyosis, Conradi–Hünermann syndrome displays the typical calcifications, and a few affected females have had asymmetric rhizomelic limb shortness, cataracts, and mental retardation. The skin lesions may have a whorled pattern of hyperkeratotic, white adherent scales with underlying red skin and palmar and plantar hyperkeratosis that disappears by 3 to 6 months of age. Biochemically, Conradi–Hünermann syndrome patients have normal or, occasionally, decreased cholesterol levels and elevated concentrations of 8-dehydrocholesterol and 8(9)-cholestenol in plasma and tissues due to a defect of 3-β-hydroxysteroid-Δ^8,Δ^7-isomerase. Deficient sterol-4-demethylase, the enzymatic step just prior to sterol-8-isomerase, is the underlying defect in CHILD syndrome. The disorder involves unilateral ichthyotic skin lesions with a sharp demarcation at the midline of the trunk; the facial area is typically spared, although the scalp may be affected. Punctate calcifications similar to those in Conradi–Hünermann syndrome occur in the epiphyses and other cartilaginous structures of the affected side (usually the right).

Ichthyosis has recently been described along with psychomotor retardation, night blindness, and dwarfism in siblings in a distinct form (1f) of carbohydrate-deficient glycoprotein (CDG) syndrome. The sialotransferrin pattern in the serum was consistent with type I. Activities of phosphomannose isomerase, phosphomannose mutase, and guanosine diphosphate (GDP)-mannose synthase were normal. A low CSF serine has been encountered in a patient with ichthyosis and neurologic disease who did not have 3-phosphoglycerate dehydrogenase deficiency.

Hyperkeratosis

Hyperkeratotic lesions are a minor, often absent sign of oculocutaneous tyrosinemia or tyrosinemia type II. The combination of ocular lesions and hyperkeratotic lesions has also been called the Richner–Hanhart syndrome, although none of Richner and Hanhart's patients ever had their tyrosine levels measured. The major manifestations of this disease are keratitis and corneal ulcers (see Chapter 21), which are frequently thought to be herpetic. The skin lesions occur on the palms and soles. They are usually discrete and hyperkeratotic, and they are often painful. Sometimes, the lesions are ulcerated. Amino acid analysis of the plasma reveals the elevated level of tyrosine, which is usually much higher than that seen in hepatorenal tyrosinemia. The symptoms are a consequence of elevated levels of tyrosine; they resolve with modest reduction in the dietary intake of phenylalanine and tyrosine. The defect occurs in the cytosolic tyrosine aminotransferase.

Ulcers of the Skin

Cutaneous ulcers, predominantly of the lower leg, are the hallmark finding of prolidase deficiency. Analysis of the urinary amino acids usually provides the diagnosis. The pattern obtained is confusing to many laboratories if technicians have never seen the peaks of the number of peptides of proline that are found. Because ulcers are unusual in childhood, the clinician should pursue this diagnosis vigorously. These ulcers also resist common symptomatic measures. Patients may, in addition, have mental retardation, ophthalmoplegia, and other skin lesions, including teleangiectases, purpuric ecchymoses, or erythematous areas of skin. Some have had splenomegaly and dysmorphic features. The ulcers may be complicated by secondary infection. Ulcers in late childhood and adolescence may also develop in classical homocystinuria that is caused by cystathionine β-synthase deficiency. These ulcers result from thromboembolic disease, usually in the lower extremities. Diagnosis is made by determining the concentrations of homocystine and methionine by amino acid analysis.

Erythematous Vesicular Dermatoses

The rash of the infant with holocarboxylase synthetase deficiency (Table 22.5) is unforgettable. It is a bright red total body eruption that is associated with alopecia totalis and is desquamative. The skin lesions are not vesicular unless they are complicated by mucocutaneous monilial infection. The usual initial presentation is the classic organic aciduria emergency (see Chapter 6) with massive ketosis and acidosis progressive to coma.

Table 22.5.   Erythematous vesicular dermatoses

Disease	Diagnostic test
Multiple carboxylase deficiency	Organic acid analysis of urine
	Assay of carboxylases of lymphocytes and fibroblasts
	Assay of holocarboxylase synthetase of lymphocytes or fibroblasts
	Assay of biotinidase of plasma
Methylmalonic aciduria	Organic acid analysis of urine
	Assay of methymalonyl-CoA mutase
	Complementation analysis in fibroblasts
Propionic acidemia	Organic acid analysis of urine
	Assay of propionyl-CoA carboxylase

Some infants die before skin lesions ever develop. Those who survive the initial neonatal episode regularly develop the dermatosis. The laboratory evaluation reveals lactic acidemia, as well as ketoacidosis; and the organic aciduria is typically that of multiple carboxylase deficiency with lactic acid, 3-hydroxyisovaleric acid, 3-methylcrotonylglycine, 3-hydroxypropionic acid, and methylcitric acid. Deficient activities of propionyl-CoA carboxylase, 3-methylcrotonyl-CoA carboxylase, and pyruvate carboxylase are readily demonstrable in the lymphocytes or fibroblasts. The fundamental defect is in holocarboxylase synthetase. The differential diagnosis includes seborrheic dermatitis.

The other form of multiple carboxylase deficiency is biotinidase deficiency. This disease produces the same type of skin lesions, but they are patchy rather than generalized and particularly are periorificial. Complication by monilial infection is very common, especially about the mouth and the eyes and in the diaper area. These patients are less likely to develop life-threatening ketoacidosis. They may present with convulsions. All are hypotonic; most progress to mental retardation if they are undiagnosed and untreated. Visual and auditory impairment are late complications.

The differential diagnosis includes acrodermatitis enteropathica. In fact, the first patients described with biotinidase deficiency carried the diagnosis of acrodermatitis enteropathica. Patients with acrodermatitis enteropathica have diarrhea. Some are zinc deficient; these may respond to treatment with zinc, but the diagnosis may be a wastebasket term. Therefore, any infant with this diagnosis should, at the least, have organic acid analysis of the urine and biotinidase of the plasma, as well as a work-up for immunodeficiency (see Chapter 25).

The typical skin lesions of propionic aciduria and methylmalonic aciduria are those of an extensive mucocutaneous candidiasis. Classically, the lesions are periorificial, but they may become quite general as satellite lesions coalesce. They are bright red and vesicular in appearance, sometimes looking like a thermal burn. These patients present with the classic organic aciduria emergency (see Chapter 6); they display anorexia, vomiting, and failure to thrive. Once diagnosed, they are managed with a high-calorie, very-low-protein dietary regimen so that they are always on the brink of malnutrition. An intercurrent infection, especially one that includes diarrhea, pushes them over the brink; and they develop kwashiorkor. This is the other dermatologic picture characteristic of these diseases. Edema, hypoproteinemia, and an eczematoid or vesicular erythematous eruption that darkens and desquamates may be found. This picture may complicate any of the organic acidurias or disorders of amino acid metabolism that are treated with protein restriction. It is rather common in maple syrup urine disease.

Infiltration of the Skin with Mucopolysaccharides

The coarse features of the mucopolysaccharidoses result largely from the deposition of mucopolysaccharides that accumulate as a result of the metabolic block. The appearance reflects the hirsutism and the infiltration of the bones of the face and head in the generalized dysostosis multiplex, but it is also conveyed by deposition in the skin. The skin does not feel different or thickened, but its thickness can readily be appreciated in places like the alae and septum of the nares. This appearance is characteristic of all the mucopolysaccharidoses. It is classic in the late infantile period in Hurler and the severe Hunter diseases. It may be subtle until adulthood in Sanfilippo disease. It is also seen in the Maroteaux–Lamy and Sly diseases. In the mucolipidoses, especially II, or I-cell disease, it may be evident in the early days of life, as it is in G_{M1}-gangliosidosis, sialidosis, and galactosialidosis. A later infantile or toddler onset is seen in mucolipidosis III, N-acetylglucosamine phosphotransferase deficiency, and in fucosidosis, mannosidosis, Salla disease, and multiple sulfatase deficiency. Aspartylglucosaminuria and some of these other disorders may present later in childhood.

Photosensitivity

Photosensitive skin lesions (Table 22.6) characterize many of the porphyrias (Fig. 22.1). The most dramatic and the earliest in onset is that of congenital erythropoietic porphyria, the disease in which pink urine and red teeth occur. These patients may also have hemolytic anemia and splenomegaly. The skin lesions are

Table 22.6.   Photosensitive skin lesions

Disease	Diagnostic test
Congenital erythropoietic porphyria	Urine (isomer I), blood, stool, uroporphyrin
	Uroporphyrinogen-III cosynthase
Hepatoerythropoietic porphyria	RBC Zn-protoporphyrin, urine, uroporphyrin
	Uroporphyrinogen decarboxylase
Porphyria cutanea tarda	Urine, ALA, PBG, uroporphyrin
	Uroporphyrinogen decarboxylase
Hereditary coproporphyria	Urine ALA, PBG, coproporphyrin
	Coproporphyrinogen oxidase
Variegate porphyria	Fecal protoporphyrin
	Protoporphyrinogen oxidase
Erythropoietic protoporphyria	Free erythrocyte protoporphyrin
	Ferrochelatase
Hartnup disease	Amino acid analysis of the urine, urinary indole derivatives

Abbreviations: ALA, δ-aminolevulinic acid; PBG, porphobilinogen; RBC, red blood cells; Zn, zinc.

vesicular and bullous. The skin appears quite fragile, and ulcers or erosions emerge. Residual scarring and alternating hyperpigmentation and depigmentation may occur. Mutilation of fingers, nasal tips, and ears may eventually happen.

Patients with variegate porphyria have abdominal and neurologic crises. Onset is from puberty to adulthood. Late changes in the skin may be pseudosclerodermatous.

In patients with hepatoerythropoietic porphyria, the homozygous form of uroporphyrinogen decarboxylase III deficiency, onset is neonatal or shortly thereafter. Patients may also have hemolytic anemia and splenomegaly, and their urine may be black or pink. The skin is fragile, developing vesicles and blisters in response to sun exposure. Hypertrichosis about the face is commonly seen. Liver disease is a complication. Patients with porphyria cutanea tarda, the heterozygous, autosomal dominant form of uroporphyrinogen decarboxylase III deficiency, present first as adults. The skin is fragile so that minor trauma leads to erosions. Patients also develop hepatic siderosis.

Patients with hereditary coproporphyria have hemolytic anemia and abdominal and neurologic crises. Onset occurs in adulthood. Drugs that increase the production of the hepatic cytochrome P450 may precipitate abdominal or psychiatric symptoms.

Pains in the extremities, similar to those of Fabry disease, may occur in erythropoietic protoporphyria; in the absence of exposure to the sun, they may occur in isolated, unexplained fashion for years. The vesicular lesions resulting from exposure to the sun usually are smaller and more patchy than those in the other porphyrias of childhood. They leave tiny areas of flat, depressed atrophy of skin that may be very subtle but that are telltale markers of the disease. Unusual late complications include biliary tract stones and hepatic failure.

Patients with Hartnup disease have a transport disorder that involves the intestine and the renal tubule. The latter provides the diagnosis because the pattern of monocarboxylic aciduria, in which small neutral amino acids, such as alanine, serine, and threonine are excreted in excess, while glycine and imino acids are normal, is unique. The failure to absorb tryptophan leads to the dermatologic picture of pellagra, but no other symptoms are seen. Cutaneous manifestations of this disease have been rare in the United States, presumably because most patients eat such a high-protein diet that they do not become deficient.

The differential diagnosis of photosensitive dermatoses includes xeroderma pigmentosa, Cockayne syndrome, Bloom syndrome, and trichothiodystrophy. Recognizing all these disorders of DNA repair is important because of their frequent complication by neoplasia.

Nodular Lesions of the Skin

These lesions are summarized in Table 22.7.

The enlarged fat pads of the patient with congenital disorders of glycosylation (CDG) syndrome are unique and thus are absolutely

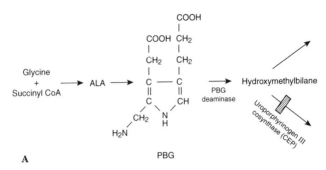

Fig. 22.1. Metabolic pathways in porphyrin/heme metabolism. The enzyme defects (*blocked arrows*) represent those that cause photosensitive lesions of the skin: uroporphyrinogen III cosynthase in congenital erythropoietic porphyria (CEP), uroporphyrinogen decarboxylase in porphyria cutanea tarda (PCT) and hepatoerythropoietic porphyria (HEP); coproporphyrinogen oxidase in hereditary coproporphyria (HCP), protoporphyrinogen oxidase in variegate porphyria (VP); and ferrochelatase in erythropoietic protoporphyria (EPP). Other abbreviations employed include ALA, δ-aminolevulinic acid; PBG, porphobilinogen; urogen, coprogen, and protogen for the respective porphyrinogens; and proto, protoporphyria.

Table 22.7. Nodular skin lesions

Disease	Diagnostic test
Congenital disorders of glycosylation (CDG) syndromes	Transferrin isoelectric focusing; phosphomannomutase
Familial hypercholesterolemia	Cholesterol, LDL cholesterol
Sitosterolemia (phytosterolemia)	Phytosterol and sitosterols in serum
Lipoprotein lipase deficiency	Triglycerides; lipoproteinelectophoresis; postheparin lipoprotein lipase
Hunter disease	Urinary glycosaminoglycans; iduronate sulfatase
Farber lipogranulomatosis	Ceramidase

Abbreviation: LDL, low density lipoprotein.

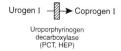

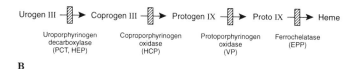

B

Fig. 22.1. *Continued*

diagnostic. Patients may come to attention early because of inverted nipples. The enlargement of the fat pads is usually evident toward the end of the first year. These pads are typically located over the upper and outer areas of the buttocks or lower back, but they may be seen elsewhere, including the lateral thighs and upper arms. The skin may feel thickened. Later, lipoatrophy may leave streaks on the lower extremities. These infants may be characterized by failure to thrive or pericardial effusions. Developmental delay is evident early, but neurodegenerative disease may occur later.

Cutaneous xanthomata along with tendinous xanthomata are seen in familial hypercholesterolemia homozygotes. This disorder of low-density lipoprotein metabolism leads to early coronary artery disease and myocardial infarction; early adult myocardial infarction occurs in heterozygotes. In homozygotes, the xanthomata are large, flat, and sometimes distinctly yellowish. A similar picture can occur in sitosterolemia, which, if untreated, also results in premature atherosclerosis and occasionally in hemolysis.

The xanthomata of patients with lipoprotein lipase deficiency are very different. They are tiny, white, difficult-to-see lesions, seldom larger than a pinhead. They occur when triglyceride levels are very high, and they disappear promptly on dietary reduction of triglycerides. These patients have chylomicronemia and do not develop vascular disease. They are subject to attacks of pancreatitis. The appearance of the blood, which looks like milky tomato soup, may provide the diagnosis.

In Hunter disease, which is unique among the mucopolysaccharidoses, localized nodular accumulations of mucopolysaccharide in the skin of the scapular area are observed.

Patients with Farber disease resulting from deficiency of ceramidase have nodular lesions in the subcutaneous tissues around joints and pressure point areas. Interphalangeal lesions, as well as those of the ankle and wrist, may occur. The patient complains of pain and stiffness of the joints and may be given a diagnosis of arthritis. Hoarseness is another feature. Development may be severely and progressively delayed. Deep tendon reflexes may be diminished or absent. Interstitial pneumonia is an infiltrative component of the disease.

DISORDERS OF THE HAIR

Hair Shaft Abnormalities

Trichorrhexis nodosa is seen in some patients with argininosuccinic aciduria. At a distance, the patient appears to have alopecia, but the abundance of very short hairs is clear on close examination. The hair shafts are fragile, and they break easily. Parents may note hair on the pillow. A longer hair under the microscope displays the characteristic nodules. The disorder is an abnormality of the urea cycle (see Chapter 6).

In Menkes disease the hair also appears abnormal on microscopic examination. The typical appearance is that of pili torti, in which the hair shaft is twisted. These patients may also have trichorrhexis nodosa or monilethrix, in which segmental narrowing of the hair shaft is seen. These hairs generally break readily as well, but the patient never appears to have alopecia. Menkes called the hair kinky, but it is not. It stands on end, brushlike. Danks referred to it as steely as, to him, it resembled steel wool. This association led to the discovery of the defect in copper metabolism because copper-deficient sheep in Australia have wool that is also described as steely. Patients suffering from Menkes disease have a devastating cerebral degenerative disorder, refractory seizures, bone lesions like those of scurvy, and elongated, tortuous cerebral arteries. Copper levels in the blood are low. The defect is in a copper-transporting adenosine-triphosphatase (ATPase) resulting from mutations on a gene on the X chromosome.

The differential diagnosis for abnormalities of the hair includes trichothiodystrophy and a kinky hair, photosensitivity, and mental retardation syndrome.

Alopecia

Alopecia totalis is the characteristic appearance of holocarboxylase synthetase deficiency (see earlier). Patients have no hair on their heads and no eyebrows, eyelashes, or lanugo hair (Table 22.8).

Patients with biotinidase deficiency have patchy alopecia in the pattern of the patient with acrodermatitis enteropathica.

Patients with porphyria, particularly those with the most destructive skin diseases, congenital erythropoietic porphyria and hepatic erythropoietic porphyria, have alopecia.

Patients with vitamin D–resistant rickets in which binding of 1,25-hydroxycalciferol receptors (type II) is defective have alopecia totalis.

Patients with organic acidurias (e.g., methylmalonic aciduria, propionic aciduria, or maple syrup urine disease) or with urea cycle defects—all of whom must be treated with strict restriction

Table 22.8. Alopecia

Disease	Diagnostic test
Multiple carboxylase deficiency	Organic acid analysis; carboxylases
Holocarboxylase synthetase deficiency	Holocarboxylase synthetase
Biotinidase deficiency	Biotinidase
Porphyrias	
Hepatoerythropoietic porphyria, porphyria cutanea tarda	RBC Zn protoporphyrin; urine uroporphyrin, uroporphyrinogen decarboxylase
Congenital erythropoietic porphyria	Blood, urine, stool uroporphyrin Uroporphyrinogen III cosynthase
Vitamin D–resistant rickets, type II	Defective binding of 1,25-hydroxycalciferol to receptor

Abbreviation: RBC, red blood cells; Zn, zinc.

of the intake of protein, in addition to patients with urea cycle diseases treated with agents, such as benzoate and phenylacetate, that create a nitrogen drain—may develop alopecia when the protein restriction is too stringent or when intercurrent infection increases demand. In fact, in the experience of the authors, hair loss is the most sensitive indicator of protein inadequacy, as it occurs many times before the level of albumin is depressed or before the occurrence of skin changes of kwashiorkor.

Miscellaneous Skin Lesions

Mottled pigmentation in exposed areas and distal erythrocyanosis of fingers and toes in response to cold have been reported, along with proximal renal tubular disease, diabetes, and cerebellar ataxia, in the presence of mitochondrial DNA deletion.

Some patients with Bartter syndrome (see Chapter 18) have been reported to have a chronic thickening of the skin with a purple-red coloration reminiscent of the erythematous skin of rats in response to a depletion of magnesium.

23 ♣ Metabolic Errors with Major Malformations

Many disorders that cause malformations do so by affecting the genes and proteins of morphogenesis. Known mechanisms include changes in the homeobox genes (HOX), the similar PAX genes, fibroblast growth factor receptor (FGFR) genes, and signaling pathways. Conversely, most disorders of intermediary metabolism do not produce distinctive malformations. However, the discovery that a classical malformation syndrome (Zellweger syndrome) was associated with a detectable change in cellular ultrastructure (absence of peroxisomes) has been followed by an intense search for the biochemical basis for this syndrome and related conditions.

This chapter focuses on the disorders of intermediary metabolism, excluding the lysosomal and peroxisomal disorders discussed in Chapters 27 and 29, in which malformations are conspicuous. The lysosomal storage disorders and mucopolysaccaridoses are the prototypical biochemical malformation syndromes. The distortion of facial, skeletal, and connective tissues at a macroscopic level can be attributed to the engorgement of intracellular lysosomes.

The disorders considered here include defects in the cholesterol biosynthesis pathway and the congenital disorders of glycosylation (CDG). All are inherited in an autosomal recessive manner. Menkes, Conradi–Hünermann–Happle, and congenital hemidysplasia, ichthyosis, and limb defects (CHILD) syndromes are X-linked.

CONGENITAL DISORDERS OF GLYCOSYLATION

The congenital disorders of glycosylation (CDG) were originally called carbohydrate-deficient glycoprotein syndromes. The name was recently changed to preserve the familiar abbreviation yet to reflect the appreciation of a broadening of this class of disorders. Glycosylation of peptides, using N- or O-linked oligosaccharides, is a common mechanism of posttranslational modification, so defects in this process affect a great number of proteins. Structural malformations and abnormal function of the brain, heart, liver, kidneys, and coagulation occur in various combinations.

At least six subtypes of CDG have been described so far. Current classification is based on defects of assembly and transfer of the oligosaccharide tree (CDG-I) and abnormalities of trimming and modifying the protein-bound oligosaccharides (CDG-II).

The form initially described, now called CDG-Ia, occurs in about one in 80,000 births. The typical patient progresses through four clinical stages. The infantile, multisystem alarming stage may be recognized in the neonatal period. The most unusual feature is uneven fat distribution, with fat pads found near the axilla, buttocks, and inguinal region even in a slender or wasted infant; however, in some infants these highly characteristic features do not develop until the second month of life. Early malformations include a high nasal bridge, a prominent jaw, large ears, and inverted nipples.

Neurologic problems include hypotonia, hyporeflexia, strabismus, roving eye movements, and ataxia. Olivoponto-cerebellar hypoplasia or atrophy may be seen on cerebral imaging. Cardiac involvement, particularly pericardial effusions and cardiomyopathy, is common. Nephrotic syndrome, hepatic failure, and life-threatening infection may occur. Severe carnitine deficiency may occur, leading to further problems with the liver, heart, and muscle.

The later stages of CDG-Ia include the childhood ataxia–mental retardation stage, in which strokelike episodes and hemorrhagic cerebral infarctions may occur; pigmentary retinal degeneration may occur in this stage, along with teenage neuropathies and atrophy of the lower limbs, general weakness and muscle atrophy, joint contractures, and scoliosis. In the adult hypogonadic stage, patients have moderate to severe intellectual impairment (IQ 40 to 60) and usually cannot walk. Ovarian failure, which is reminiscent of the late complications of galactosemia, occurs in females.

Initial laboratory findings may include the discovery of apparent hypothyroidism on newborn screening. Unlike congenital hypothyroidism, this is the result of a deficiency of thyroid-binding globulin (TBG). These patients, like others with TBG deficiency, are euthyroid. Many other plasma proteins are also deficient, including antithrombin III (AT III), α-1-acid glycoprotein, α-1-antitrypsin and α-1-antichymotrypsin, ceruloplasmin, ferritin, and complement C1, C3a, and C4a. The disturbance of hemeostasis is reflected in abnormal coagulation studies by an unusual pattern of prominent decreases of AT III, factor XI, and proteins C and S.

The diagnosis is made by isoelectric focusing of serum transferrin. Several bands, predominantly those of proteins with four or five sialic acid residues, are usually seen. Impaired synthesis of oligosaccharide side chains results in deficiency of the penta- and tetrasialo-transferrin species and in an increase in asialo- and disialo-forms. Abnormalities of transferrin isoelectric focusing occur in all forms of CDG.

In CDG-Ib, no malformations are seen, and psychomotor development is normal. The clinical picture is mainly gastrointestinal, with failure to thrive, protein-losing enteropathy, and diarrhea having prominence. Hepatic fibrosis and coagulopathy may occur; some patients present with hypoglycemia.

The rare forms, CDG-Ic, -Id, -Ie, and -IIa, have been found in only a few patients. The severe phenotypes that have been recognized so far will likely be expanded to include more subtle problems. In CDG-Ic, hypotonia, esotropia, and developmental delay are noted early. Recurrent edema of the eyelids is also observed. Infections are frequent; they are accompanied by seizures after 11 months. Magnetic resonance imaging (MRI) shows slight atrophy of cerebrum and cerebellum. "Atrophic retinal pigmentation" and abnormalities of coagulation occur.

CDG-Id involves microcephaly, minimal psychomotor development, and severe epilepsy. A high-arched palate and abnormality of the uvula may be seen. One child had optic atrophy and an iris coloboma. In patients with CDG-Ie, dysmorphic features include microcephaly, downslanting palpebral fissures, a high and narrow palate, telangiectases and hemangiomas, mild limb shortening (especially of the arms), small hands, dysplastic nails, and failure to thrive despite adequate caloric intake. Intractable seizures, the absence of mental development, cortical blindness, hyperreflexia, and profound hypotonia occur. In CDG-IIa the mental retardation is severe, and dysmorphic features occur; but the neuropathology and cerebellar changes of CDG-Ia are not present.

Pathway

Mannose is a common constituent of many oligosaccharide side chains. It must be provided as guanosine diphosphate (GDP) mannose. Isomerization of fructose-6-phosphate to mannose-6-phosphate is catalyzed by phosphomannose isomerase (PMI). Mannose-6-phosphate is converted to mannose-1-phosphate by phosphomannomutase 2 (PMM2) and is then transferred to guanine nucleotide, forming GDP-mannose. Mannose from GDP-mannose is added to the growing oligosaccharide chain or is transferred to dolichol phosphate to form dolichol-phosphate-mannose, the donor of mannose for O- and C-mannosylation in the lumen of the endoplasmic reticulum (ER).

Oligosaccharide "trees" of seven sugars are formed on a lipid dolichol-pyrophosphate backbone on the outer surface of the ER membrane. The oligosaccharide tree is then flipped into the lumen of the ER, where four mannoses and three glucoses are added. From there, it is transferred to a peptide chain, and three glucoses and one mannose are removed. The glycoprotein is transported to the Golgi apparatus, where further modification occurs. Defects in this process result from deficient activity of the enzymes involved in the synthesis of precursors or the assembly of the mature structures. The consequence is the production of many proteins lacking appropriate carbohydrate side chains.

Deficiency of phosphomannose isomerase (PMI) leads to CDG-Ib. This disorder can be successfully treated with oral mannose.

Patients with CDG-Ia have deficient activity of PMM2, which converts mannose-6-phosphate to mannose-1-phosphate, which is the immediate precursor of GDP-mannose. Deficient PMM activity can be documented in cultured fibroblasts. At this point, all mutations found have been in PMM2; no deficiency of PMM1 has been discovered.

CDG-Ie results from impaired formation of dolichol-phosphate-mannose because of deficiency of dolichol-phosphate-mannose synthetase (DPM1). CDG-Id and CDG-Ic are due to defects in the intraluminal addition of mannose and glucose respectively; the defects are in the genes hALG3 and (presumably) hALG6.

Approximately 20% of the patients with a CDG-I pattern on isoelectric focusing have normal activities of PMM and the other known enzymes; they are lumped together as CDG-Ix, suggesting that other enzyme defects remain to be unraveled. Mannose has been proposed as a therapy for CDG-Ia, but clinical results have been disappointing.

DISORDERS OF THE CHOLESTEROL BIOSYNTHESIS PATHWAY

The malformation syndromes due to disorders of cholesterol biosynthesis currently include mevalonic aciduria, desmosterolosis, the X-linked dominant Conradi–Hünermann–Happle and CHILD syndromes, and the Smith–Lemli–Opitz syndrome, which is the most common. Cholesterol is a major component of membranes. Its role in fetal development includes an important covalent interaction with the sonic hedgehog protein, which may help to explain why disruptions of cholesterol synthesis can lead to congenital malformations. The biosynthetic pathway is shown in Fig. 23.1.

Mevalonic Aciduria

Children with mevalonic aciduria have a characteristic facial appearance that includes dolichocephaly, frontal bossing, low-set and posteriorly rotated ears, long eyelashes, blue sclerae, and cataracts. Growth failure and developmental delay, along with hypotonia and ataxia, often occur. Hepatosplenomegaly, lymphadenopathy, anemia, and malabsorption may be found. Febrile episodes with vomiting, diarrhea, arthralgia, a morbilliform rash, and an elevated erythrocyte sedimentation rate and creatine kinase concentration often lead to investigations for infection and immune dysfunction. At this point, increased IgD may be found. Urinary organic acid analysis shows mevalonic acid, and the activity of mevalonate kinase in cultured skin fibroblasts is decreased. Mutations in the mevalonate kinase gene have recently been shown to cause hyperimmunoglobulinemia D and periodic fever syndrome (HIDS); mevalonic aciduria, a malformation syndrome, can thus be seen as a severe form of that disorder. Intermittent corticosteroids and the antioxidants ubiquinone, vitamin E, and vitamin C have been used to treat mevalonic aciduria.

Desmosterolosis

Facial features in infants with desmosterolosis include macrocephaly, a hypoplastic nasal bridge, thickening of the alveolar ridges, and gingival nodules, all of which resemble a lysosomal storage disorder. Congenital heart disease and ambiguous genitalia (in genetic males) may be seen. Rhizomelic limb shortening, reminiscent of chondrodysplasia punctata, may also occur. Analysis of plasma reveals the accumulation of desmosterol. Deficient activity of 3β-hydroxysterol-Δ^{24}-reductase can be demonstrated in cultured skin fibroblasts.

Conradi–Hünermann–Happle Syndrome

Conradi–Hünermann–Happle syndrome, an X-linked dominant condition with chondrodysplasia punctata, called CDPX2, is confined to females and is characterized by a mosaic of normal and affected regions in various tissues. It is thought to be lethal in

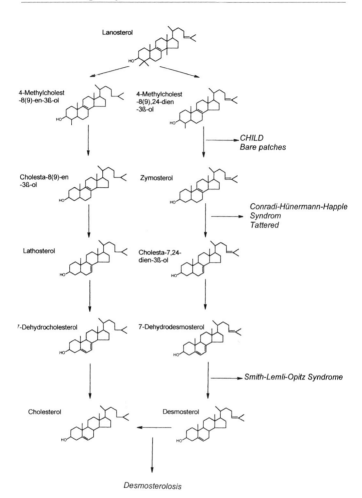

Fig. 23.1.   Distal pathway of cholesterol biosynthesis. The initial steps
in the synthesis of cholesterol involve the formation of mevalonic acid
from acetyl-CoA, catalyzed by a sequence of three enzymes. The last of
these, 3-hydroxy-3-methylglutaryl-CoA reductase, is the rate-limiting
step of cholesterol synthesis. The phosphorylation of mevalonic acid
catalyzed by the mevalonate kinase is defective in mevalonic aciduria
and in hyperimmunoglobulinemia D and periodic fever syndrome
(HIDS). The phosphorylation of mevalonic acid is followed by the
synthesis of nonsterol isoprenoids, isopentyl-, geranyl-, and farnesyl-
pyrophosphates. The last is converted into squalene, followed by
cyclization into lanosterol. The final modification of the sterol nucleus
follows one of two distinctive pathways depicted in the figure. The

males. Rhizomelic limb shortening, which is usually asymmetric, occurs, as do patches of ichthyosis, follicular atrophoderma, and alopecia. The hair is generally coarse, and it lacks luster. The facial features include flattening of the midface and cataracts. Biochemically, CDPX2 patients have normal or, occasionally, decreased cholesterol levels and elevated concentrations of 8-dehydrocholesterol and 8(9)-cholestenol that can be detected by gas chromatography mass spectrometry (GC-MS) sterol analysis in plasma and tissues. A defect in cholesterol synthesis at the locus for 3-β-hydroxysteroid-Δ^8,Δ^7-isomerase can be demonstrated in cultured skin fibroblasts (Fig. 23.1). This gene encodes the emopamil-binding protein. The mosaicism in this X-linked condition may be due to expression of the different X chromosomes (lyonization) following conception of an XX fetus carrying the mutation or to a half-chromatid mutation early in embryonic development that leads to somatic mosaicism on a clonal basis. To allow the abnormal cells to survive, the presence of normal cells appears to be a necessity. Thus, affected males are miscarried and all patients are female.

Other forms of chondrodysplasia punctata with pre- and postnatal growth, retardation, ichthyosis, cataracts, and variable mental retardation are the X-linked recessive form chondrodysplasia punctata X1 (resulting from deficiency of arylsulfatase E), the autosomal dominant Conradi–Hünermann syndrome (defect not yet known), and rhizomelic chondrodysplasia punctata (RCDP), which can result from several defects of plasmalogen synthesis or peroxisome enzyme import (see Chapter 29). Warfarin embryopathy is a teratogenic form of chondrodysplasia punctata that is caused by drug inhibition of arylsulfatase E.

CHILD Syndrome

In CHILD syndrome the skin and skeletal system are usually (some authorities suggest always) involved. A unilateral erythematous exfoliative dermatosis that stops at the midline is seen; it was originally called ichthyosis but which is now classified on the basis of skin cell kinetics as psoriasis. The right side is the one

◄───────────────────────────────────

location of enzyme defects leading to specific malformation syndromes is indicated, as are two known animal models. The "tattered" mouse phenotype resembling CDPX2 results from an X-linked semidominant mutation of the emopamil binding protein gene encoding for the sterol-Δ^8-isomerase; the "bare patches" that the mouse mutant suffers result from a deficiency of the NAD(P)H steroid dehydrogenase-like subunit of the sterol-4-demethylase complex, the enzymatic step just prior to sterol-8-isomerase.

1: CHILD syndrome due to defects in the sterol-4-demethylase

2: Conradi–Hünermann–Happle syndrome due to defects sterol-Δ^8-isomerase

3: Smith–Lemli–Opitz syndrome due to defects in 7-dehydrocholesterol-reductase

4: Desmosterolosis due to defects in 3β-hydroxysterol-Δ^{24}-reductase

most likely to be involved. Usually the face is spared. Some skin lesions (including hyperkeratosis, acanthosis, verruciform xanthomatous changes, and inflammation) follow the lines of Blaschko. Punctate calcifications of the epiphyses of vertebrae and long bones, calcification of airway cartilage, and renal hypoplasia may occur. Cataracts are not part of the CHILD syndrome. Since all patients are female, the disease appears to be lethal in males, and the inheritance is X-linked dominant. This syndrome usually results from deficient activity of sterol-4-demethylase, caused by mutations in the gene on the X-chromosome encoding the NAD[P]H steroid dehydrogenase-like protein (NSDHL) subunit (Fig. 23.1). Plasma sterol analysis shows increased 4-methylsterols. In two CHILD syndrome patients, the same sterol pattern that occurs in CDPX2 patients has been found; later, mutations in the gene for 3-β-hydroxysteroid-Δ^8,Δ^7-isomerase, the enzyme that is also deficient in Conradi–Hünermann–Happle syndrome, were also observed. The mechanism, which causes strikingly asymmetric malformations in one condition and patchy distribution in the other, is not yet understood.

Smith–Lemli–Opitz Syndrome

Smith–Lemli–Opitz syndrome (SLO) is the most common of the disorders of the cholesterol pathway, as it occurs in between one in 20,000 to one in 40,000 births. Although low plasma cholesterol was noted in the 1980s, its significance as a diagnostic clue was not initially appreciated. A better understanding of the biochemistry of this condition has resulted in the cessation of classification as either a milder (type I) or a more severe (type II) form.

The importance of cholesterol in morphogenesis is demonstrated by the problems that occur when cholesterol is deficient. The mildest malformation is syndactyly of toes 2 and 3. More severe features include microcephaly with bifrontal narrowing, ptosis, a short nose with anteverted nostrils, a broad nasal tip, low-set ears, micrognathia, and cleft palate. Postaxial polydactyly of the hands; short, proximally placed thumbs; and overlapping fingers may be present. Genital abnormalities in males may range from mild hypospadias to ambiguous genitalia. Prenatal and postnatal growth retardation is common, and intellectual impairment may be severe. Various malformations of the heart, lung, liver, kidneys, adrenal gland, pancreas, and brain may also exist. Intrauterine or early neonatal death may occur in the severe form of this disorder, in which mesomelic shortening of the limbs may be seen. Holoprosencephaly with midline clefting and ocular hypotelorism can also occur in severe SLO, which may be undiagnosed unless the specific metabolic defect is sought.

Serum cholesterol levels correlate inversely with severity but may be in the normal range once dietary sources of cholesterol are introduced. The fundamental defect is in 7-dehydrocholesterol reductase, the last step of cholesterol synthesis (Fig. 23.1). The levels of 7-dehydrocholesterol and 8-dehydrocholesterol in serum, measured by GC-MS in many laboratories, are significantly elevated. The mechanism of altered morphogenesis is not completely understood, but it may involve abnormalities of the hedgehog signaling pathway.

Treatment strategies include both cholesterol supplementation and the reduction of pathologic sterol metabolites. Cholesterol therapy, sometimes used with ursodeoxycholic acid, appears to improve the disposition and motor function of some patients, who then learn to walk and regain speech; some patients have even been able to say how much better they felt after the initiation of cholesterol supplementation. Remarkable results have been obtained following treatment with 3-hydroxy-3-methylglutaryl-CoA reductase inhibitors that block cholesterol biosynthesis. In SLO children this remedy leads to a surprising increase of cholesterol levels, as well as to improvement of clinical manifestations. Providing cholesterol to the growing brain, reducing pathologic metabolites, and repairing the damage caused in embryonic life remain major challenges.

MENKES SYNDROME

Menkes syndrome, an X-linked recessive disorder of copper metabolism, typically presents in boys in the neonatal period. Delivery may be premature, and initial findings often include hypothermia and hypoglycemia. The physical features include pudgy cheeks and sagging jowls and lips. The scalp hair and eyebrows are hypopigmented with sparse, stubby, and broken hairs. The hair was originally described by Menkes as kinky, but in reality, it looks wiry, similar to steel wool; under microscopic examination it has the appearance of a flat, twisting ribbon. X-rays show Wormian bones along the cranial sutures, metaphyseal spurs, and osteoporosis, which may eventually lead to fractures.

Menkes syndrome results from abnormalities of the MNK gene, which codes for an intracellular copper-transporting ATPase, ATP7A. This protein is similar to ATP7B, which is deficient in Wilson disease. In Menkes disease the copper transporter is abnormally expressed in many tissues but not in the liver. In contrast, in Wilson disease the deficiency is in the separate hepatic copper transporter (see Chapter 16). Deficient copper transport by ATP7A impairs the synthesis of several copper-containing enzymes. These include lysyl oxidase (essential for collagen and elastin cross-linking), dopamine β-hydroxylase, cytochrome C oxidase, tyrosinase, and superoxide dismutase, as well as ceruloplasmin.

The secondary deficiencies of these cuproenzymes account for the symptoms of Menkes syndrome, including poor bone formation and osteoporosis, lax joints and skin, tortuous blood vessels (especially cerebral), diverticuli of the bladder, blood pressure instability and hypotension, and hypopigmentation. Subdural hematomas are common.

The course in untreated boys is one of neurologic deterioration. Survival beyond 2 to 3 years of age is rare. Treatment using copper histidinate attenuates Menkes syndrome, slowing the progression of neurologic symptoms. Treatment with copper histidinate must be begun as early as possible. Inducing of labor at 8 months to begin early therapy is one way of doing so.

The physical findings of treated Menkes syndrome resemble an allelic, milder defect of copper transport, called Ehlers–Danlos syndrome type IX or the occipital horn syndrome. Patients with this condition have the connective-tissue aspects of Menkes syndrome, but neurologic deterioration is minimal or absent.

Clinical findings lead to suspicion of Menkes syndrome. The serum copper and ceruloplasmin levels are low within a week of birth. Studies of radioisotopic copper accumulation in cultured fibroblasts and biopsy of tissues in order to assay copper content (high in intestinal tissue, low in liver) can confirm the diagnosis. No common mutation has been identified, so molecular diagnosis is difficult. Large deletions and smaller mutations have been reported.

Heterozygous female carriers of a mutant MNK gene may show the patchy involvement of skin and hair, and copper studies can help detect carriers. Neurologic and vascular complications do not occur in heterozygotes.

MULTIPLE ACYL-COA DEHYDROGENASE DEFICIENCY

Multiple acyl-CoA dehydrogenase deficiency, which is also called glutaric aciduria type II, is due to a deficiency of either electron-transfer flavoprotein (ETF) or ETF dehydrogenase; it causes deficient electron transfer from the electron donor $FADH_2$ to coenzyme Q that funnels into the respiratory chain. A mild impairment of this process leads to predominant hepatic and muscle disease. A characteristic organic acid pattern, sometimes called ethylmalonic-adipic aciduria, is seen; and various short- and medium-chain acylcarnitines are present in the blood.

Severe impairment of ETF or ETF dehydrogenase results in significant physical abnormalities and overwhelming metabolic decompensation with a poor prognosis. The physical findings can include macrocephaly with a high forehead, craniotabes, large anterior fontanelle, ocular hypertelorism, epicanthic folds, short nose, and long philtrum. Renal cortical cysts are often present. Abdominal wall defects and anomalous external genitalia have been reported. Structural brain malformations, including heterotopias, may occur. An unpleasant and characteristic acrid odor (see Chapter 4) may be prominent. Acidosis, cardiomyopathy, liver dysfunction, and epileptic encephalopathy may be overwhelming even on the first day because the metabolic decompensation in this disorder is among the most rapid.

AMINO ACID DISORDERS

Maternal Phenylketonuria

Maternal phenylketonuria (PKU) is an excellent example of biochemical teratogenesis. Children of mothers with PKU are obligate heterozygotes and may be affected by PKU if the father is a heterozygote; however, the real danger in this situation is not from PKU in the infant (which would be detected by newborn screening) but from prenatal damage caused by high maternal concentrations of phenylalanine. Birth defects caused by inadequately treated maternal PKU include mental retardation, microcephaly, facial dysmorphism, and congenital cardiac defects, especially ventricular septal defects. Toxicity from phenylalanine is likely to occur if the mother's level is more than 400 μM, which is relatively low when one considers that persons who have phenylalanine levels in that range on a normal diet may have never been treated. Active transport across the placenta increases phenylalanine levels in the child to 1.5 times that of the mother.

These complications can only be avoided if a woman with PKU who is contemplating pregnancy adheres to a strict PKU diet before conceiving and if she is carefully monitored throughout the pregnancy. Pregnancy itself, and the nausea and poor appetite that often occur in early pregnancy, make this situation especially challenging.

Most women with PKU in developed countries who are in their reproductive years have been previously identified by newborn screening programs; however, occasionally a woman with undiagnosed PKU is discovered through the birth of a baby with the maternal PKU syndrome.

Homocystinuria

Homocystine is the dimeric form of the amino acid homocysteine. It accumulates with mixed disulfides of homocysteine in cystathionine β-synthase deficiency, which is the principal cause of homocystinuria. Subtle or prominent physical manifestations may occur (principally, a Marfanoid appearance). This condition is not generally recognized until school age. Progressive myopia, tall stature and slender build, scoliosis, prominent livido reticularis, lenticular dislocation (usually downward, in contrast with the usual upward dislocation of Marfan syndrome), narrow hands and feet, and osteoporosis may occur. These findings are apparently due to effects of homocysteine on collagen, fibrillin, and other connective-tissue substances. Vessels may become occluded (not typical of Marfan syndrome) as a consequence of increased platelet "stickiness" caused by increased plasma homocysteine. Vascular occlusion may result in subtle cortical atrophy, or major cerebral vascular thrombosis. Mental retardation and epilepsy may occur. Some of the manifestations of Marfan syndrome, such as aortic dilatation and mitral valve prolapse, do not usually occur in homocystinuria. Total plasma homocyst(e)ine levels determine the diagnosis. A simple first step is the urine nitroprusside test (Brand test), but a negative result does not conclusively rule out homocystinuria. Roughly half of all patients with homocystinuria due to cystathionine β-synthase deficiency become essentially normal biochemically if they receive pyridoxine supplementation, sometimes with folic acid and betaine. Mild hyperhomocystinemia and homocystinuria may occur with defects of metabolism or availability of vitamin B_{12}, folate, or pyridoxine and in renal failure.

METABOLIC ERRORS WITH SUBTLE MALFORMATIONS

The following conditions have been reported to have some subtle dysmorphisms, but the primary and most obvious problem is the biochemical derangement.

Infants with propionic aciduria may have inverted nipples or other nipple abnormalities. These patients, as well as patients with other organic acidurias, particularly glutaric aciduria type I and methylmalonic aciduria, may have a slightly unusual facial appearance. The combination of muscular hypotonia and increased facial fat (presumably brown fat) results in slightly droopy cheeks, particularly in infants and young children. In addition, frontal bossing and a relatively large head (up to macrocephaly) may be seen. A similar facial appearance can be observed in children with congenital lactic acidosis (due to pyruvate dehydrogenase or oxidative phosphorylation defects), who may also have increased body hair (especially on the back and limbs) and long (or darker) eyelashes. Agenesis of the corpus callosum occurs in children with deficient energy production and in those with nonketotic hyperglycinemia.

ADDITIONAL READING

Bankier A. Menkes disease. *J Med Genet* 1995;32:213–215.

Freeze HH. Disorders in protein glycosylation and potential therapy: tip of an iceberg? *J Pediatr* 1998;133:593–600.

Jaeken J, Carchon H. What's new in congenital disorders of glycosylation? *Europ J Paediatr Neurol* 2000;4:163–167.

Kelley RI. RSH/Smith-Lemli-Opitz syndrome: mutations and metabolic morphogenesis. (Editorial) *Am J Hum Genet* 1998;63:322–326.

Kelley RI. Inborn errors of cholesterol biosynthesis. *Adv Pediatr* 2000; 47:1–53.

Patterson MC. Screening for "prelysosomal disorders": carbohydrate deficient glycoprotein syndromes. *J Child Neurol* 1999;14(Suppl 1): S16–S22.

24 ♣ Hematologic Abnormalities

Abnormalities in one or more components of the hematologic system occur in a variety of inborn errors of metabolism. In some they may serve as signals to alert the clinician to the presence of an underlying metabolic disease. In others, such as the enzymopathies that produce hemolytic anemia, the abnormal hematology is the disease. In some, as in the hypersplenism of Gaucher disease, they represent an important complication that must be monitored and treated appropriately in a patient whose diagnosis had been made earlier on the basis of other manifestations.

The mechanisms by which metabolic disease causes a hematologic abnormality vary. Storage of lipids, as in Gaucher disease, leads to enlargement of the spleen and the pancytopenia of hypersplenism. Intrinsic abnormalities of erythrocyte enzymes, such as glucose-6-phosphate dehydrogenase, lead to hemolytic anemia. The organic acidurias in which accumulation of CoA esters is seen inhibit the maturation of marrow elements, most notably polymorphonuclear leukocytes; but they may also produce thrombocytopenia or pancytopenia. Megaloblastic anemia results from diseases in which the absorption or transportation of cobalamin or its conversion to methylcobalamin is interrupted. It may also result from abnormalities in folate metabolism.

NEUTROPENIA, THROMBOCYTOPENIA, ANEMIA, PANCYTOPENIA

Effects on hematologic function are prominent manifestations of metabolic imbalance in the organic acidurias, particularly propionic aciduria, methylmalonic aciduria, and isovaleric aciduria (Table 24.1). An ontogeny exists, whereby neonatal infants up to the age of 4 to 6 weeks may present with pancytopenia. Those under a year of age may have both neutropenia and thrombocytopenia, while neutropenia may accompany metabolic imbalance in any age group. The other concomitants of metabolic imbalance are ketoacidosis and life-threatening emergency illness (Chapter 6). Patients may be hypotonic, and they may also demonstrate failure to thrive. Any patient with an acute life-threatening illness and this hematologic picture should be tested with an organic acid analysis of the urine or an acylcarnitine profile of the blood to establish the specific type of organic aciduria. Rarely, the pancytopenia may present without the acute ketoacidosis (especially in the neonatal period). At least two of the authors' patients were diagnosed by an alert hematologist who sent a urine sample from such an infant for organic acid analysis. At the same time, the clinician must remember that the hematology results from metabolic imbalance and the accumulation of the CoA esters behind the block. A patient whose organic aciduria is under good metabolic control and who suddenly develops neutropenia should be investigated for sepsis; the clinician must not assume that this always results from the abnormal metabolism.

Neutropenia is also seen in glycogenosis type Ib. These patients are usually diagnosed early because of the hypoglycemia. The

Table 24.1.   Metabolic disorders with neutropenia, thrombocytopenia, or pancytopenia

Hematologic manifestation	Disorder	Diagnostic test
Neutropenia	Organic acidurias:	
	Propionic aciduria	Urinary organic acids
	Methylmalonic aciduria	Urinary organic acids
	Isovaleric acidemia	Urinary organic acids
	Glycogenosis Ib	Glucagon test, enzyme assay of biopsied liver, mutation analysis
	Lysinuric protein intolerance	Amino acid analysis, plasma and urine
	Aspartylglu-cosaminuria	Urinary HPLC, paper chromatography, or TLC
Neutropenia and thrombocytopenia	Organic acidurias in infancy	Urinary organic acids
Thrombocytopenia	Cobalamin C disease	Urinary methyl-malonate; homocys-teine in blood or urine
Pancytopenia	Organic aciduria, neonatal	Urinary organic acids
	Transcobalamin II deficiency	Urinary methyl-malonate; homo-cysteine in blood or urine
	Pearson mt DNA deletion	mt DNA
	Mevalonic aciduria	Urinary organic acids
	Gaucher disease	Lysosomal enzyme assay
	Methylcobal-amin—Cbl E + G disease	Homocysteine in blood or urine; methionine in plasma

Abbreviations: HPLC, high-performance liquid chromatography; mt DNA, mitochondrial DNA; TLC, thin-layer chromatography.

metabolic picture of hypoglycemia, hypercholesterolemia, hyper-triglyceridemia, lactic acidemia, and hyperuricemia is virtually diagnostic. Of course, hepatomegaly is also prominent, and no glycemic response to glucagon occurs (see Chapter 11, "Glucagon Stimulation"). The Ib variety is usually diagnosed by enzyme assay of biopsied liver. The glucose-6-phosphatase activity is defective in the usual assay but normal when the preparation is frozen and then thawed or when it is treated with detergents. The fundamental defect is in the glucose-6-phosphate translocase. Neutrophils have been shown to be abnormal with the uptake of glucose, and this may be employed to test for Ib. These patients do have repeated infections and may develop inflammatory bowel disease.

Hematologic abnormalities have been reported in a group of patients with prominent consanguinity who had lysinuric protein intolerance. The appearance of the marrow resembled Niemann-Pick disease with sea-blue histiocytes but normal sphingomyelinase.

Neutropenia and repeated infections may be seen in aspartyl-glucosaminuria. Vacuolated lymphocytes are found in the blood; marrow cells and hepatocytes are also vacuolated. Diagnosis usually rests on the demonstration of the key compound in the urine.

Isolated thrombocytopenia may be seen in cobalamin C disease, in which methylmalonic aciduria, homocystinuria and homo-cystinemia are found. More often, this disease presents with megaloblastic anemia (Table 24.2). This is also true of transcobalamin II deficiency and cobalamin E and G disease, but in their most advanced form in which platelet transfusions are necessary to sustain life, pancytopenia and an acellular marrow may be seen.

In Pearson syndrome the mitochondrial DNA depletion presents with severe, transfusion-dependent anemia and a characteristic marrow appearance of vacuolated erythrocyte precursors and sideroblasts detectable with Prussian blue stain. Thrombocytopenia and neutropenia are variable.

In Gaucher disease the effects on the marrow are those of hypersplenism, and the diagnosis is usually well established long before their appearance. Monitoring the hematology is important because a splenectomy may be required, especially for thrombocytopenia. Enzyme replacement therapy should avert that if begun early.

MEGALOBLASTIC ANEMIA

Megaloblastic anemia (see Table 24.2), neutropenia, and hypersegmented leukocytes are early characteristics of orotic aciduria. Infectious complications are common, and they vary widely. Cellular immunity may be impaired. Sparse hair and hypoplastic nails are common, as is failure to thrive. Patients have been detected because of crystalluria and precipitated orotic acid in the urine.

Megaloblastic anemia results from defective transportation or metabolism of B_{12} in transcobalamin II disease, cobalamin C disease (cbl C), pernicious anemia and Immerslund disease. In all of these but cbl C disease, levels of B_{12} in the blood are low. In all, the formation of both methylcobalamin and adenosylcobalamin

Table 24.2. Metabolic disorders with megaloblastic anemia

Disorder	Diagnostic test
Orotic aciduria	Urinary orotic acid, organic acids
Transcobalamin II deficiency	Urinary methylmalonate, homocysteine in blood and urine
Cobalamin C disease	Urinary methylmalonate, homocysteine in blood and urine
Pernicious anemia, intrinsic factor deficiency	Urinary methylmalonate, homocysteine in blood and urine, B_{12}, Schilling test
Imerslünd disease (B_{12} malabsorption)	Urinary methylmalonate, homocysteine in blood and urine, B_{12}, Schilling test
Methionine synthase deficiency	Homocysteine in blood and urine
Cobalamin E, G disease	Homocysteine in blood and urine
Folate malabsorption	Folate
Glutamate formimino transferase deficiency	Urinary FIGLU
Dihydrofolate reductase deficiency	Hepatic dihydrofolate reductase
Lesch–Nyhan disease	Erythrocyte HPRT

Abbreviations: B_{12}, vitamin B_{12}; FIGLU, formiminoglutamic acid; HPRT, hypoxanthine phosphoribosyl transferase.

is defective, and methylmalonic aciduria and homocystinuria/ homocystinemia are observed. Cbl C patients also have global developmental delay and neurologic dysfunction. Homocystinemia without methylmalonic aciduria is found in methionine synthase deficiency and in cbl E and G diseases. Megaloblastic anemia is also seen in disorders of folate metabolism, in which activity of dihydrofolate reductase or glutamate formininotransferase are deficient. In the latter, formiminoglutamic acid (FIGLU) excretion is increased. Patients also have neurologic dysfunction and developmental delay. Patients with folate malabsorption generally have mouth ulcers as well.

In Lesch-Nyhan disease, megaloblastic anemia is evanescent, is usually mild, and is self-limited. In exceptional cases it may be severe enough to require treatment. In these patients abnormal purine metabolism leads to neurologic dysfunction, abnormal behavior, and hyperuricemia (see Chapter 28).

HEMOLYTIC ANEMIA

Hemolytic anemia and the immediate consequences of red cell breakdown, such as hyperbilirubinemia, splenomegaly, and biliary stones, are the only manifestations of a number of disorders with defective erythrocyte glycolytic enzymes. The classic disorder is glucose-6-phosphate dehydrogenase deficiency (Table 24.3), but an extensive list of enzymes with defective activity can lead to hemolysis. This is also a major manifestation of the hemoglobinopathies. Additionally, neurologic manifestations are seen in triosephosphate isomerase deficiency and phosphoglycerol kinase deficiency, in which crises of hemolysis occur in conjunction with neurologic crises, such as hemiplegia or coma. Hemolysis is also characteristic of congenital erythropoietic porphyria (see Chapter 22).

Table 24.3.   Metabolic or molecular disease in which there is hemolytic anemia

Disorder	Diagnostic test
Glucose-6-phosphate dehydrogenase (G6PD) deficiency	Enzyme assay—RBC
Hexokinase deficiency	Enzyme assay—RBC
Glucose phosphate isomerase deficiency	Enzyme assay—RBC
Phosphofructokinase (PFK) deficiency	Enzyme assay—RBC
2,3-Diphosphoglycerate mutase deficiency	Enzyme assay—RBC
Triosephosphate isomerase deficiency	Enzyme assay—RBC
Phosphoglycerate kinase (PGK) deficiency	Enzyme assay—RBC
Pyruvate kinase (PK) deficiency	Enzyme assay—RBC
Glutathione synthetase deficiency	Enzyme assay—RBC
γ-Glutamylcysteine synthetase deficiency	Enzyme assay—RBC
Hemoglobinopathies	RBC hemoglobin electrophoresis, DNA diagnosis
Congenital erythropoietic porphyria	Urinary uroporphyrin
Neonatal hemochromatosis	Hepatic or buccal iron
Wilson disease	Plasma ceruloplasmin, hepatic copper
Abetalipoproteinemia	Acanthocytes, low ESR, lipoprotein electrophoresis
Wolman disease	Vacuolated lymphocytes, enzyme assay
Lecithin cholesterol acyltransferase (LCAT) deficiency	Lipoprotein electrophoresis, enzyme assay

Abbreviations: ESR, erythrocyte sedimentation rate; RBC, erythrocytes.

Disorders, such as neonatal hemochromatosis and Wilson disease, in which early liver malfunction is the major feature often display early hemolysis. In abetalipoproteinemia, hemolytic anemia accompanies ataxia, peripheral neuropathy, retinitis pigmentosa, and acanthocytosis. Acanthocytosis and hemolytic anemia are also early signs in Wolman disease. In this condition, extreme failure to thrive is associated with vomiting, diarrhea, and abdominal distension; calcified adrenals are found. In this disorder, the deficient enzyme is the lysosomal lipase. In lecithin cholesterol acyltransferase (LCAT) deficiency, hemolytic anemia accompanies proteinuria and corneal opacities.

VACUOLATED LYMPHOCYTES AND ABNORMAL CELLS IN THE BONE MARROW

Examination of blood smears for vacuolated lymphocytes by an experienced hematologist or an examination of the bone marrow for typical storage cells or foam cells often provides the first substantive diagnosis of a lysosomal storage disease, including disorders of complex lipid catabolism and the mucopolysaccharidoses (see Chapter 29). Mucolipidoses are also detectible in this way. The term I-cell disease, which is used for mucolipidosis II or N-acetylglucosaminyl (GlcNAc) phosphotransferase deficiency, symbolizes the fact that the disease was first recognized as a disorder in which cytoplasmic inclusions were seen in cultured fibroblasts.

Among the lipid storage diseases, vacuolated lymphocytes are seen in all subtypes of Niemann-Pick disease and in G_{M1} gangliosidosis, Wolman disease, the ceroid lipofuscinoses, galactosialidosis, mucolipidosis II and III, sialidosis, α-mannosidosis, fucosidosis, and aspartylglucosaminuria. They are also seen in Salla disease, the lysosomal transport disorder in which lysosomal storage of sialic acid occurs because of a defect in the transporter responsible for removing it from the lysosome. These patients present with hypotonia, nystagmus, and ataxia, as well as with developmental delay. Coarse features do not appear until adulthood. The early findings are sufficiently nonspecific so that, unlike typical storage diseases, vacuolated lymphocytes may be the only real clue to the diagnosis.

Vacuoles of stored glycogen may be seen in Pompe disease, but the more common infantile form is usually diagnosed from an assay for the defective glucosidase in an infant presenting with major cardiac muscle disease.

In the mucopolysaccharidoses, the abnormal microscopic appearance is that of the polymorphonuclear neutrophils, which contain metachromatic granules known as Alder-Reilly, or Reilly, bodies. These may be visualized better in histocytes of the bone marrow.

25 ❧ Approach to the Patient with Immunologic Problems

A number of children with inherited metabolic diseases have immunologic problems that result in increased susceptibility to infection. In some, infections are secondary to chronic disease, malnutrition, or poor control of swallowing and the resulting aspiration. In most metabolic defects the immunologic abnormalities are secondary to the metabolic derangement. Immune defects can occur in one or more of the major components of the immune system: T cells, B cells (including immunoglobulins), phagocytes (e.g., neutrophils, monocytes, macrophages, and natural killer [NK] cells), and complement. Primary metabolic immunodeficiency diseases include adenosine deaminase deficiency or purine nucleoside phosphorylase deficiency. Other inherited diseases with severely compromised immunity include inborn errors of cobalamin and folate metabolism, organic acidurias, and disorders of carbohydrate metabolism. In most of these, correction of the metabolic defect results in normal immune function.

A wide range of immune defects has been identified in association with inherited metabolic diseases; sometimes, the defect is found only in single case reports, and in others it is a constant manifestation. In clinical practice, the following two situations arise: (a) the patient presents with a known metabolic disorder accompanied by immunologic problems that are recognized manifestations of the disease; or (b) the patient presents with immunologic deficiencies and a metabolic disorder is sought. Metabolic defects lead to symptoms such as chronic or recurrent infection, infection with unusual agents, or poor response to treatment. Laboratory examination for immunodeficiency should be performed on patients with these complaints (Table 25.1). A clinically significant immunodeficiency presents with both an unusual history of infection and corresponding, confirmatory laboratory tests. Other patients may have milder manifestations; they may only have laboratory evidence of immunologic abnormalities. Inborn errors of metabolism can be associated with single or combined T-cell or B-cell, phagocyte, and/or NK-cell immunodeficiencies. In patients presenting with immunologic problems in which an underlying metabolic disorder has to be ruled out, specific laboratory investigations should be performed (Table 25.2).

INHERITED METABOLIC DISEASES ASSOCIATED WITH T-CELL IMMUNODEFICIENCY

Purine nucleoside phosphorylase is required for normal catabolism of purines. In purine nucleoside phosphorylase (PNP) deficiency, substrates that affect the immune and nervous systems accumulate. The disease is associated with severe immunodeficiency, and it represents the most important metabolic disease to be associated with clinically relevant, isolated T-cell immunodeficiency. Some patients also have reduced levels of immunoglobulins and B cells, but B-cell function is normal in most patients. The number of T cells is greatly reduced, which leads to lympho-

Table 25.1. Diagnostic tests in patients with a known metabolic disorder and frequent or recurrent infection

History
Physical examination
CBC with differential
Sedimentation rate
Urine analysis
Chest roentgenography
Immune work-up:
  B-cell disorders
    Quantitative immunoglobulins
    Isohemagglutinin
    Specific antibody titers
  T-cell disorders
    Skin tests for tetanus, mumps, and monilia (>3 years of age)
    Lymphocyte count/differentiation
    Lymphocyte stimulation
  Thymus on roentgenographic studies
  Phagocyte disorders
    Granulocyte count
    Nitro blue tetrazolium (NBT) test
    Neutrophil function tests

Abbreviation: CBC, complete blood count.

Table 25.2. Routine and specific investigations for differential diagnosis of inherited metabolic diseases in patients with immunologic problems

Urine
  Purines and pyrimidines
  Organic acids
  Amino acids
  Orotic acid
  Oligosaccharides
  Reducing substances/sugars
  Copper
  Uric acid per creatinine
Plasma/serum
  Lactate
  Copper
  Zinc
  Very-long-chain fatty acids
  Folic acid
Enzyme studies
  Galactose-1-phosphate uridyl transferase

penia and cutaneous anergy. Recurrent infections are usually obvious by the end of the first year. In rare instances, onset may be delayed up to the age of six years. The patient's susceptibility to viral diseases, such as varicella, measles, cytomegalovirus, and vaccinia, is enhanced. Severe pyogenic or fungal infections also occur. T-cell dysfunction may worsen during the course of the disease. Affected patients may have autoantibodies and autoimmune hemolytic anemia. Neurological symptoms include abnormal motor development, ataxia, and spasticity. The World Health Organization (WHO) classifies PNP deficiency as a primary immunodeficiency.

Lysinuric protein intolerance is characterized by defective transport of the dibasic amino acids lysine, arginine, and ornithine in the intestine and the renal tubules. Biochemically, this defect results in decreased levels of these amino acids in the plasma and increased levels in urine, which leads to interference with the urea cycle and which also results in hyperammonemia. Intestinal protein intolerance, failure to thrive, and osteoporosis, as well as progressive encephalopathy that results from the hyperammonemia, mark the disease. The highest prevalence is found in Finland. In patients with lysinuric protein intolerance, decreases in the CD4$^+$ T-cell number, lymphopenia, and leukopenia have been reported in addition to decreased leukocyte phagocytic activity. In this condition, as in PNP deficiency, varicella infection may be characterized as having an especially severe clinical course.

Impaired T-cell function has been also described in Menkes disease. This disorder is caused by a defect in a membrane copper transport channel that interferes with the absorption of copper from food and its distribution to the cells, and it results in generalized copper deficiency. Clinical symptoms of classical Menkes disease include neonatal hypothermia, unconjugated hyperbilirubinemia, mental retardation, seizures, typical facies, "kinky" hair, and abnormalities of the connective tissue and bone. Immunologic problems or infections are rare, but pulmonary infection secondary to inhalation may prove lethal.

Thymic hypoplasia and defective T-cell function has been noted in some patients with Zellweger syndrome, which is one of the most severe disorders of peroxisome biogenesis. In this syndrome, which is characterized by extreme muscular hypotonia, seizures, liver dysfunction, dysmorphic skeletal and eye abnormalities, failure to thrive, and early death due to the progressive encephalopathy, immunologic problems present only as a minor part; thus they are not usually of high clinical relevance.

INHERITED METABOLIC DISEASES ASSOCIATED WITH B-CELL IMMUNODEFICIENCY

Excessive nucleotide degradation that leads to nucleotide depletion syndrome because of increased activity of 5′-nucleotidase has been reported in a syndrome that is characterized by immunodeficiency, megaloblastic anemia, and a developmental disorder similar to autism. The first reported patient, a 3-year-old girl, presented with recurrent sinusitis, developmental retardation (particularly of speech), seizures, ataxia, alopecia, megaloblastic anemia, and aggressive behavior. Biochemically, an increased catabolism of purine and pyrimidine nucleotides was demonstrated in the patient. Neither cobalamin nor folic acid metabolism was affected. Immunoglobulin G (IgG) levels were found to be decreased. Whether the increased nucleotidase activity was the primary cause or was secondary is not actually known, but the symptoms appeared to result from pyrimidine nucleotide depletion because supplementation with pyrimidine nucleoside led to significant improvement in clinical symptoms.

Transcobalamin II is necessary for intestinal absorption of cobalamin and transport to tissues. Deficiency of transcobalamin II leads to severe megaloblastic anemia with hypocellular bone marrow, leukopenia, thrombocytopenia, vomiting, failure to thrive, diarrhea, and lethargy. A frequent finding in transcobalamin II deficiency is the presence of hypogammaglobulinemia, particularly of IgG. Less often, levels of IgA and IgM are decreased. A failure to produce specific antibodies against diphtheria or poliomyelitis has been found in several patients. Although phagocytic killing is generally normal, a specific impairment of neutrophils against *Staphylococcus aureus* was reported in a single patient. The clinical symptoms and immunological abnormalities usually resolve after cobalamin supplementation.

Propionic aciduria is a member of the classical organic acidurias. It is caused by deficiency of propionyl-CoA carboxylase, a biotin-dependent enzyme. In its long-term course, the major clinical symptoms, besides the recurrent metabolic decompensations, include mental retardation, an extrapyramidal movement disorder, and osteoporosis. In some patients with propionic aciduria, decreased levels of IgG and IgM, as well as B-cell lymphopenia, have been observed during periods of metabolic acidosis; patients often suffer from extensive monilial dermatosis that also involves the scalp. These defects may be corrected following improvement of the metabolic status.

INHERITED METABOLIC DISEASES ASSOCIATED WITH COMBINED T- AND B-CELL IMMUNODEFICIENCY

Adenosine deaminase (ADA) deficiency is the most well-characterized metabolic disease associated with immunodeficiency; it has been classified as a primary immunodeficiency by WHO. ADA deficiency accounts for up to 50% of patients who suffer from autosomal recessive severe combined immunodeficiency (SCID) disease. ADA converts adenosine and deoxyadenosine to inosine and deoxyinosine respectively. With ADA deficiency, the resulting accumulation of deoxyadenosine and adenosine may lead to lymphocyte toxicity. The severity of the disease correlates directly with the accumulation of toxic metabolites and inversely with residual adenosine deaminase expression. The multiple, recurrent infections are usually more severe than in PNP deficiency, and they rapidly become life-threatening. Typical laboratory findings include lymphopenia (usually less than 500 total lymphocytes per mm³) that involves both the B- and T-cells, as well as hypogammaglobulinemia.

Whereas IgM deficiency may be detected early, IgG deficiency manifests only after the age of 3 months when the maternal supply has been exhausted. Further immunologic abnormalities include a deficiency of antibody formation following specific immunization and an absence or a severe diminution of the lymphocyte proliferation induced by mitogens. This condition is progressive since residual B- and T-cell function, which may be found at birth, disappears later. Only a few patients with delayed (up to 3 years of age) or late (up to 8 years of age) onset have been reported.

Infections are caused by a broad variety of microorganisms. Localized infections predominate in the skin and the respiratory tract, as well as in the gastrointestinal tract, where they often lead to intractable diarrhea and malnutrition. In patients older than 6 months of age, the hypoplasia or apparent absence of lymphoid tissue may constitute a diagnostic sign. In approximately half of the affected patients, bony abnormalities include prominence of the costochondral junctions, which is seen roentgenographically as cupping and flaring. In some affected patients, neurologic abnormalities, including spasticity, head lag, movement disorders, and nystagmus, are found. Injection with bovine ADA that has been conjugated to polyethylene glycol (PEG-ADA) results in the normalization of T-cell number and of many cellular and humoral responses. Bone marrow transplantation has been very successful in some patients. Gene therapy has been performed in a small number of patients, but interpretation of the results is difficult because PEG-ADA therapy was continued.

The disturbance of zinc homeostasis in acrodermatitis enteropathica results from a partial block in intestinal absorption. Reduced zinc absorption leads to the functional impairment of many zinc metalloenzymes that are involved in major metabolic pathways. Symptoms usually start in infancy, and the most dramatic clinical feature is a characteristic skin rash. In many patients with zinc deficiency states, impaired humoral and cell-mediated immune responses can be demonstrated. Secondary infections, usually with *Candida* or *Staphylococci,* are common. Mucosal lesions include gingivitis, stomatitis, and glossitis. Other symptoms include diarrhea, failure to thrive, alopecia, irritability, and mood changes. Zinc therapy leads to clinical remission.

Biotin is a cofactor for carboxylation of 3-methylcrotonyl-CoA, propionyl-CoA, acetyl-CoA and pyruvate. Therefore, biotinidase deficiency and holocarboxylase synthetase deficiency result in multiple carboxylase deficiency, which may also be caused by acquired biotin deficiency. This has resulted from ingestion of avidin in raw eggs and, theoretically, can be caused by long-term intestinal sterilization. Multiple carboxylase deficiency presents clinically as an organic aciduria. Symptoms include lactic acidosis, muscular hypotonia, seizures, ataxia, psychomotor retardation, skin rashes, hair loss, and immune system defects. Immunologic dysfunction affecting both the B- and T-cell lines has been reported in several children with biotinidase deficiency. Symptoms in these patients include mucocutaneous candidiasis; the absence of delayed hypersensitivity, assessed by a skin test and *in vitro* lymphocyte responses to Candida challenge; decreased IgA levels; poor antibody formation in response to pneumococcal immunization; subnormal amounts of T-lymphocytes; reduced leukocyte killing of *Candida*; lack of myeloperoxidase activity in neutrophils; impaired lymphocyte suppressor activity; and decreased prostaglandin E_2 production *in vitro*. One child with biotinidase deficiency was initially diagnosed with SCID and was treated with bone marrow transplantation; however, the symptoms were not ameliorated until biotin was given. In general, findings with biotinidase deficiency are often inconsistent, and treatment with biotin corrects both the immunologic and the metabolic abnormalities.

Hereditary orotic aciduria is an inborn error of pyrimidine metabolism that is characterized by growth retardation, developmental delay, and megaloblastic anemia; it is unresponsive to cobalamin and folic acid. Hereditary orotic aciduria is caused by deficiency of uridine-monophosphate synthetase (see Fig. 28.2). Lymphopenia and increased susceptibility to infections, including candidiasis, bacterial meningitis and fatal varicella, have been observed with hereditary orotic aciduria. Immunologic abnormalities vary and include low T-cell numbers, an impaired delayed-type hypersensitivity (DTH) response, reduced T-cell mediated killing, and decreased levels of IgG and IgA.

Deficiency of intestinal folic acid absorption leads to megaloblastic anemia, psychomotor retardation, seizures, and ataxia. Recurrent infections are an occasional clinical feature of this condition. Immunologic abnormalities vary but can include decreased levels of IgM, IgG, and IgA, as well as decreased proliferation in response to phytohemagglutinin (PHA) and pokeweed mitogen (PWM).

Deficiency of α-mannosidase leads to the accumulation of mannose-rich oligosaccharides in neural and visceral tissues. The disease is termed α-mannosidosis, a lysosomal storage disease, and is characterized by progressive mental retardation, deafness, cataracts, corneal clouding, dysostosis multiplex, progressive ataxia, hernias, and hepatomegaly (Chapter 29). Many patients with α-mannosidosis experience recurrent infections. Immunologic abnormalities may include decreased IgG levels, impaired lymphoproliferation to PHA, defective chemotaxis, phagocytosis, and bactericidal killing. Pancytopenia resulting from antineutrophil antibodies has been reported in one patient.

Leukopenia occurs in approximately 50% of patients with methylmalonic aciduria (MMA), another classical organic aciduria that affects branched-chain amino acid metabolism. Immunologic abnormalities associated with MMA include neutropenia, pancytopenia, decreased B- and T-cell numbers, low IgG levels, and impaired phagocyte chemotaxis. Specific lack of responsiveness to the Candida antigen has been observed and results in extensive dermatosis. In addition, methylmalonic acid inhibits bone marrow stem-cell growth *in vitro*.

INHERITED METABOLIC DISEASES ASSOCIATED WITH PHAGOCYTE IMMUNODEFICIENCY

Galactosemia results from galactose-1-phosphate uridyl transferase deficiency; it is characterized by jaundice, hepatomegaly, nuclear cataracts, mental disability, and difficulties with feeding. In this metabolic disease granulocyte chemotaxis is impaired; bactericidal activity, however, is usually not affected. Neonates with galactosemia are at an increased risk for life-threatening sepsis from *Escherichia coli. In vitro* exposure of neutrophils from affected neonates to galactose results in impaired function.

Glycogen storage diseases (GSD) types Ib and Ic present with hepatomegaly, hypoglycemia, acidosis, and growth failure. The conditions are clearly distinguished from GSD type Ia by the recurrence of severe bacterial infections and immunologic abnormalities that result from neutropenia and defective leukocyte function. Neutrophil function is variable, and in most patients, random movement, chemotaxis, microbial killing, and respiratory burst are diminished. In contrast, monocytes have decreased respiratory burst but usually display normal random and directed motility. T-cell, B-cell, and NK-cell functions are normal. In most patients, recurrent or chronic bacterial infections represent a major clinical problem. The impact of these infections is increased because of the decreased number of neutrophils (usually below 1500/µL) and by defective neutrophil and monocyte functioning. Bone marrow examination shows hypercellularity. GSD type Ib and GSD type Ic are now referred to as glycogen storage disease type I non-a because both are caused by mutations in the glucose-6-phosphate translocase gene. This gene encodes a microsomal transmembrane protein that is expressed in numerous tissues, including monocytes and neutrophils. Frequently observed symptoms, such as inflammatory bowel disease similar to that occurring in Crohn disease, oral lesions, and perianal abscesses, are presumably related to defective neutrophil function. Neutrophil cell counts and some, but not all, neutrophil functions improve following subcutaneous treatment with granulocyte colony-stimulating factor.

X-linked cardioskeletal myopathy (Barth syndrome) is characterized by a congenital dilated cardiomyopathy and mitochondrial myopathy with growth failure. In most patients moderate to severe neutropenia is a persistent feature that leads to serious, recurrent bacterial infections.

Glutathione synthetase deficiency causes severe metabolic acidosis and hemolytic anemia. Over the course of the disease, progressive neurological symptoms may develop, including psychomotor retardation, seizures, ataxia, and spasticity. In nearly 10% of patients with glutathione synthetase deficiency, recurrent bacterial infections resulting from impaired bacterial killing have been reported. The patient's neutrophils fail to assemble microtubules during phagocytosis, which leads to damage of the membranous structures. However, the patient's susceptibility to these infections is relatively mild. Treatment with vitamins C and E can restore abnormal immunologic functions.

Pearson syndrome is characterized by exocrine pancreatic and liver dysfunction, failure to thrive, and neuromyopathy. This metabolic disease is caused by large deletions and duplications in the mitochondrial DNA. In addition to anemia and thrombocytopenia, neutropenia is frequently found.

Defective monocyte oxidative metabolism has been reported in a single patient with Smith-Lemli-Opitz syndrome. However, in general, frequent infections are not a problem in this disease unless the patient is severely malnourished.

In isovaleric aciduria, as in propionic aciduria and MMA, neutropenia and pancytopenia can occur during periods of acidosis. Neonatal sepsis can lead to early death. The bone marrow contains large numbers of immature cells, which suggests an arrest of maturation. Pancytopenia is commonly found in branched-chain organic acidurias. The underlying mechanism is not clear, but is probably related to the accumulation of CoA esters of organic acids.

Phagocyte dysfunction is associated with other, previously discussed inborn errors of metabolism, including acrodermatitis enteropathica, methylmalonic aciduria, propionic aciduria, lysinuric protein intolerance, or α-mannosidosis, in some patients.

INHERITED METABOLIC DISEASES ASSOCIATED WITH NK-CELL IMMUNODEFICIENCY

Lysinuric protein intolerance is one of the few inborn errors of metabolism in which at least one instance of NK-cell immunodeficiency has been reported. Other syndromes, such as Chédiak-Higashi syndrome, Sutor syndrome, Griscelli syndrome, or xeroderma pigmentosum, also manifest deficiency of NK-cell function.

ADDITIONAL READING

Ming JE, Stiehm ER, Graham JM Jr. Syndromes associated with immunodeficiency. *Adv Pediatr* 1999;46:271–351.

V

Selected Groups of Metabolic Diseases

26 ♣ Organic Acid Analysis: Approach to the Diagnosis of Organic Acidurias

Analysis of ninhydrin negative, non-amino organic acids by gas chromatography mass spectrometry (GC-MS) has allowed the identification of increasing numbers of recessively inherited disorders of small molecule intermediary metabolism. These disorders have been referred to as organic acidurias, organic acidemias, organic acid disorders, or organoacidopathies. As organic acids constitute key metabolites of virtually all the pathways of small molecule metabolism (Fig. 26.1), quantitative organic acid analysis has become the most powerful tool in the diagnostic work-up of a patient who is suspected of suffering from an inherited metabolic disease. Disease types elucidated in this manner represent a spectrum of metabolic abnormalities.

The earliest discoveries among the organic acidurias resulted from the pursuit of abnormalities of amino acid degradation. Diseases that were recognized earlier, such as maple syrup urine disease and phenylketonuria, were discovered by amino acid analysis in which detection is facilitated by the purple color produced by the reaction between amino acids and ninhydrin. With recognition of the fact that the first step of amino acid degradation involves the removal of the amino group responsible for this reaction, additional analytical techniques were developed for ninhydrin-negative organic acids. These led to the detection of many metabolic defects of amino acid degradation that lay distal to the initial step, including isovaleric, propionic, and methylmalonic acidurias. In some disorders, the accumulating metabolite may become evident without any technical equipment because of the characteristic smell of the patient or the body fluids, especially during metabolic decompensation (see Chapter 4, "Unusual Odor"). The most useful approach combines gas chromatography and mass spectrometry (GC-MS).

Researchers soon realized that analysis by GC-MS disclosed the accumulation of compounds that indicated the existence of abnormalities in fatty acid oxidation or carbohydrate metabolism. The spectrum of diseases detectable by organic acid analysis is still growing (see Fig. 26.1).

CLINICAL PRESENTATIONS

The range of clinical and biochemical manifestations and findings in organic acidurias is extensive (Tables 26.1 and 26.2) as they differ considerably depending on the pathway involved, the extent of residual enzyme activity, and additional individual genetic and environmental factors. Organic acid analysis should be performed in every patient who presents with symptoms of unexplained intoxication or encephalopathy.

In classic organic acidurias, acute episodes of life-threatening acidosis occur early in infancy. Defects of fatty acid oxidation classically present with hypoketotic hypoglycemia, hepatic failure,

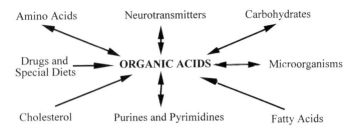

Fig. 26.1.   Organic acids in small molecule intermediary metabolism.

and/or (cardio-)myopathy. In contrast, in mevalonic aciduria, the impairment of cholesterol and nonsterol isoprene biosynthesis results in a severe multisystem disorder with extreme failure to thrive and dysmorphic features. *N*-acetylaspartic aciduria (Canavan disease) and 4-hydroxybutyric aciduria are examples of *cerebral organic acid disorders* in which disturbed metabolism results only in neurological disease.

The classic organic acidurias, which result from defects in pathways of amino acid degradation, present a few days after birth as progressive irritability or drowsiness in a healthy full-term newborn who had an unremarkable pregnancy and perinatal adaptation. However, life-threatening disease may occur as soon as a few hours after birth, or the initial metabolic decompensation may first be seen late in infancy or after. Sometimes, children with a mild form are repeatedly admitted with unusual severe reactions to common infections, especially gastroenteritis, and homeostasis is restored by glucose and electrolyte infusions without the realization of the existence of the underlying metabolic disease. In such patients, routine chemical results may not arouse suspicion between crises.

Most typically, a young infant who is exhibiting vomiting or refusal to feed then quickly deteriorates. The initial diagnosis is usually perinatal infection or intracranial hemorrhage. Metabolic derangement, such as metabolic acidosis, hypoglycemia, and leukopenia, does occur with infection, but the physician should remember that septicemia, following an uneventful pregnancy and delivery from a healthy mother, may be as rare as an inborn error of metabolism. Therefore, seeking the latter should have an equal priority from the onset of the crisis. A presumptive diagnosis of a classic neonatal organic aciduria within 24 to 48 hours of the onset of symptoms may be indispensable for successful treatment and a satisfactory outcome.

Highest consideration should be given to the possibility of inborn errors of metabolism, especially of organic acidurias and disorders of ammonia detoxification, with the baby of parents who previously lost a child with early symptoms similar to those exhibited by the new infant. The same consideration should be made

Table 26.1.   Clinical presentation of organic acidurias

Intoxication
Kussmaul tachypnea/acidotic breathing
Peculiar smell
Refusal of/adverse reaction to feeding
Protracted episodic vomiting
Erroneous diagnosis of pyloric stenosis (with acidosis)
Reye-syndrome presentation
Hepatomegaly/liver failure
Rhabdomyolysis
Sudden infant death syndrome (SIDS) or near miss SIDS

Acute encephalopathy
Coma
Seizures (myoclonic, intractable)
Acute profound dyskinesia
Pseudotumor cerebri
Cerebral/intraventricular hemorrhage in full-term babies
Strokelike episodes

Chronic encephalo(myelo)pathy
Progressive psychomotor deterioration
Macrocephaly
Ataxia (progressive)
Hypotonia
Dystonia, athetosis
Myoclonus
Seizures (myoclonic, intractable)
Peripheral neuropathy
Pyramidal signs—"cerebral palsy"
Pronounced deficiency of speech
Congenital cerebral malformations

Multisystem disease
Failure to thrive
Pancreatitis
Hepatosplenomegaly
Nephromegaly with renal cysts
Osteoporosis and fractures
Myopathy and/or cardiomyopathy
Recurrent severe infections
Anemia (nonimmune hemolytic or megaloblastic)
Myeloproliferative syndrome

Table 26.2. Routine clinical chemical indices of organic acidurias

Metabolic acidosis
Increased anion gap
Hypoketotic hypoglycemia
Hyperglycemia
Ketosis and ketonuria (especially suggestive in newborns)
Lactic acidosis
Hyperammonemia
Hyperuricemia
Hypertriglyceridemia
Increase of transaminases
Increased creatine kinase
Myoglobinuria
Granulocytopenia, thrombocytopenia, anemia

for a symptomatic sibling of a victim of sudden infant death syndrome. Other relevant information from the family history includes the occurrence of acute fatty liver in pregnancy, which is reported in mothers carrying a fetus that is affected by defects of long-chain fatty acid degradation. A vegan diet in a nursing mothers that results in B_{12} deficiency may cause a progressive encephalopathy with methylmalonic aciduria and homocystinuria in her infant.

A substantial number of patients with organic acidurias have presentations that are quite different from the classic picture. Severe decompensation may be present at birth in disorders of impaired oxidative phosphorylation, such as glutaric aciduria type II, and with defects of the respiratory electron transport chain. Recurrent acute presentation alternating with unremarkable clinical and routine chemical features is the rule for patients with disorders of fatty acid oxidation (see Chapter 6, "Work-up of the Child Suspected of Having a Disorder of Fatty Acid Oxidation"). During the first months, these patients usually receive regular, frequent feeding, so the disorder remains hidden. Its appearance is triggered by prolonged fasting, usually as a result of intermittent infection. In a young infant metabolic decompensation may occur so acutely that it results in sudden cardiac and respiratory arrest and the infant's death. More often the clinical picture is that of hypoketotic hypoglycemia. In some patients with disordered fatty acid oxidation, rapidly evolving liver disease is reflected by acute hepatomegaly, cytolysis, or hepatic failure. Chronically progressive myopathy may manifest as muscular hypotonia, exercise intolerance, muscle pain, or recurrent episodes of myolysis and myoglobinuria. In disorders of fatty acid oxidation, routine chemical tests and specific investigations, such as organic acid analysis, may be completely unremarkable in between episodes. Slowly progressive depletion of free carnitine and elevation of acylcarnitines usually develop. Characteristic acylcarnitine patterns can be determined by tandem mass spectrometry from blood spots or body fluids (see Chapter 9).

The other two main categories of clinical presentation of organic acidurias are chronic progressive neurological disease and fluctuating multisystem manifestations (see Table 26.1). In chronic encephalopathy nonspecific symptoms, such as developmental delay or epilepsy, may be the presenting complaint, but examination will usually reveal other, more characteristic findings, including ataxia, myoclonus, extrapyramidal signs, metabolic stroke, or macrocephaly. Routine clinical chemistry is often unrevealing; elevations of diagnostic metabolites by organic acid analysis may be small and thus be missed by semiquantitative organic acid analysis or organic acid screens. This is often found in vitamin responsive disorders or glutaryl-CoA dehydrogenase deficiency. Important diagnostic clues can be derived from neuroimaging studies. Magnetic resonance imaging (MRI) or computerized tomography (CT) scans may reveal characteristic neuropathological changes, such as progressive disturbances of myelination, cerebellar atrophy, frontotemporal atrophy, hypodensities, and/or infarcts of the basal ganglia. Symmetrical (fluctuating) imaging changes that apparently are independent from defined regions of vascular supply are especially suggestive of organic acid disorders or disorders of oxidative phosphorylation (see Chapter 13). Chronic subdural effusions, hematomas, and retinal hemorrhages in infants and toddlers are distinctive findings in glutaryl-CoA dehydrogenase deficiency; they should not automatically be attributed to child abuse.

Multisystem involvement, especially with muscular, hepatic, or pancreatic diseases, should prompt organic acid analysis. Nephromegaly or renal cysts suggest glutaric aciduria type II or peroxisomal disorders. Nonprogressive psychomotor retardation, hypotonia in infancy, epilepsy, failure to thrive, or recurrent infections should be investigated for the usual causes if they are isolated findings before organic aciduria is considered.

ROUTINE LABORATORY INVESTIGATIONS

Patients with the classic organic acidurias display metabolic acidosis and massive ketosis during exacerbations. The pH and the bicarbonate concentration are low, and the anion gap is increased. Hematologic evaluation may reveal leukopenia, thrombocytopenia, and occasionally, pancytopenia. Glucose concentrations can be either low or high. Hyperammonemia occurs frequently in the initial neonatal crisis. If it leads to hyperventilation, the pH may be normal or may even be increased. In these instances an increased anion gap still may point toward the existence of an organic aciduria versus a urea cycle disorder. Hyperammonemia rarely occurs after early infancy except in propionic aciduria. Lactic acid may be increased (see Table 26.2.) Testing for ketonuria is especially useful. In neonates with organic acidurias, pronounced ketonuria is seen, whereas it is rarely observed in newborns suffering from nonmetabolic diseases, even if they are very sick. It is rare even in infants with neonatal diabetes.

In patients with disorders of fatty acid oxidation, hypoglycemia is the classic presentation. If no ketonuria is found at the same time, the diagnosis is straightforward; however, testing for ketones in the urine may confuse the picture. The presence of a positive test does not exclude such a defect. Quantitative assessment of 3-hydroxybutyrate and of free fatty acids with or without aceto-acetate should document that the hypoglycemia is hypoketotic in such a manner that the ratio of free fatty acids to 3-hydroxybutyrate is elevated. In a patient who is examined after the resolution of the acute crisis, a controlled fast (see Chapter 11, "Monitored Prolonged Fast") may be required to document this situation. Concentrations of uric acid are increased during the acute crisis, as is the level creatine kinase. Elevations of transaminases and/or myoglobinuria may be documented.

SPECIALIZED INVESTIGATIONS

Specimens

Organic acid analysis is best when it is performed on early morning urine samples. In comparison with an untimed random sample, the morning urine is more concentrated and abnormalities of metabolism are more readily recognized. Of course, analysis at the time of acute metabolic decompensation is most revealing. Accurate and complete information regarding clinical status, any dietary manipulations, and medication should be provided for optimal interpretation of the results of organic acid analysis. The strength of organic acid analysis—detecting abnormalities of pathways of small molecule metabolism, metabolic imbalances due to dietary manipulation, and products of microorganisms (see Fig. 26.1)—is also its greatest weakness. Subtle abnormalities, especially in partial or vitamin-responsive inborn errors of metabolism, can be missed by qualitative organic acid screens or are misinterpreted as nonspecific. Optimal results require a successful interplay between the clinician and the biochemical genetics laboratory.

Experience with organic acid analysis of body fluids other than urine is limited. As most acidic metabolites are excreted in the urine, it is the preferred diagnostic sample. Theoretically, the study of organic acids in the cerebrospinal fluid (CSF) might define disorders of cerebral metabolism that are not evident systemically, analogous to nonketotic hyperglycinemia or defects of biogenic amine metabolism. A few individual patients, in whom diagnostic elevations of specific organic acids were found only in CSF, have been identified in this way. This analysis appears warranted as an additional specialized diagnostic procedure when used in parallel with enzymatic or molecular investigations in children who are suspected of having glutaric aciduria type I or a disorder of biotin metabolism and in whom repeated urinary analyses have been unrevealing. Analysis of lactic acid in the CSF, even when the analysis of the blood is normal, is often useful in patients with mitochondrial disease. Another obvious indication for organic acid analysis of the CSF is the postmortem analysis of a patient with a suspected organic acidemia when no urine sample is available. In this circumstance CSF is the next best material for analysis. Plasma, vitreous fluid, and bile are additional possibilities for obtaining a diagnosis and giving genetic counsel.

Analytical results are only as good as the sample that is to be analyzed. For organic acid analysis samples should be kept frozen after collection. At room temperature some important groups of acids, particularly oxo acids, are unstable and may be lost. For prolonged storage periods, samples should be kept at $-80°C$ instead of at $-20°C$. Samples should be shipped on dry ice and should be sent early in the week to avoid the loss of dry ice over the weekend. For shipment from some places, recording the volume of the sample, lyophilizing it, and sending it dry may be preferable. Such samples are stable, and they can be sent by regular mail. Sample preservation that utilizes 2 to 3 drops of chloroform and unfrozen shipping, even by express mail, may result in a loss of diagnostic metabolites. Urine can also be applied to neonatal screening card paper and can be sent for organic acid analysis by regular mail. In such samples, extremely high elevations of diagnostic metabolites (e.g., for most organic acidurias caused by defects in amino acid, fatty acid, or glucose catabolism) will still be diagnosable. Smaller metabolite abnormalities are, however, not reliably detectable this way.

The most important source of artifacts in organic acid analysis is bacterial contamination of the sample, which can be minimized by proper handling of specimens. Microorganisms can alter concentrations of organic acids in either direction by eliminating organic acids characteristic of inborn errors of metabolism or by producing metabolites the mimic organic acidurias. Unusual bowel flora or a urinary tract infection can likewise lead to abnormal organic acid excretion in the urine. Elevated concentrations of lactic acid and Kreb cycle intermediates, especially 2-oxoglutaric acid and succinic acid, that are caused by bacterial contamination may be mistakenly interpreted as an indication of mitochondrial disorders. The most common cause of elevated 2-oxoglutaric acid is a urinary tract infection.

Analytical Procedures and Interpretation

The method of choice for organic acid analysis is quantitative GC-MS of the urine. International standards of quality control are being developed, and established programs of proficiency testing exist. If the referring clinician is in doubt, he or she should discuss the patient and the results with an experienced biochemical genetics laboratory. Often, a repeat analysis is recommended, and sometimes, additional tests like fasting and/or loading studies may be indicated (see Chapter 11, "Function Tests").

The interpretation of organic acid analysis depends on key diagnostic metabolites, as well as on characteristic patterns of abnormalities. Repeated analyses may be necessary, especially during an exacerbation of metabolic decompensation. However, characteristic metabolites may also become masked with severe metabolic decompensation and ketosis. This is particularly true in 2-oxothiolase (beta-ketothiolase) deficiency, in which key metabolites may be absent during episodes of ketosis.

Some patients with organoacidopathies may exhibit only slight elevations of diagnostic metabolites that may not be conclusive or even detectable by currently used organic acid analysis. This is particularly true of disorders in which the elevations of methylmalonate and homocysteine are small, such as defects of cobalamin metabolism, and of 4-hydroxybutyric aciduria and N-acetylaspartic aciduria (Canavan disease). In the latter two disorders, ordinary organic acid analysis consistently underestimates the actual concentrations. Specific organic acids, such as 4-hydroxybutyric acid or mevalonic acid, can be accurately quantified by stable isotope dilution internal standard assays (Table 26.3). This is also the method of choice for prenatal diagnosis of many disorders in which direct metabolite analyses of amniotic fluid provides much more rapid and precise diagnosis than does enzymatic analysis of cultured amniocytes. However, concentrations in amniotic fluid are much lower than in urine, and the diagnosis must be ascertained from investigation of a single sample.

In addition to the diagnoses of organic acidurias, elevations of acidic metabolites can be diagnostic for inherited disorders of neurotransmitter metabolism (e.g., vanillacetic acid in aromatic L-amino acid decarboxylase deficiency; dihydrothymine, dihydrouracil, thymine, uracil, orotate, or xanthine in disorders of purine and pyrimidine metabolism; increased concentrations of 2-hydroxy-sebacic acid in peroxisomal disorders; or increased concentrations of homovanillic and vanillylmandelic acids in neuroblastoma).

Table 26.3.   Stable isotope dilution internal standard assays useful in the diagnostic work-up of specific organic acidurias

Compound	Suspected disease
N-acetylaspartic acid	Canavan disease
Glutaric acid and 3-hydroxyglutaric acid	Glutaryl-CoA dehydrogenase deficiency
4-Hydroxybutyric acid	Succinate semialdehyde dehydrogenase deficiency
3-Hydroxyisovaleric acid	Multiple carboxylase deficiencies, isovaleric acidemia, 3-methylcrotonyl-CoA carboxylase deficiency
Methylmalonic acid	Disorders of B_{12} metabolism, including dietary deficiency and transcobalamin II deficiency; methylmalonyl CoA mutase deficiency
Succinylacetone	Hepatorenal tyrosinemia

ADDITIONAL READING

Hoffmann GF, Fehy P. Organic acid analysis. In: Blau N, Duran M, Gibson KM, Blaskovics ME, eds. *Physicians' guide to the laboratory diagnosis of inherited metabolic disease,* 2nd ed. Heidelberg: Springer, 2002.

Hoffmann GF, Gibson KM. Disorders of organic acid metabolism. In: Moser HW, ed. *Handbook of clinical neurology: neurodystrophies and neurolipidoses.* Elsevier Science Publishers 1996;66:639–660.

Jakobs C, ten Brink H, Stellard F. Prenatal diagnosis of inherited metabolic disorders by quantitation of characteristic metabolites in amniotic fluid: facts and future. *Prenatal Diagnosis* 1990;10: 265–271.

27 ♣ Markers of Peroxisomal Function: Approach to Peroxisomal Disorders

Peroxisomes are indispensable for the synthesis of bile acids, cholesterol, and lipids, including plasmalogens and other phospholipids that are present in highest concentrations in the brain, heart, and muscle. Impairments of these biosynthetic pathways result in progressive multisystem disease. Peroxisomes are also critical for the oxidation of very-long-chain fatty acids and related substances, such as phytanic acid. In addition, peroxisomes accommodate many oxygen-dependent reactions, and peroxisomal catalase protects against H_2O_2.

Peroxisomal disorders can be subclassified as follows: generalized defects of peroxisome biogenesis, such as Zellweger syndrome, infantile Refsum disease, and neonatal adrenoleukodystrophy, and defects of individual peroxisomal metabolic enzymes, such as hyperoxaluria type I, Refsum disease, and X-linked adrenoleukodystrophy. However, this widely used classification is not optimal for a clinical and diagnostic approach to peroxisomal disorders. Symptoms and disease courses in patients with generalized versus specific peroxisomal disorders are often indistinguishable, and they may vary tremendously within the same group. Table 27.1 provides a modified grouping of peroxisomal disorders on the basis of the simple, comprehensive diagnostic approach outlined below.

CLINICAL PRESENTATIONS

Peroxisomal disorders present in many different ways, including dysmorphisms and relentless neural degeneration in infancy or early childhood, short-limbed dwarfism, adrenal failure, spinocerebellar degeneration, or renal stones.

The prototypic disorder of peroxisomal biosynthesis is Zellweger syndrome, which was originally described as a cerebrohepatorenal disease. Usually, it is first seen as a dysmorphic syndrome. Affected infants have craniofacial abnormalities, including a prominent high forehead and flat occiput with wide fontanels and cranial sutures, abnormal helices of the ear, a low and broad nasal bridge, epicanthal folds, and hypoplastic supraorbital bridges. Many patients are macrocephalic. In addition, patients experience hepatomegaly, hepatic fibrosis, and renal cysts. Cerebral manifestations, including widespread demyelination and hypomyelination, periventricular rarefaction, microcalcifications, and gray matter abnormalities, are extensive. Neurophysiological assessments (VEP [visual evoked potentials], ERG [electroretinogram], BAER [brainstem auditory evoked response]) become abnormal (see Chapter 13). Many infants show little evidence of psychomotor development. Patients often feed poorly, and the severity of the hypotonia may suggest a diagnosis of myopathy. Profound hypotonia is also a characteristic early finding in neonatal adrenoleukodystrophy in which seizures, hepatic fibrosis, and atrophy of the adrenals occur. Ocular abnormalities include cataracts, nystagmus, optic atrophy, and pigmentary degeneration of the retina. This feature, along with sensorineural deafness and anosmia, is particularly characteristic of infantile Refsum disease.

In contrast, rhizomelic chondrodysplasia punctata is a proximal short-limbed dwarfism in which punctate calcific stippling of the epiphyses occurs and is often associated with ichthyosis, cataracts, and severe developmental delay. Adrenoleukodystrophy is an X-linked disease in which the typical neurodegenerative disease is associated with adrenal insufficiency. However, individual patients may be exclusively Addisonian or leukodystrophic. Adult Refsum disease develops in later childhood and adolescence; it is characterized by pigmentary degeneration of the retina, ataxia, polyneuropathy, sensorineural deafness, and anosmia. Regression of mental functions may or may not be seen.

Hyperoxaluria type I is like none of the disorders discussed above. It presents with nephrocalcinosis, urolithiasis, and renal failure. Furthermore, glutaryl-CoA oxidase deficiency appears to be a relatively benign metabolic condition that only predisposes the patient to an increased susceptibility to hyperketotic hypoglycemia in early childhood. After detection by organic acid analysis, this deficiency must be differentiated from glutaric acidurias types I and II.

In summary, the clinical manifestations of peroxisomal disorders vary widely. Variant, milder phenotypes are dominated by neurological manifestations. Patients may begin a neurodegenerative course after a period of normal development. An important clue can be white matter abnormalities that are consistent with the pathologic appearance of sudanophilic leukodystrophy. Therefore, peroxisomal disorders should be included in the differential diagnosis of infants and young children who suffer from severe hypotonia and seizure disorders but not in patients with mental retardation only.

ROUTINE LABORATORY INVESTIGATIONS

Infants may have elevated transaminases and a tendency to hypoglycemia, which may be a hint to the differential diagnosis. More suggestive is hypocholesterolemia and increased concentrations of iron and transferrin in the serum. Organic acid analysis in patients with peroxisomal diseases may show dicarboxylic aciduria—characteristically an elevation of 2-hydroxysebacic acid—which reflects impaired peroxisomal beta-oxidation.

SPECIALIZED INVESTIGATIONS

The decisive marker for peroxisomal diseases, with the exception of rhizomelic chondrodysplasia punctata, is the elevation of very-long-chain fatty acids (VLCFA) in serum or cultured fibroblasts. Their concentrations can be reliably determined by gas chromatography, following elaborate preparation of the sample, or more simply by gas chromatography and mass spectrometry (GC-MS) because of its superior sensitivity and specificity. VLCFA are found consistently and reliably elevated in all disorders of peroxi-

Table 27.1. Diagnostic grouping of peroxisomal disorders

| | Biochemical diagnosis | | |
	Very-long-chain fatty acids	Plasmalogens	Additional tests
A. Disorders of peroxisome biogenesis and peroxisomal ß-oxidation (elevations of very-long-chain fatty acids)			
1. Disorders of peroxisome biogenesis			
a. Zellweger syndrome	⇑	⇓	⇑ bile acid intermediates; ⇑ phytanic and pristanic acids; ⇑ pipecolic acid
b. Infantile Refsum disease			See below
c. Neonatal adrenoleukodystrophy			
2. Defects of peroxisomal ß-oxidation			
a. Bifunctional protein deficiency	⇑	Normal	⇑ phytanic and pristanic acids
b. Pseudo-Zellweger (peroxisomal thiolase deficiency)	⇑	Normal	⇑ pristanic acid
c. Pseudoneonatal adrenoleukodystrophy (acyl-CoA oxidase deficiency)	⇑	Normal	⇑ pristanic acid

3. Defective activity of very-long-chain acyl-CoA synthetase	⇑	Normal	—
4. X-linked adrenoleukodystrophy and variants	⇑	Normal	—
B. Defects of plasmalogen synthesis			
1. Chondrodysplasia punctata	Normal	⇒	⇑ phytanic acid
2. Dihydroxyacetonephosphate acyltransferase deficiency	Normal	⇒	—
3. Alkyl-dihydroxyacetonephosphate synthase deficiency	Normal	⇒	—
C. Single peroxisomal disorders with variant phenotypes			
1. Refsum disease	Normal	Normal	⇑ phytanic acid
2. Hyperoxaluria type I	Normal	Normal	⇑ glyoxylic and oxalic acids
3. Dihydrocholestanoic and trihydrocholestanoic acidemia	Normal	Normal	⇑ bile acid intermediates
4. Glutaryl-CoA oxidase deficiency	Normal	Normal	⇑ glutaric acid

Table 27.2.   Summary of biochemical markers of peroxisomal disorders

Analysis	Results
Routine clinical chemistry	⇊ cholesterol; ⇊ glucose; ⇑ transaminases; ⇑ serum iron; ⇑ transferrin (in plasma or serum)
Very-long-chain fatty acids	⇑⇑⇑ (in plasma, serum, or cultured fibroblasts)
Ratio of C26/C22	⇑⇑⇑
Plasmalogens	⇊⇊ (in whole blood or erythrocyte membranes)
Phytanic and pristanic acids	⇑ (in plasma or serum, levels dependent on dietary intake)
Bile acids	⇑ individual metabolites (differentiation in plasma or urine
Pipecolic acid	⇑ (in urine, plasma, or bile by GC-MS or fast atom bombardment mass spectrometry)
Organic acids	Dicarboxylic aciduria, often characteristic ⇑ of 2-hydroxysebacic acid (in urine by GC-MS)

Abbreviations: GC-MS, gas chromatography mass spectrometry. Number of arrows indicates degree of increase or decrease.

some biogenesis, as well as in single defects of transport or beta-oxidation of VLCFA (Table 27.2). The ratio of C26 to C22 is the most sensitive index. Additional biochemical investigations for peroxisomal disorders in patients with normal levels of VLCFA are seldom warranted.

In patients with a presumptive diagnosis of rhizomelic chondrodysplasia punctata or its variants, measuring plasmalogens in erythrocytes should be the initial evaluation. If the levels are abnormally decreased, a demonstration of increased phytanic acid in plasma will provide the diagnosis of classical rhizomelic chondrodysplasia punctata. The increase in phytanic acid distinguishes this disorder from the single enzyme defects dihydroxyacetone-phosphate acyltransferase and alkyl-dihydroxyacetonephosphate synthase, which can also produce the clinical and radiologic features of rhizomelic chondrodysplasia punctata. If the plasmalogens are normal, other disorders with punctate calcifications, such as chromosomal aberrations, Warfarin embryopathy (which should be evident from the prenatal history), and X-linked chondrodysplasia punctata due to defects of sterol biosynthesis, must be considered.

A few defects of individual peroxisomal enzymes, such as hyperoxaluria type I, present with quite different clinical and biochemical phenotypes (Group C in Table 27.1). Their diagnosis requires special biochemical investigations, which must be initiated as follow-up to the presumptive clinical diagnosis.

ADDITIONAL READING

Al-Essa MA, Ozand PT. *Atlas of common lysosomal and peroxisomal disorders.* Riyadh: King Fahd National Library Cataloging-in-Publication Data, 1999.

Wanders RJA, Schutgens RBH, Barth PG. Peroxisomal disorders: a review. *Journal of Neuropathology and Experimental Neurology* 1995;54:726–739.

Wanders RJA, Barth PG, Schutgens RBH, Heymans HSA. Peroxisomal disorders: post- and prenatal diagnosis based on a new classification with flowcharts. *International Pediatrics* 1996;11:203–214.

28 ♣ Purines and Pyrimidines: Approach to Diseases of Nucleotide Metabolism

Purines and pyrimidines are the building blocks of nucleic acids and of many cofactors of intermediary metabolism. Inosine monophosphate occupies a central point in the multistep synthesis of purines and in conversions to adenosine monophosphate or guanosine monophosphate. The common end product of purine catabolism, uric acid, is quantitatively excreted in the urine.

Pyrimidines are synthesized from carbamylphosphate, which condenses with aspartate and proceeds using orotic acid to yield the central uridine monophosphate. The other two nucleotides, cytidine monophosphate and thymine monophosphate, are derived from uridine monophosphate, and degradation products are dispersed into intermediary metabolism. The synthesis of carbamyl phosphate is also a central element of ureagenesis (see Fig 6.6). Additional waste nitrogen in the form of ammonia leads to increased production of carbamylphosphate, which is reflected in an increase of orotic acid and orotidine in urine (see Chapter 11, "Allopurinol tests," under "Function tests").

CLINICAL PRESENTATIONS

Diseases of purine and pyrimidine metabolism may affect all living cells. Abnormalities are especially evident in the rapidly dividing tissues. As of now, 24 different genetic disorders are known, of which 14 cause significant clinical disease. Although different combinations of clinical symptoms of varying degrees can be observed, three organ systems are prominently affected: the kidneys, bone marrow, and brain (Table 28.1). Overproduction or disturbed degradation of purines results in the accumulation of large amounts of uric acid or its even less soluble precursor, xanthine (Fig. 28.1). Patients develop dysuria, hematuria, crystalluria, or urinary tract calculi. Plain roentgenograms of the abdomen are usually negative since purine stones are radiolucent. Arthritis can also be directly attributed to increased tissue concentrations of uric acid. The pathophysiology with regard to muscle symptoms, from cramps to wasting, is not yet understood. Immune deficiency and megaloblastic anemia occur in disorders in which the metabolism of either purines or pyrimidines is affected.

A wide variety of neurological manifestations that result from defects in purine and pyrimidine metabolism have been observed. Diseases of purine metabolism can cause abnormal muscle tone, dystonia, and ataxia, in addition to psychomotor retardation. Behavioral abnormalities, which are sometimes reminiscent of autism or a pervasive developmental disorder, are prominent; they can range up to the compulsive, aggressive, severe self-injurious behavior of classic Lesch-Nyhan disease. A number of patients, especially those with diseases of pyrimidine metabolism, present with nonspecific psychomotor retardation or seizure disorders

(text continues on page 339)

Table 28.1. Organ system–based symptomatology of diseases of purine and pyrimidine metabolism

	Kidney	Immune/blood	CNS	Main symptoms	Additional symptoms
PRPPS	+	–	+	Urolithiasis	Gout; deafness
ASL	–	–	++	Developmental delay; seizures	Short stature; muscle wasting
AMPDA	–	–	–	Mostly asymptomatic; myopathy; muscle cramps	–
ADA	–	+++	+	Severe combined immune deficiency	Diarrhea; failure to thrive; candidiasis
PNP	–	++	+	Immune deficiency due to T-cell dysfunction; hemolytic anemia	Diarrhea; failure to thrive; candidiasis
XO	++	–	–	Urolithiasis	Arthropathy; myopathy
Mb-Cof. and isolated SO	+	–	+++	Severe developmental delay; seizures	Dislocation of lenses
HPRT	++	–	++	Urolithiasis; spastic diplegia; involuntary movements; self-injurious behavior	Gout; tophi; short stature
APRT	++	–	–	Urolithiasis	–

continued

Table 28.1. *Continued.*

	Kidney	Immune/blood	CNS	Main symptoms	Additional symptoms
UMPS	(+)	++	+	Megaloblastic anemia; urolithiasis; developmental delay	Heart defects; strabismus
UMH	–	++	–	Hemolytic anemia	Splenomegaly
Pyr. Nucl. Depl. Dis.	–	+	++	Seizures; developmental delay; abnormal behavior	–
DPD	–	–	+	Sometimes asymptomatic; seizures; developmental delay; sensitivity to 5-fluorouracil	–
DHP	–	–	+	Sometimes asymptomatic; seizures; developmental delay	–

Legend: The following symbols indicate the severity of disease: – = not affected; + = affected; ++ = severely affected; +++ = leading to death in infancy or early childhood.

Abbreviations: ADA, adenosine deaminase; AMPDA, muscle adenosine monophosphate deaminase; APRT, adenine phosphoribosyltransferase; ASL, adenylosuccinate lyase (adenylosuccinase); CNS, central nervous system; DHP, dihydropyrimidine amidohydrolase (dihydropyrimidinase); DPD, dihydropyrimidine dehydrogenase; HPRT, hypoxanthine-guanine phosphoribosyltransferase; Mb-Cof., molybdenum cofactor; PNP, purine nucleoside phosphorylase; PRPPS, phosphoribosylpyrophosphate synthetase; Pyr. Nucl. Dis, pyrimidine nucleotide depletion disease due to cytosolic 5'-nucleotidase superactivity; SO, sulfite oxidase; UMH, uridine monophosphate hydrolase (pyrimidine-5'-nucleotidase); UMPS, uridine monophosphate synthetase (multienzyme catalyzing orotate phosphoribosyltransferase and orotidine-5'-monophosphate decarboxylase activities, see Fig. 28.2); XDH (XO), xanthine oxidase (xanthine dehydrogenase).

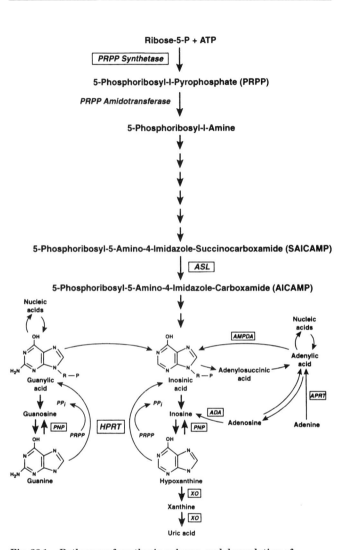

Fig. 28.1. Pathways of synthesis, salvage, and degradation of Purines. The enzymatic steps in boxes indicate the sites of the commonly encountered disorders of purine metabolism. Abbreviations: ADA, adenosine deaminase; AMPDA, muscle adenosine monophosphate deaminase; APRT, adenine phosphoribosyltransferase; ASL, adenylosuccinate lyase (adenylosuccinase); ATP, adenosine 5'-triphosphate; HPRT, hypoxanthine-guanine phosphoribosyltransferase; PNP, purine nucleoside phosphorylase; PP_i, inorganic pyrophosphate (diphosphate); XO, xanthine oxidase (xanthine dehydrogenase).

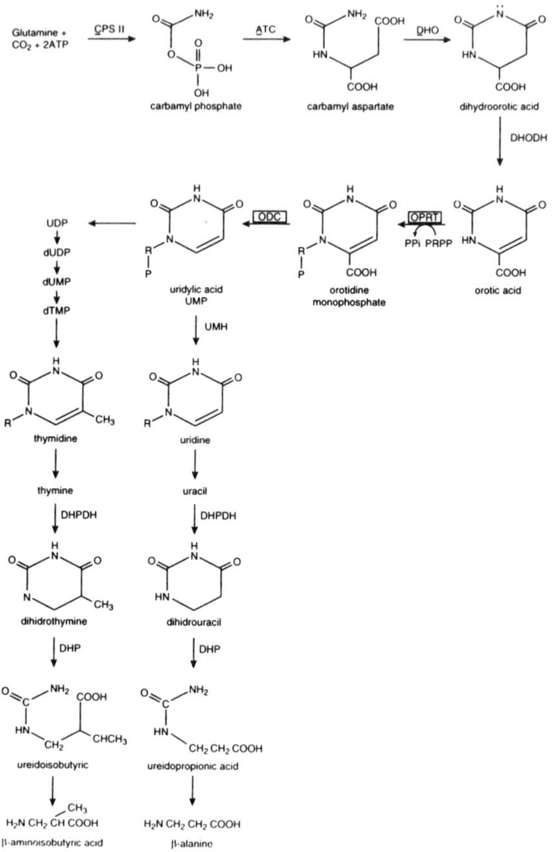

Fig. 28.2. Pathways of synthesis and degradation of pyrimidines. The enzymatic steps in boxes indicate the sites of the defect in hereditary orotic aciduria. The two enzymatic activities, carbamyl phosphate synthetase and aspartate transcarbamylase, reside within a single polypeptide chain, which is coded by the gene uridine monophosphate synthetase. The activities of the six enzymes of *de novo* biosynthesis are coded by three genes. The first protein catalyses the first three enzymatic steps of the pathway, namely carbamylphosphate synthetase (CPS II), aspartate transcarbamylase (ATC), and dihydro-orotase (DHO). The abbreviation CAD can also used to refer to the whole enzyme. The second gene codes for dihydroorotate dehydrogenase (DHODH) and the third for the last two steps, which are orotate phosphoribosyltransferase (OPRT) and orotidine-5'-monophosphate decarboxylase (ODC) activities. Abbreviations: ATP, adenosine 5'-triphosphate; DHP, dihydropyrimidine amidohydrolase (dihydropyrimidinase); DHPDH, dihydropyrimidine dehydrogenase; dTMP, deoxythymidylic acid (thymidine 5'-monophosphate); dUDP, deoxyuridine 5'-diphosphate; dUMP, deoxyuridine 5'-monophosphate; PP, pyrophosphate; PRPP, 5-phospho-α-D-ribosyl-l-pyrophosphate; UDP, uridine 5'-diphosphate; UMH, uridine monophosphate hydrolase; UMP, uridine 5'-monophosphate.

(Fig. 28.2). Heterozygotes and homozygotes for dihydropyrimidine dehydrogenase or dihydropyrimidinase deficiency are at risk for the development of severe neurological abnormalities during chemotherapy with 5-fluorouracil.

ROUTINE LABORATORY INVESTIGATIONS

Uric acid is the only routine clinical chemical determination that points specifically to defects of purine metabolism. None currently exist for the pyrimidines. In interpreting values of uric acid in plasma or serum, the clinician must remember that children have an especially high clearance capacity for uric acid and that, consequently, they can keep serum levels within normal ranges even with a pathologically increased endogenous production. Therefore, urinary concentrations of uric acid give more reliable results. For diagnostic purposes, a random urine sample should be promptly analyzed for uric acid and creatinine. Age-related control ranges are given in Table 28.2.

Table 28.2. Uric acid excretion in control subjects

Age (years)	<2	2–4	4–8	8–10	10–12	>12
Upper limit Ua/Crea	<2*	<1.5	<1.3	<1.1	<1.0	<0.8
Lower limit Ua/Crea	<0.5*	<0.5	<0.4	<0.3	<0.3	<0.3

* In very young infants, especially during the first week of life, the standard deviation is extremely high (99th percentile between approximately 0.2 and 2.8).
Abbreviations: Crea, creatinine; Ua, uric acid.
Table 2 gives estimates of uric acid/creatinine ratios in morning urine samples (Kaufman), which can be taken as a possible hint to either elevated or reduced excretion of uric acid. A few facts have to be borne in mind when interpreting uric acid excretion in spot urine samples in general and when using this table in particular:
The numbers are estimated from a continuously falling curve with varying standard deviations at different ages. This means they represent "forced mean values" for the given age group and give an approximation of the normal range of uric acid excretion. Patients with Lesch-Nyhan syndrome (HPRT deficiency) seem to lie clearly above those upper limits always. In patients with either "borderline findings" with this proposed uric acid/creatinine ratio or with high clinical suspicion of primary or secondary disturbances of uric acid metabolism, a determination of the 24-hour excretion corrected for body surface is probably more accurate. Wilcox calculates this with $520 \pm 147/1.73$ m^2/24hours (mean ± 1 SD) based on several previous publications. As an alternative, correction of uric acid excretion for creatinine clearance gives a constant value between 3 and 40 years of age: 0.34 ± 0.11 mg/dL of glomerular filtrate (mean ± 1 SD) according to Wilcox. Glomerular filtrate is estimated from simultaneous measurement of serum creatinine (S_{cr}), urinary creatinine (U_{cr}), and urinary uric acid (U_{ua}) in patients who fasted overnight. All values are in mg/dL, using the following equation:
$[(U_{cr}) \times (S_{cr})]/(U_{cr})$ = uric acid excreted in mg/dL of glomerular filtrate.

SPECIALIZED INVESTIGATIONS

Specimens

All but two defects of purine and pyrimidine metabolism show abnormalities on analysis of the urine (Table 28.3). However, several pitfalls that range from obtaining the sample to the analytical procedure must be considered. A major one arises from the propensity of microorganisms to consume purines and pyrimidines. Although more precise information can be obtained from 24-hour samples, they should not be the primary diagnostic specimens. The primary specimen should be an early morning urine sample, which is promptly frozen and is sent to the laboratory on dry ice. Frozen transport is necessary not only to avoid bacterial growth but also to stabilize labile metabolites, such as succinylaminoimidazole carboxamide ribonucleoside (SAICAR), the marker metabolite of adenylosuccinate lyase deficiency. If frozen transport is impossible, the urine specimen should be preserved with a few drops of thymol or chloroform (acidic additives may not be used) or it should be lyophilized and sent dry.

In the authors' experience, the excretion of SAICAR shows considerable diurnal variation, but it is highest in the morning urine. Excretion of purines and pyrimidines is highly influenced by dietary manipulations, another reason for preferring an early morning urine specimen. Finally, subjects should refrain from intake of methylxanthines (e.g., chocolate, coffee, tea, and licorice) for at least 24 hours prior to taking the sample. When collecting a 24-hour sample for detailed analysis of purines and pyrimidines, a urinary tract infection or bacteriuria must be excluded first; during collection each portion should be frozen immediately and then added to the batch already stored in the freezer.

Analytical Procedures

Most purine and pyrimidine metabolites can be reliably analyzed in urine by high performance liquid chromatography (HPLC) with ultraviolet (UV) detection. However, a number of analytical pitfalls can lead to misdiagnosis. An elegant and complete analysis of purine and pyrimidine metabolites is achieved by nuclear magnetic resonance (NMR) spectroscopy, which is not widely available now but may become more so in the future. Defects in the degradation of purines and pyrimidines, such as xanthine oxidase, dihydropyrimidine dehydrogenase, dihydropyrimidinase and ureidopropionase deficiencies, are suspected on the basis of the presence of marker metabolites (see Table 28.3) on organic acid analysis. Such elevations should be carefully looked for during the investigation of urinary organic acids in the diagnostic work-up. The final verification of any suspected defect of purine and pyrimidine metabolism requires enzymatic or molecular investigations.

Specific Logistics of Diagnostic Procedures

Myoadenylate deaminase deficiency can be the cause of mild nonprogressive myopathy that presents with muscle cramps and pains during exercise. The metabolic defect can be assumed by

Table 28.3. Urinary biochemical findings in diseases of purine and pyrimidine metabolism

	PRPPS	ASL	AMPDA	ADA	PNP	XO	Mb-Cof	SO	HPRT	APRT	UMPS	UMH	Pyr. Nucl. Depl. Dis.	DPD	DHP
Uric Acid	↑				↓	↓	↓		↑				↓		
Xanthine						↑	↑								
Hypoxanthine	↑					↑	↑		↑						
Orotic Acid											↑				
Uracil														↑	↑
Thymine														↑	↑
Dihydrouracil														↓	↑
Dihydrothymine														↓	↑
Succinyladenosine		↑													
SAICAR		↑													
Adenine				↑						↑					
2-Desoxyadenosine				↑											
2,8-Dihydroxyadenosine										↑					

continued

Table 28.3. *Continued.*

	PRPPS	ASL	AMPDA	ADA	PNP	XO	Mb-Cof	SO	HPRT	APRT	UMPS	UMH	Pyr. Nucl. Depl. Dis.	DPD	DHP
Guanine															
Inosine				↑											
2-Desoxyguanosine				↑											
2-Desoxyinosin				↑											
Special Investigations	1)			2)		3)	3)	3)	3)			4)	5)		

Abbreviations: ADA, adenosine deaminase; AMPDA, muscle adenosine monophosphate deaminase; APRT, adenine phosphoribosyltransferase; ASL, adenylosuccinate lyase (adenylosuccinase); DHP, dihydropyrimidine amidohydrolase (dihydropyrimidinase); DPD, dihydropyrimidine dehydrogenase; HPRT, hypoxanthine-guanine phosphoribosyltransferase; Mb-Cof, molybdenum cofactor; PNP, purine nucleoside phosphorylase; PRPPS, phosphoribosylpyrophosphate synthetase, Pyr. Nucl. Depl. Dis; pyrimidine nucleotide depletion disease due to cytosolic 5'-nucleotidase superactivity; SAICAR, succinylaminoimidazole carboxamide ribonucleoside; SO, sulfite oxidase; UMH, uridine monophosphate hydrolase (pyrimidine-5'-nucleotidase); UMPS, uridine monophosphate synthetase (multienzyme catalyzing orotate phosphoribosyltransferase and orotidine-5'-monophosphate decarboxylase activities, see Fig. 28.2); XO, xanthine oxidase (xanthine dehydrogenase).

The following refer to special investigations:
1) Absence of an increase of ammonia in the forearm ischemia test (see Chapter 11, "Function Tests, Forearm Ischemia Test").
2) Elevated dATP in erythrocytes.
3) Sulfite test in fresh urine. Elevations of S-sulfocysteine, taurine, and thiosulfate; reductions of sulfate and cysteine in body fluids. Detectable by amino acid analysis and ion chromatography.
4) Diagnostic abnormalities are found only in erythrocytes: UV-spectrum of nucleotides, elevated glutathione. Nucleotides by high pressure liquid chromatography (HPLC).
5) Incorporation of pyrimidine precursors into nucleotides in intact fibroblasts.

the absence of an increase of ammonia in the forearm ischemia test (see Chapter 11, the "Forearm Ischemia Test," under "Function tests") and can be ascertained by enzyme analysis of a muscle biopsy.

Two disorders are diagnosable only by whole-cell incubation studies *in vitro* (i.e., analysis of nucleosides and nucleotides in fresh red blood cells or cultured fibroblasts); these are uridine-monophosphate hydrolase deficiency and pyrimidine nucleotide depletion disease due to cytosolic 5′-nucleotidase superactivity. In the latter, the diagnosis is suspected on the basis of the demonstration of lowered uric acid in serum or urine of a child who suffers from an autistic-like developmental disorder.

FUTURE PERSPECTIVES

The extreme variability of the clinical symptoms and the bioanalytical problems with detecting diseases of purine and pyrimidine metabolism still hampers their diagnosis in affected patients. In the authors' experiences, mild or oligosymptomatic manifestations may occur quite frequently and, presumably, many of them remain undiagnosed. Even diseases like adenosine deaminase or molybdenum cofactor deficiencies, which are generally considered as presenting with severe disease from early infancy, have been recognized in school-age children or even adults who have had a relatively mild clinical course.

As many diseases of purine and pyrimidine metabolism are associated with seizure disorders and/or nonspecific mental retardation, investigations for purines and pyrimidines may prove more valuable than does screening for amino or organic acid disorders; they should be considered in the diagnostic work-up of such patients. The authors consider purine and pyrimidine analysis to be one of the few indications for specialized metabolic analyses in patients with nonspecific neurological symptoms. Thus, selective screening for purines and pyrimidines is a valuable addition to existing biochemical genetics laboratory programs but does require special care and logistics in all areas ranging from sample collection to interpretation of results.

ADDITIONAL READING

Gresser U, ed. *Molecular genetics, biochemistry and clinical aspects of inherited disorders of purine and pyrimidine metabolism.* Heidelberg: Springer, 1993.

Kaufman JM, Greene ML, Seegmiller JE. Urine uric acid to creatinine ratio—a screening test for inherited disorders of purine metabolism. *J Pediatr* 1968;73:583–592.

Page T, Yu A, Fontanesi J, Nyhan WL. Developmental disorder associated with increased cellular nucleotidase activity. *Proc Natl Acad Sci U S A* 1997;94:11601–11606.

Wevers RA, Engelke UFH, Moolenaar SH, et al. ¹H-NMR spectroscopy of body fluids: inborn errors of purine and pyrimidine metabolism. *Clin Chem* 1999;45:539–548.

Wilcox WD. Abnormal plasma uric acid levels in children. *J Pediatr* 1996;128:731–741.

29 ♣ Storage Disorders

Lysosomal storage disorders comprise a group of over 40 different diseases that are caused by genetic defects of lysosomal enzymes, resulting in the accumulation of incompletely digested substrates within the lysosome, and, consequently, in the increasing impairment of cellular function. As cells become filled with storage material, the whole organ may enlarge. Although different predominances of involvement are characteristic for individual disorders, the three systems primarily affected are the connective tissue, nervous tissue, and parenchymatous organs. However, the idea that all lysosomal storage disorders generally cause visceromegaly and characteristic skeletal changes is a misconception. A substantial number affect predominantly, or even exclusively, the central nervous system, causing chronic progressive neurologic and psychiatric dysfunction. Inheritance is autosomal recessive with the exceptions of mucopolysaccharidosis type II (Hunter disease) and Fabry disease, a sphingolipidosis in which the affected genes are located on the X-chromosome.

CLINICAL PRESENTATIONS

Lysosomal storage disorders cause chronic progressive symptoms. They do not cause acute metabolic crises. Because of the substantial clinical overlap and the characteristic differences, a rationale, stepwise diagnostic approach can be used (Table 29.1). The age of manifestation may vary greatly depending on the underlying disorder and on the amount of residual enzyme activity. Some disorders present at birth with facial dysmorphy and visceromegaly, especially cardiomegaly. Nonimmunologic *hydrops fetalis* should be carefully investigated for a diagnosis of a storage disorder.

However, most affected children appear completely normal at birth and continue to develop normally for variable time span, which may be only a few weeks or can be up to adulthood. If storage takes place in the connective tissue, *coarse facial features,* skin, and skeletal changes will develop slowly, but they may go unrecognized for surprisingly long periods. Striking facial dysmorphia accompanies infantile sialidosis, mucopolysaccharidoses I and VII, mucolipidosis II, and G_{M1} gangliosidosis. Macroglossia and gingival hyperplasia may accompany severe facial changes; they are especially prominent in G_{M1} gangliosidosis.

Dysostosis multiplex is a classic feature of the roentgenographic appearance, which results from progressive involvement of cartilage and bone. A roentgenographic search for the presence of dysostosis multiplex (hand, pelvis, spine) is one of the key investigations in the diagnosis of lysosomal storage disorders; it may even be more reliable than some of the chemical tests used for screening. With this feature, the shafts of all bones widen. The cortical walls thicken early in the course of the disease, but later they become thin as the medullary cavity dilates. Osteopenia with secondary fractures may be seen. Lack of normal modeling and tubulation characterizes the bones. Epiphyseal centers are poorly developed. The bones of the upper extremities become short and stubby, and they taper toward the ends, often with enlargement of the mid-portions. The metacarpals are broad at their distal ends and taper at their proximal ends. With the thickened and bullet-shaped phalanges, this gives the roentgenographic appearance of a claw hand. In the lower extremities, coxa valga, small femoral heads, and a poorly developed pelvis may be observed. The lower ribs are broad and spatulate; and the lateral portion of the clavicle is hypoplastic, or it can even be absent. The vertebrae are hypoplastic and are scalloped posteriorly and beaked anteriorly. At the thoracolumbar junction especially, anterior vertebral wedging, leading to a thoracolumbar gibbus, may occur. Further aspects of skeletal involvement include progressive macrocephaly, short stature, pectus carinatum, kyphosis, hypoplasia of the odontoid that leads to atlantoaxial subluxation, spinal cord compression, and hydrocephalus. Finally, these children become immobile with stiff and contracted joints.

Visceromegaly is another hallmark of lysosomal storage disorders. *Hepatosplenomegaly* may be impressive, and it should be sought by ultrasonography of the abdomen and the heart. A protuberant abdomen and umbilical hernias may be seen. Isolated hepatomegaly or splenomegaly requires an extended differential diagnosis. Splenomegaly is more characteristic of storage diseases than is hepatomegaly. Hepatosplenomegaly may precede the late hematological complications of hypersplenism. *Cardiac involvement* is far more serious. Acute cardiomyopathy and endocardial fibroelastosis may be present in infancy, leading to intractable arrhythmias and *cardiac failure;* and, if they are present prenatally, they cause nonimmunologic hydrops fetalis. Cardiac murmurs and valvular disease may result from storage in the mitral, aortic, tricuspid, or pulmonary valves and can progress to congestive cardiac failure. Thickening of the valves of the coronary arteries leads to angina pectoris and myocardial infarction. Endothelial disease in Fabry disease leads to coronary or cerebrovascular occlusion. Patients may also die of pneumonia. Primary pulmonary involvement is prominent in the sphingolipidosis and lipid storage disorders, Niemann-Pick disease (types A, B, and C), Gaucher disease (types I and II), multiple sulfatase deficiency, and Wolman disease. Diarrhea from infiltration of the autonomic innervation of the intestine occurs in several disorders (e.g., in mucopolysaccharidosis type II [Hunter disease] and the Chediak-Higashi syndrome). This infiltration is severe in Wolman disease, leading to intractable diarrhea and vomiting. In these infants failure to thrive dominates the clinical picture, and the underlying lysosomal storage disorders may not be considered for a long time. While the diagnosis of a lipid storage disorder will be evident on laparotomy, calcifications of the adrenals are the diagnostic hallmark of Wolman disease. Calcifications may be seen on plain roentgenogram of the abdomen as fine-stippled or discrete, punctate calcifications.

(*text continues on page 350*)

Table 29.1.   Differential findings in lysosomal storage diseases

Nomenclature	Enzyme defect	Hydrops fetalis	Coarse facial features Dysostosis multiplex
Mucopolysaccharidoses			
Type I, Hurler disease	α-L-Iduronidase	–	++
Type II, Hunter disease	Iduronate-2-sulfatase	–	++
Type III, Sanfilippo disease	Four diff. enzymes in the degradation of heparan sulfate (→ types A–D)	–	(+)
Type IV, Morquio disease	Galactose-6-sulfatase → type A β-Galactosidase→ type B	(+)	+
Type VI, Maroteaux–Lamy disease	N-Acetylgalactosamine-4-sulfatase	–	+
Type VII, Sly disease	β-Glucuronidase	(+)	+
Multiple sulfatase deficiency (Austin disease)	Sulfatases	(+)	++
Oligosaccharidoses			
Aspartylglucosaminuria	Aspartylglucosaminase	–	+
Fucosidosis	α-Fucosidase	–	++
α-Mannosidosis	α-Mannosidase	–	++
β-Mannosidosis	β-Mannosidase	–	+
Schindler disease	α-N-Acetylgalactos-aminidase	–	–
Sialidosis I	Sialidase	(+)	–
Sialidosis II (Mucolipidosis I)	Sialidase	(+)	++
Mucolipidoses			
Mucolipidosis II, I-cell disease	N-Acetylglucos-aminylphosphotransferase	–	++
Mucolipidosis III, Pseudo-Hurler	N-Acetylglucos-aminylphosphotransferase	–	+
Mucolipidosis IV	Unknown	–	–

Hepatosplenomegaly	Cardiac involvement Cardiac failure	Mental deterioration	Myoclonus	Spasticity	Peripheral neuropathy	Cherry-red spot	Corneal clouding	Angiokeratomata	Vacuolated lymphocytes	↑GAG (urine)	↑Pathologic oligosaccharides
++	+	++	–	–	–	–	++	–	–	+	–
+	+	++	–	–	–	–	–	–	–	+	–
(+)	–	++	–	+	–	–	–	–	–	(+)	–
(+)	(+)	–	–	–	–	–	(+)	–	–	(+)	–
+	+	–	–	–	–	–	++	–	–	+	–
+	(+)	+	–	–	–	–	+	–	–	+	–
++	+	++	–	++	–	(+)	++	–	–	+	–
(+)	(+)	+	–	–	–	–	(+)	(+)	+	–	+
(+)	+	++	+	+	–	–	–	(+)	+	–	+
+	–	++	–	(+)	–	–	++	(+)	+	–	+
(+)	–	+	–	+	+	–	–	(+)	–	–	+
–	–	+	+	+	–	–	–	–	–	–	+
–	–	–	++	+	+	++	(+)	–	+	–	+
+	+	++	(+)	–	–	++	–	+	+	–	+
+	++	++	–	–	–	–	(+)	–	+	–	–
(+)	–	(+)	–	–	–	–	+	–	+	–	–
+	–	(+)	–	–	–	–	–	–	–	–	–

continued

Table 29.1.   *Continued.*

Nomenclature	Enzyme defect	Hydrops fetalis	Coarse facial features Dysostosis multiplex
Sphingolipidoses			
Fabry disease	α-Galactosidase	–	–
Farber disease	Ceramidase	–	–
Galactosialidosis	β-Galactosidase and sialidase	(+)	++
G$_{M1}$ gangliosidosis	β-Galactosidase	(+)	++
G$_{M2}$ gangliosidosis (Tay–Sachs disease, Sandhoff disease)	β-Hexosaminidases A and B	–	–
Gaucher type I	Glucocerebrosidase	–	–
Gaucher type II	Glucocerebrosidase	(+)	–
Gaucher type III	Glucocerebrosidase	(+)	–
Niemann–Pick type I (= A & B)	Sphingomyelinase	(+)	–
Metachromatic leukodystrophy	Arylsulfatase A	–	–
Krabbe disease	β-Galactocerebrosidase	–	–
Lipid storage disorders			
Niemann–Pick type II (= C & D)	Intracellular cholesterol transport	–	–
Wolman disease	Acid lipase	(+)	–
Ceroid lipofuscinosis, infantile (Santavuori–Hantia)	Palmitoyl-proteinthioesterase (CLN1)	–	–
Ceroid lipofuscinosis, late infantile (Jansky–Bielschowsky)	Pepstatin-insensitive pepti-didase (CLN2). Variants in Finland (CLN5), Turkey (CLN7), and Italy (CLN6)	–	–
Ceroid lipofuscinosis, juvenile (Spielmeyer–Vogt)	CLN3, membrane protein	–	–
Ceroid lipofuscinosis, adult (Kufs, Parry)	CLN4, probably heterogeneous	(+)	–

Hepatosplenomegaly	Cardiac involvement Cardiac failure	Mental deterioration	Myoclonus	Spasticity	Peripheral neuropathy	Cherry-red spot	Corneal clouding	Angiokeratomata	Vacuolated lymphocytes	↑GAG (urine)	↑ Pathologic oligosaccharides
−	+	−	−	−	−	−	+	++	−	−	−
(+)	++	+	−	−	+	(+)	−	−	−	−	−
++	+	++	(+)	+	−	+	+	+	+	−	+
+	(+)	++	−	(+)	−	++	+	+	−	−	+
(+)	−	++	+	+	−	++	−	−	−	−	+
+	−	−	−	−	−	−	−	−	−	−	+
+	−	++	+	+	−	−	−	−	−	−	+
+	−	+	(+)	(+)	−	−	−	−	−	−	+
++	−	+	(+)	−	−	(+)	(+)	−	+	−	−
−	−	++	−	+	++	(+)	−	−	−	−	−
−	−	++	−	+	++	(+)	−	−	−	−	−
(+)	−	+	−	−	−	(+)	−	−	+	−	−
+	(+)	−	−	−	−	(+)	−	−	+	−	−
−	−	+	+	+	−	−	−	−	+	−	−
−	−	+	+	+	−	−	−	−	+	−	−
−	−	+	−	(+)	−	−	−	−	(+)	−	−
−	−	+	−	−	−	−	−	−	(+)	−	−

continued

Table 29.1.   *Continued.*

Nomenclature	Enzyme defect	Hydrops fetalis	Coarse facial features Dysostosis multiplex
Lysosomal glycogen storage			
Glycogenosis type II, Pompe disease	α-1,4-Glucosidase	–	–
Lysosomal transport disorders[a]			
Sialic acid storage disease, Salla disease	Sialin (SLC17A5)	–	–
Cystinosis	Cystine transporter	–	–
Unclassified lysosomal disorders			
Chediak–Higashi syndrome	Lysosomal trafficking regulator LYST	–	–

Legend: ++ = prominent; + = often present, (+) = inconstant or occurring later in the disease course; – = not present.
Abbreviations: diff., different; GAG, glycosaminoglycans.

In the majority of disorders, storage occurs in the central nervous system causing progressive *mental deterioration.* This is the most important manifestation. Many children have normal development initially for a variable time period. The developmental delay or regression may be very subtle at the onset. In some children the downhill course appears to accelerate once it has become obvious.

Seizures are uncommon in the mucopolysaccharidoses, although they regularly occur in the oligosaccharidoses and sphingolipidoses. Severe seizures are often associated with fast regression until the patient reaches a vegetative state after one or two years. *Myoclonus,* if present, points more specifically toward an underlying neurometabolic disorder. It occurs in oligosaccharidoses and sphingolipidoses, and it is a hallmark of the infantile and late infantile ceroid lipofuscinoses, Jansky-Bielschowsky disease, and Spielmeyer-Vogt disease. Polyspikes evoked by single flashes of

Hepatosplenomegaly	Cardiac involvement Cardiac failure	Mental deterioration	Myoclonus	Spasticity	Peripheral neuropathy	Cherry-red spot	Corneal clouding	Angiokeratomata	Vacuolated lymphocytes	↑GAG (urine)	↑Pathologic oligosaccharides
+	++	−	−	−	−	−	−	−	+	−	+
(+)	−	+	(+)	−	+	−	−	−	+	−	+
−	−	−	−	−	−	−	(+)	−	−	−	−
++	−	+	−	−	−	−	−	−	−	−	−

[a] For completeness the Cbl F defect should be mentioned in this group, as it is caused by deficient release of cobalamin from the lysosome. However, it results in combined methylmalonic aciduria and homocystinuria and no histologically detectable storage in lysosomes.

light are characteristic of the late infantile form. Children with G_{M2}-gangliosidosis may display hyperacusis, which is considered to correspond to acoustic myoclonus.

Neurologic features can include *spasticity,* increased deep tendon reflexes, and a positive Babinski sign. Spasticity is especially severe with rigidity and opisthotonus in type II Gaucher disease (infantile) and Krabbe disease. In metachromatic leukodystrophy, deep tendon reflexes initially are diminished or can even be absent. They become exaggerated later in the course of the disease.

In Krabbe disease and metachromatic leukodystrophy, progressive *peripheral neuropathy* is prominent. Peripheral nerve involvement is also a feature in some oligosaccharidoses, such as Farber and sialic acid storage diseases. Bulbar and pseudobulbar palsies cause difficulties with feeding, resulting in aspiration pneumonia, a common cause of death in metachromatic leukodystrophy. Cerebellar involvement and ataxia are regular features of sialidosis type I, Niemann-Pick type C, metachromatic leukodystrophy, the juvenile G_{M1} gangliosidosis, and the juvenile ceroid lipofuscinosis. Some patients develop Parkinson-like features. Prominent extrapyramidal involvement is usually not a feature of lysosomal storage disorders, except for Niemann-Pick type C and the ceroid lipofuscinoses.

Some lysosomal storage disorders predispose the patient to deviant, especially aggressive behavior. This tendency is prominent in the mucopolysaccharidoses types II and III (Hunter and Sanfilippo diseases) and in patients with α-fucosidosis. These patients are often stubborn, fearless, and unresponsive to discipline. Their eating habits may be unusual, and pica is common. Others, however, remain well-adapted or continue to be quite pleasant children despite their unusual appearance. An example of this occurs with the mucopolysaccharidosis type I (Hurler disease). Especially with late onset and, consequently, slowly progressing disease courses, patients may initially present with psychiatric diagnoses such as dementia, psychosis, or emotional illness. Depression and chronic alcoholism have been seen. With adult onset metachromatic leukodystrophy, psychotic changes may resemble those of schizophrenia. The diagnosis depends mainly on the recognition of the additional progressive neurologic features. However, some patients remain undiagnosed and eventually die in psychiatric institutions.

Vision and hearing may be affected in different ways by lysosomal storage disorders. During the diagnostic work-up and follow-up, patients should be regularly seen by an ophthalmologist. *Corneal clouding* giving a steamy or ground-glass appearance is present in many disorders, as are lens opacities. Some patients develop glaucoma. A *cherry-red spot* that is sometimes surrounded by snowflakelike storage material can be visualized early by fundoscopy. In looking for it, remember that the white degeneration of the macula is larger and more impressive than the red foveal spot in the middle. Together, they look like a fried egg. This is caused as lipid storage in the ganglion cells obscures the choroidal vessels behind them. In the fovea, where few ganglion cells are found, the vascularity of the choroid is seen as the red spot. With time, the spot may become darker or brownish in color. Optic atrophy develops in the two lysosomal storage disorders that lead to leukodystrophy (i.e., Krabbe disease and metachromatic leukodystrophy) and in the neuronal ceroid lipofuscinoses. The late infantile and juvenile forms of the latter are the only storage disorders that result in retinitis pigmentosa. Mild retinopathy may also develop in mucolipidosis III. Most of these ophthalmological manifestations result in progressive loss of vision and, finally, in blindness. Sensorineural or mixed conductive and neural deafness also develops in many disorders, which eventually causes hearing loss in addition to the blindness. A very specific ophthalmological finding is the vertical supranuclear ophthalmoplegia that is pathognomonic of Niemann-Pick type II (both C and D). The patients may complain that their eyes became stuck when they look up.

Cutaneous manifestations should be specifically looked for when one suspects a lysosomal storage disorder. *Angiokeratomata* are small, dark red teleangiectasias. They do not blanch with pressure and may be mistaken for petechiae. With time, some become papular and may feel rough to the touch. They are characteristic of Fabry disease; a few may be seen in other disorders (see Table 29.1). Ichthyosis is seen in multiple sulfatase deficiency, and it is due to steroid sulfatase deficiency. Brownish-yellow discoloration of the skin and xanthomas may develop in Niemann-Pick disease type A.

A few clinical findings are virtually specific to those individual storage disorders, and, if recognized, aid the diagnosis tremendously. Chronic renal disease, of which the earliest sign is proteinuria, occurs in Fabry disease. Examination of the urine may reveal red cells, casts, and birefringent lipid globules that form Maltese crosses both within and outside cells and are best seen under polarizing microscopy. Severe joint involvement that is frequently confused with rheumatoid arthritis is prominent in Farber disease and mucolipidosis III. Renal tubular acidosis develops in sialidosis type II.

LABORATORY INVESTIGATIONS

The search for *vacuolated lymphocytes* should be one of the primary investigations for lysosomal storage disorders. They are best seen in a blood smear that is done at the patient's bedside and may go unrecognized when blood from an ethylene diamine tetraacetate (EDTA) tube is used for the smear following transport to the laboratory. If the smear is negative or doubtful, bone marrow aspirates or biopsies of affected organs may reveal the storage material. Histochemistry and chemical analysis may permit the identification of the storage material. Electron microscopy allows the ultrastructure of the material to be examined and its location within the individual cells and different cell types to be studied. In some disorders (e.g., in Niemann-Pick types A and C, Wolman disease, cholesterol ester storage disease and glycogen storage disease II), storage in the lymphocytes is small and discrete and thus is only recognized by experienced examiners. In glycogen storage disease II, glycogen is the storage material. Although no storage can be demonstrated in lymphocytes in mucopolysaccharidoses, coarse metachromatic granules (Alder-Reilly granules) may be found in polymorphonuclear and other leukocytes; they are particularly prominent in Type I (Hurler disease), Type VI (Maroteaux-Lamy disease), Type VII (Sly disease), and multiple sulfatase deficiency. Giant granules in leukocytes occur in the Chediak-Higashi syndrome. Eosinophils are abnormal in multiple sulfatase deficiency, Salla disease, and the infantile G_{M1} gangliosidosis.

A SEQUENTIAL APPROACH TO THE DIAGNOSIS
OF LYSOSOMAL STORAGE

In a baby born with nonimmunologic *hydrops fetalis,* mucopolysaccharides and oligosaccharides are determined in the urine. Lymphocytes, the bone marrow, and liver are investigated for storage cells. Fibroblast cultures are established. Depending on the results of these initial investigations, enzymatic studies are initiated. Glycogen storage disease type IV can also present with congenital hydrops, as can a variety of hematologic diseases, such as the Pearson marrow syndrome.

If *coarse facial features* and *dysostosis multiplex* are the presenting features, mucopolysaccharides and oligosaccharides are investigated in the urine. In mucopolysaccharidosis type IV (Morquio disease) and in type III (Sanfilippo disease), total glycosaminoglycans can be normal; but differentiation by electrophoresis reveals the pathological excretion of keratan sulfate. Tests for total glycosaminoglycans, therefore, are not sufficient for the investigation of mucopolysaccharidoses; and electrophoretic studies should be performed, if the disorder is clinically suspected. Positive urinary results for either mucopolysaccharides and oligosaccharides point to an investigation of specific enzymes. Some clinicians prefer to begin with a battery of lysosomal hydrolase assays. If the urinary investigations are negative, they are repeated, and the lymphocytes are investigated for vacuoles. If these are found, the activities of α-neuraminidase (sialidosis type II) and *N*-acetylglucosaminylphosphotransferase (mucolipidoses II or III) are determined. Patients with mucolipidoses II or III may also have corneal clouding. If urinary findings are normal and no vacuolated lymphocytes are seen, the bone marrow should be investigated for storage cells, and enzyme analyses of sialidase and *N*-acetylglucosaminylphosphotransferase (mucolipidoses II and III) should be ordered. Progressive skeletal changes that are reminiscent of dysostosis multiplex and that are accompanied by a coarse face, gingival hyperplasia, and unaffected mental development are also seen in juvenile hyaline fibromatosis. This rare recessive disorder is characterized by the development of painful contractions of all extremities, osteolyses, and subcutaneous tumors. Diagnosis is made by a histological examination of the tumors, which reveals subepithelial fibrous and connective tissue with small vessels embedded in a periodic acid-Schiff stain (PAS) positive matrix.

Hepatosplenomegaly is an important characteristic for storage disorders. Once it is detected in a child, additional clinical signs, such as macroglossia, should be sought. If they are present, they help differentiate from other causes of hepatosplenomegaly by making a storage disorder virtually certain. The diagnostic workup for storage disorders in a patient with hepatosplenomegaly may also start with the investigation of mucopolysaccharides and oligosaccharides in the urine. Positive results are followed up with confirmatory enzymatic studies. If mucopolysaccharides and oligosaccharides are negative, the lymphocytes are investigated for vacuoles. If this test is negative, the bone marrow should be investigated for storage cells. If storage cells are found, corneal clouding is sought with a slit lamp. If both are present, N-acetylglucosaminylphosphotransferase is determined in order to make a diagnosis of mucolipidoses II or III. If corneal clouding is not present, other potential enzymes that should be determined are sphingomyelinase (Niemann-Pick disease), acid lipase (Wolman disease), and cholesterol uptake and storage (Niemann-Pick disease). If neither pathological urinary screening results nor storage cells are found but peripheral neuropathy is, the activity of ceramidase is determined to confirm a diagnosis of Farber disease. Histologic, histochemical, electron microscopic, and chemical examinations of biopsied liver may be required.

If a *cherry-red spot* is detected as the first clinical symptom, the determination of oligosaccharides in the urine should be carried out. Mucopolysaccharides do not need to be determined. Many clinicians order the direct determinations of relevant enzymes, particularly for the activity of hexosaminidase. Leukodystrophy and peripheral neuropathy make Krabbe disease the likely diagnosis and suggest the assay of β-galactosidase. If "only" leukodystrophy is present, the clinician should determine arylsulfatase A to search for metachromatic leukodystrophy. If peripheral neuropathy is present without leukodystrophy, the diagnosis may be Farber disease; for confirmation, ceramidase is determined. If storage cells are present but no leukodystrophy or peripheral neuropathy is found, sphingomyelinase should be determined for a diagnosis of Niemann-Pick type I; acid lipase, for Wolman disease; and cholesterol uptake and storage, for Niemann-Pick type II.

Progressive mental deterioration, which is the picture of neurodegenerative disease with no associated clinical findings, has a broad differential diagnosis with lysosomal storage disorders as only one of many possible causes. Clearly, stationary mental retardation is no indication for investigating for these disorders. For the former the pattern of investigation may follow the previous outline of urinary mucopolysaccharides and oligosaccharides, vacuolated lymphocytes, evidence of leukodystrophy on magnetic resonance imaging (MRI) (arylsulfatase A deficient metachromatic leukodystrophy), or peripheral neuropathy (ceramidase-deficient Farber disease). If neither pathological urinary findings nor storage cells are seen, a skin biopsy should be conducted, primarily for Batten disease. To make this diagnosis, the biopsy must contain the deeper layers of the skin. Storage of gangliosides and mucopolysaccharides should be investigated in fibroblasts, and, if this test is positive, it establishes a diagnosis of mucolipidosis IV.

Sometimes *storage cells* are accidentally discovered during the investigation of a blood smear in a patient with no clinical signs of a lysosomal storage disorder. In these instances, the same pattern of investigation, starting with urinary mucopolysaccharides and oligosaccharides and vacuolated lymphocytes, is useful. If, following these, no additional positive findings are seen, the investigation can be concluded; however, some clinicians prefer to order a battery of lysosomal hydrolases.

ADDITIONAL READING

Al-Essa MA, Ozand PT. *Atlas of common lysosomal and peroxisomal disorders.* Riyadh: King Fahd National Library Cataloging-in-Publication Data, 1999.

Applegarth DA, Dimmick JE, Hall JG, eds. *Organelle diseases. Clinical features, diagnosis, pathogenesis and management.* London: Chapman & Hall, 1997.

Nyhan WL, Ozand PT. *Atlas of metabolic diseases.* London: Chapman & Hall, 1998.

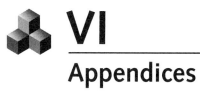

VI

Appendices

Appendix A Differential Diagnosis of Suggestive Signs and Symptoms

Adapted and extended from Nyhan WL, Ozand PT. *Atlas of Metabolic Diseases.* London: Arnold, 1998.

ALOPECIA

An(hypo)hidrotic ectodermal dysplasia
Biotin deficiency
Cartilage hair hypoplasia
Conradi–Hünermann syndrome
Multiple carboxylase deficiency (holocarboxylase synthetase and biotinidase deficiencies)
Trichorrhexis nodosa-arginosuccinic aciduria
Vitamin D-dependent rickets-receptor abnormalities

ANGIOKERATOMAS

Fabry disease
Fucosidosis
Galactosialidosis
G_{M1} gangliosidosis
Sialidosis

ARTHRITIS

Alkaptonuria
Farber disease
Gaucher type I
Gout–hypoxanthine-guanine phosphoribosyl transferase (HPRT) deficiency (Lesch-Nyhan disease); phosphoribosylprophos-phate synthetase (PRPPS) overactivity
Homocystinuria
I-cell disease (mucolipidosis II)
Lesch-Nyhan disease
Mucolipidosis III
Mucopolysaccharidosis (MPS) IS (Hurler) or IIS (Scheie)

BLEEDING TENDENCY

Abetalipoproteinemia
α1-Antitrypsin deficiency
Congenital disorders of glycosylation (CDG)
Chediak-Higashi syndrome
Fructose intolerance
Gaucher disease
Glucogenoses types I & IV
Hermansky-Pudlak syndrome
Tyrosinemia type I

CARDIOMYOPATHY

Congenital muscular dystrophy
Disorders of fatty acid oxidation
Electron transport chain disorders
Glycogenosis type III
Hemochromatosis
D-2-Hydroxyglutaric aciduria
3-Methylglutaconic aciduria (Barth syndrome)
Mucopolysaccharidoses
Pompe disease

CATARACTS—LENTICULAR

Cerebrotendinous xanthomatosis
Electron transport chain disorders
Fabry disease
Galactokinase deficiency
Galactosemia (uridyl transferase deficiency)
Homocystinuria
Hyperornithinemia (Ornithine aminotransferase deficiency)
Lowe syndrome
Lysinuric protein intolerance
Mannosidosis
Mevalonic aciduria
Multiple sulfatase deficiency
Peroxisomal disorders

CEREBRAL CALCIFICATION

Abnormalities of folate metabolism
Adrenoleukodystrophy
Aicardi-Goutiere syndrome
Biopterin abnormalities
Cockayne syndrome
G_{M2} gangliosidosis
L-2-Hydroxyglutaric aciduria
Mitochondrial disorders

CHERRY RED MACULAR SPOTS

Galactosialidosis
G_{M1} gangliosidosis
Mucolipidosis I
Multiple sulfatase deficiency
Niemann-Pick disease
Sandhoff disease
Sialidosis
Tay-Sachs disease

CHONDRODYSPLASIA PHENOTYPES

Conradi–Hünermann syndrome
Peroxisomal disorders
Warfarin embryopathy

CORNEAL OPACITY

Cystinosis
Fabry disease
Fish-eye disease
Galactosialidosis
G_{M1} gangliosidosis
Hurler disease (MPS I)
I-cell disease
Mannosidosis
Mucolipidosis III
Multiple sulfatase deficiency

CORPUS CALLOSUM AGENESIS

Adrenocorticoprophic hormone (ACTH) deficiency
Aicardi syndrome
Mitochondrial disorders (especially pyruvate dehydrogenase deficiency)
Nonketotic hyperglycinemia
Peroxisomal disorders

DERMATOSIS

Acrodermatitis enteropathica
Biotinidase deficiency
Holocarboxylase synthetase deficiency

DERMATOSIS-ICHTHYOSIS

Congenital hemidysplasia, ichthyosis, and limb defects (CHILD) syndrome
Gaucher disease
Krabbe disease
Multiple sulfatase deficiency
Refsum disease
Sjögren-Larsson syndrome
X-linked ichthyosis (steroid sulfatase deficiency)

DIABETES MELLITUS—ERRONEOUS DIAGNOSIS

3-Oxothiolase deficiency
CDG
Isovaleric aciduria
Methylmalonic aciduria
Propionic aciduria

DIARRHEA

Abetalipoproteinemia
Acrodermatitis enteropathica
Congenital chloride diarrhea
Congenital lactase deficiency
Congenital microvillous atrophy
Electron transport chain disorders (especially Pearson syndrome)
Enterokinase deficiency
Glucose galactose malabsorption
Johanson-Blizzard syndrome

Lactase deficiency
Lysinuric protein intolerance
Shwachman-Diamond syndrome
Sucrase deficiency
Wolman disease

DYSOSTOSIS MULTIPLEX

Galactosialidosis
Generalized G_{M1} gangliosidosis
Hunter disease (MPS II)
Hurler disease, Hurler-Scheie disease (MPS I)
Maroteaux-Lamy syndrome (MPS VI)
I-cell disease (mucolipidosis II)
Mucolipidosis III
Multiple sulfatase deficiency
Sanfilippo disease (MPS III)
Sly disease (MPS VII)

ECTOPIA LENTIS (DISLOCATION OF THE LENS)

Homocystinuria
Marfan syndrome
Sulfite oxidase deficiency
Weill-Marchesani syndrome

ELEVATED CEREBROSPINAL FLUID PROTEIN

CDG
L-2-Hydroxyglutanic aciduria
Kearns-Sayre syndrome
Krabbe disease
Mitochondrial encephalomyopathy, lactic acidemia, and
    stroke-like episodes (MELAS)
Myoclonic epilepsy with ragged-red fibers (MERRF)
Metachromatic leukodystrophy
Multiple sulfatase deficiency
Neonatal adrenoleukodystrophy
Refsum disease

ENCEPHALOPATHY (ACUTE ENCEPHALITIS-LIKE)

Urea cycle disorders
Glutaric aciduria type I
Methylmalonic aciduria
Mitochondrial disorders
Propionic aciduria

ENCEPHALOPATHY (ACUTE STROKE)

CDG
Ethylmalonic aciduria
Fabry disease
Homocystinuria
MELAS
Menkes disease

Methylene tetrahydrofolate reductase deficiency
Purine nucleoside phosphorylase deficiency

ENCEPHALOPATHY (ACUTE STROKE-LIKE)

Carbamyl phosphate synthetase deficiency
Chédiak-Higashi syndrome
CDG
Glutaric aciduria type I
Isovaleric aciduria
MELAS
Methylmalonic aciduria
Ornithine transcarbamylase deficiency
Propionic aciduria

ENCEPHALOPATHY (RAPIDLY PROGRESSIVE)

Adenylosuccinase deficiency
Atypical homocystinuria
Atypical phenylketonuria (pterin defects)
Sulfite oxidase (molybdenum cofactor) deficiency

EXERCISE INTOLERANCE

Defects of glycogenolysis
Disorders of fatty acid oxidation
Mitochondrial disorders
Myoadenylate deaminase deficiency
Lipoamide dehydrogenase deficiency

HAIR ABNORMALITIES

Argininosuccinic aciduria
Kinky hair, photosensitivity, and mental retardation
Menkes disease (pili torti, trichorrhexis nodosa, monilethrix)
Pili torti: isolated, with deafness or with dental enamel hypo-
  plasia, MIM 261900
Trichothiodystrophy: trichorrhexis nodosa, ichthyosis, and neu-
  rological abnormalities (Pollit syndrome) MIM 27550

HEMOLYTIC ANEMIA

Defects of glycolysis
5-Oxoprolinuria
Purine and pyrimidine disorders
Wilson disease

HEPATIC CIRRHOSIS

α_1-Antitrypsin deficiency
Cholesteryl ester storage disease
Cystic fibrosis
Electron transport chain disorders, especially the mitochondrial
  DNA depletion syndrome
Fructose intolerance
Galactosemia
Gaucher disease

Glycogenosis type IV
Hemochromatosis
Hepatorenal tyrosinemia
Hypermethioninemia
Niemann-Pick disease
Phosphoenolpyruvate carboxykinase deficiency
Wilson disease
Wolman disease

HYDROPS FETALIS

CDG
Galactosialidosis
Gaucher disease
G_{M1} gangliosidosis
Mucolipidosis II (I-cell disease)
Neonatal hemochromatosis
Niemann-Pick disease
Niemann-Pick type C disease
Pearson syndrome (anemia)
Sialidosis
Sly syndrome (MPS VII)
Wolman disease

HYPOPHOSPHATEMIA

Fanconi syndrome (cystinosis)
MELAS
Pearson syndrome
X-linked hypophosphatemic rickets

HYPOURICEMIA

Fanconi syndrome (cystinosis)
Isolated renal tubular defect (Dalmation dog model)
Molybdenum cofactor deficiency
Purine nucleoside phosphorylase deficiency
Wilson disease
Xanthine oxidase deficiency

INVERTED NIPPLES

Tetrahydrobiopterin (BH_4) synthesis disorders
CDG
Isolated-dominant (MIM163610)
Menkes disease
Propionic aciduria
Weaver syndrome

ISOLATED DEFICIENCY OF SPEECH AS PRESENTATION IN METABOLIC DISEASES

Ethylmalonic aciduria
D-Glyceric aciduria
Histidinemia
3-Methylglutaconyl-CoA hydratase

LEIGH SYNDROME

Biotinidase deficiency
Electron transport chain disorders (complex 1)
Fumarase deficiency
3-Methylglutaconic aciduria
Pyruvate carboxylase deficiency
Pyruvate dehydrogenase complex deficiency
Sulfite oxidase deficiency

LEUKOPENIA WITH OR WITHOUT THROMBOPENIA AND ANEMIA

Abnormalities of folate metabolism
Isovaleric aciduria
Johanson-Blizzard syndrome
Methylmalonic aciduria
3-Oxothiolase deficiency
Pearson syndrome
Propionic aciduria
Shwachman-Diamond syndrome
Transcobalamin II deficiency

MACROCEPHALY

Canavan disease
Glutaric aciduria type I
Hurler disease (MPS I)
4-Hydroxybutyric aciduria
D-2-Hydroxyglutaric aciduria
L-2-Hydroxyglutaric aciduria
3-Hydroxy-3-methylglutaric (HMG)-CoA lyase deficiency
Krabbe disease
Mannosidosis
Multiple acyl-CoA dehydrogenase deficiency
Multiple sulfatase deficiency
Neonatal adrenoleukodystrophy
Pyruvate carboxylase deficiency
Tay-Sachs disease

MEGALOBLASTIC ANEMIA

Cobalamin metabolic errors: methylmalonic aciduria and homo-
cystinuria
Abnormalities of folate metabolism
Mevalonic aciduria
Orotic aciduria
Pearson syndrome
Transcobalamin II deficiency

MYOCARDIAL INFARCTION-CEREBRAL VASCULAR DISEASE

Familial hypocholesterolemia
Fabry disease
Homocystinuria

Menkes disease
Methylene tetrahydrofolate reductase deficiency

ODD OR UNUSUAL ODOR

Dimethylglycinuria
Glutaric aciduria type II
Hepatorenal tyrosinemia
Isovaleric aciduria
Maple syrup urine disease (MSUD)
Phenylketonuria
Treatment with high doses of carnitine
Treatment of a urea cycle disorder with phenylacetate
Trimethylaminuria

OPTIC ATROPHY

Peroxisomal disorders

OSTEOPOROSIS AND FRACTURES

Adenosine deaminase deficiency
Gaucher disease
Glycogenosis I
Homocystinuria
I-cell disease (mucolipidosis II)
Infantile Refsum disease
Lysinuric protein intolerance
Menkes disease
Methylmalonic aciduria
Propionic aciduria

PAIN AND ELEVATED SEDIMENTATION RATE

Fabry disease
Familial hypercholesterolemia
Gaucher disease

PANCREATITIS

Cytochrome C oxidase deficiency
Glycogenosis type I
Hereditary dominant, with or without lysinuria
Homocystinuria
3-Hydroxy-3-methylglutaryl (HMG)-CoA lyase deficiency
Hyperlipoproteinemia types I and IV
Isovaleric aciduria
Lipoprotein lipase deficiency
Lysinuric protein intolerance
MELAS
Methylmalonic aciduria
MSUD
Pearson syndrome
Propionic aciduria
Regional enteritis (Crohn)
Trauma

PARALYSIS OF UPWARD GAZE

Leigh and Kearns-Sayre syndromes
Niemann-Pick type C disease

PERIPHERAL NEUROPATHY

CDG
Metachromatic leukodystrophy
Methylene tetrahydrofolate reductase deficiency
Mitochondrial disorders
Refsum disease
Vitamin E deficiency

POLYCYSTIC KIDNEYS

CDG
Glutaric aciduria type II
Zellweger syndrome

RAGGED RED FIBERS

Mitochondrial DNA mutations
Menkes disease

RAYNAUD SYNDROME

Fabry disease

RENAL CALCULI

Adeninephosphoribosyltransferase (APRT) deficiency
Cystinuria
Hypoxanthine-guanine phosphoriboryl transferase (HPRT)
  deficiency (Lesch-Nyhan disease)
Oxaluria
PRPPS synthetase abnormalities
Wilson disease
Xanthine oxidase deficiency

RENAL FANCONI SYNDROME

Cystinosis
Electron transport chain disorders
Galactosemia
Hepatorenal tyrosinemia
Lysinuric protein intolerance
Wilson disease
Lowe syndrome
Glycogenosis I and III
Idiopathic

REYE SYNDROME PRESENTATION

Abnormalities of gluconeogenesis
Disorders of fatty acid oxidation
Disorders of the urea cycle
Electron transport chain disorders
Fructose intolerance
Organic acidurias

SCOLIOSIS
CDG
Homocystinuria

SENSORINEURAL DEAFNESS
Biotinidase deficiency
Canavan disease
Kearns-Sayre syndrome and other electron transport chain
   disorders
Peroxisomal disorders
PRPPS synthetase abnormality
Refsum disease

SPASTIC PARAPARESIS
Argininemia
Biotinidase deficiency
Hyperammonemia, hyperonithinemia, homocitrullinuria (HHH)
   syndrome
Metachromatic leukodystrophy
Pyroglutamic aciduria
Sjögren-Larsson syndrome

VOMITING AND ERRONEOUS DIAGNOSIS
OF PYLORIC STENOSIS
Ethylmalonic-adipic aciduria
Galactosemia
HMG-CoA lyase deficiency
D-2-Hydroxyglutaric aciduria
Isovaleric aciduria
Methylmalonic aciduria
3-Oxothiolase deficiency
Phenylketonuria
Propionic aciduria

XANTHOMAS
Cerebrotendinous xanthomatosis
Familial hypercholesterolemia
Lipoprotein lipase deficiency
Niemann-Pick disease
Sitosterolemia

Appendix B ❖ Disease References

Table B.1. Disease Reference

Disease name	Enzyme/protein	Gene locus	EC number/protein	OMIM
DISORDERS OF INTERMEDIARY METABOLISM				
Aminoacidopathies				
Phenylketonuria (PKU)	Phenylalanine 4-monooxygenase/ phenylalanine hydroxylase	12q24.1	1.14.16.1	261600
Tyrosinemia type II	Tyrosine aminotransferase	16q22.1–q22.3	2.6.1.5	276600
Tyrosinemia type III	4-Hydroxyphenylpyruvate dioxygenase	12q24-qter	1.13.11.27	276710
Hawkinsinuria	4-Hydroxyphenylpyruvate hydroxylase		1.14.2.2	140350
Tyrosinemia type I	Fumarylacetoacetate	15q23–q25	3.7.1.2	276700
Alkaptonuria (AKU)	Homogentisate 1,2-dioxygenase	3q21–q23	1.13.11.5	203500
Hyperleucine-isoleucinemia or hypervalinemia	Branched-chain aminotransferase 1, cytosolic	12p12	2.6.1.42	113520
Hyperleucine-isoleucinemia or hypervalinemia	Branched-chain aminotransferase 2, mitochondrial	19q13	2.6.1.42	113530
Hyperleucine-isoleucinemia	One of the branched-chain aminotransferases?			238340
Hypervalinemia	One of the branched-chain aminotransferases?			277100
Maple syrup urine disease (MSUD) type Ia	Branched-chain keto acid dehydrogenase (lipoamide) E1 component alpha chain	19q13.1–q13.2	1.2.4.4 ODBA	248600

Disease	Enzyme/protein	Location	EC	OMIM
MSUD type Ib	Branched-chain keto acid dehydrogenase (DH) (lipoamide) E1 component beta chain	6p21–22	1.2.4.4 ODBB	248611
MSUD type II	Dihydrolipoamide branched-chain transacylase (E2 component)	1p31	2.3.1. ODB2	248610
	Methionine adenosyltransferase I	10q22	2.5.1.6	250850
No disease known	Methionine adenosyltransferase II	2p11.2	2.5.1.6	601468
Deficiency of	Adenosylhomocysteinase/ S-adenosylhomocysteine hydrolase	20cen-q13.1	3.3.1.1	180960
Homocystinuria	Cystathionine-beta-synthase	21q22.3	4.2.1.22	236200
Cystathioninuria	Cystathionine gamma-lyase	16	4.4.1.1	219500
Hypertryptophanemia				600627
Hyperlysinemia, saccharopinuria, lysine intolerance	Saccharopine dehydrogenase/ lysine:alpha-ketoglutarate reductase		1.5.1.7	238700 247900 268700
Histidinemia	Histidine ammonialyase	12q22–q24.1	4.3.1.3	235800
Urocanase deficiency	Urocanate hydratase/urocanase		4.2.1.49	276880
Hydroxyprolinemia	4-Hydroxyproline oxidase			237000
Hyperprolinemia type I	Proline dehydrogenase	22q11.2	1.5.99.8	239500
Hyperprolinemia type II	1-Pyrroline-5-carboxylate dehydrogenase/ aldehyde dehydrogenase 4	1p36	1.5.1.12	239510
Gyrate atrophy of choroid and retina	Ornithine-oxo-acid aminotransferase/ ornithine aminotransferase	10q26	2.6.1.13	258870

(continued)

Table B.1. *Continued.*

Disease name	Enzyme/protein	Gene locus	EC number/protein	OMIM
Organic acidurias				
Isovaleric aciduria (IVA)	Isovaleryl-CoA dehydrogenase	15q14–q15	1.3.99.10	243500
3-Methylcrotonylglycinuria	3-Methylcrotonyl-CoA carboxylase		6.4.1.4	210200
3-Methylglutaconic aciduria type I	3-Methylglutaconyl-CoA hydratase		4.2.1.18	250950
3-Methylglutaconic aciduria type II; Barth syndrome	Tafazzin	Xq28	TFZ	302060 300069 300183
3-Methylglutaconic aciduria type III		19q13.2–q13.3		258501
3-Methylglutaconic aciduria type IV				250951
3-Hydroxy-3-methylglutaric aciduria	3-Hydroxy-3-methylglutaryl (HMG)-CoA lyase	1pter-p33	4.1.3.4	246450
Deficiency of Tiglic aciduria	2-Methylbutyryl-CoA dehydrogenase			275190
Deficiency of	2-Methyl-3-hydroxybutyryl-CoA dehydrogenase		1.1.1.178	
Ketothiolase deficiency	Mitochondrial acetoacetyl-CoA thiolase	11q22.3–q23.1	2.3.1.9	203750
Deficiency of	Cytosolic acetoacetyl-CoA thiolase	6q25–q27	2.3.1.9	100678

Disease	Enzyme/Protein	Location	EC Number	OMIM
Methacrylic aciduria	3-Hydroxyisobutyryl-CoA deacylase			250620
3-Hydroxyisobutyric aciduria	3-Hydroxyisobutyrate dehydrogenase		1.1.1.31	236795
Propionic aciduria type I	Propionyl-CoA-carboxylase, alpha chain	13q32	6.4.1.3	232000
Propionic aciduria type II	Propionyl-CoA-carboxylase, beta chain	3q21–q22	6.4.1.3	232050
Methylmalonic aciduria (Mut^0/Mut$^-$ defects)	Methylmalonyl-CoA mutase	6p21	5.4.99.2	251000
2-Ketoadipic aciduria				245130
2-Aminoadipic aciduria				204750
Glutaric aciduria type I (GA I)	Glutaryl-CoA dehydrogenase (GCD/GCDH)	19p13.2	1.3.99.7	231670
Deficiency of	Holocarboxylase synthetase	21q22.1	6.3.4.10	253270
Deficiency of	Biotinidase	3p25	3.5.1.12	253260
D-2-Hydroxyglutaric aciduria				600721
L-2-Hydroxyglutaric aciduria				236792
Disorders of ammonia detoxification				
Deficiency of	Carbamoylphosphate synthetase I	2q35	6.3.4.16	237300
Deficiency of	Ornithine carbamoyltransferase	Xp21.1	2.1.3.3	311250
Citrullinemia	Argininosuccinate synthetase	9q34	6.3.4.5	215700
Argininosuccinic aciduria	Argininosuccinatlyase	7cen–q11.2	4.3.2.1	207900
Argininemia	Arginase I	6q23	3.5.3.1	207800
Deficiency of	N-acetylglutamate synthetase		2.3.1.1	237310
Hyperammonemia, hyper-ornithinemia, homocitrullinuria (HHH) syndrome	Ornithine transporter	13q14		238970 603861

(continued)

Table B.1. *Continued.*

Disease name	Enzyme/protein	Gene locus	EC number/protein	OMIM
Disorders of amino acid transport				
Lowe oculocerebrorenal syndrome		Xq26.1	OCRL	309000
Dibasic aminoaciduria I				222690
Dibasic aminoaciduria II, lysinuric protein intolerance		14q11.2	*SLC7A7* gene	222700 603593
Hartnup disease, neutral amino acid transport defect		11q13		234500
Cystinuria type I	Renal amino acid transporter, heavy subunit	2p16.3	*SLC3A1* gene	220100 104614
Cystinuria type II/III	Renal amino acid transporter, light subunit	19q13.1	*SLC7A9* gene	600913 604144
Histidinuria				235830
Glucoglycinuria				138070
Methionine malabsorption				250900
Disorders of peptide metabolism				
Deficiency of	Gammaglutamylcysteine synthetase	6p12	6.3.2.2	230450
5-Oxoprolinuria	5-Oxoprolinase		3.5.2.9	260005

Disease	Protein/Enzyme	Location		OMIM
Glutathionuria	Gamma-glutamyl transferase	22q11.1–q11.2	2.3.2.2	231950
Pyoglutamic aciduria, 5-oxoprolinuria	Glutathione synthetase	20q11.2	6.3.2.3	266130, 231900
Prolidase deficiency	Peptidase D	19cen-q13.11	3.4.13.9	170100
Homocarnosinosis	Homocarnosinase			236130
Carnosinemia	Serum carnosinase	18q21.3		212200
Disorders of mitochondrial fatty acid oxidation and ketogenesis				
Carnitine deficiency	Carnitine transporter	5q33.1	OCN2	212140 603377
Deficiency of	Carnitine palmitoyltransferase I, liver	11q13	2.3.1.21	255120 600528
Deficiency of	Carnitine-acylcarnitine translocase	3p21.31		212138
Deficiency of	Carnitine palmitoyltransferase II	1p32	2.3.1.21	255110 600649 600650
Multiple acyl-CoA DH deficiency	Electron transfer flavoprotein (ETF), alpha chain	15q23–q25	ETFA	231680
Multiple acyl-CoA DH deficiency	Electron transfer flavoprotein, beta chain	19q13.3	ETFB	130410
Multiple acyl-CoA DH deficiency	ETF-CytQ oxidoreductase	4q32-qter	1.5.5.1	231675
VLCAD deficiency	Very-long-chain acyl-CoA dehydrogenase	17p11.2-11.1	1.3.99.-	201475
LCHAD deficiency	Mitochondrial trifunctional protein, alpha chain	2p23	ECHA	600890

(continued)

Table B.1. *Continued.*

Disease name	Enzyme/protein	Gene locus	EC number/protein	OMIM
LCHAD deficiency	Mitochondrial trifunctional protein, beta chain	2p23	ECHB	143450
MCAD deficiency	Medium-chain acyl-CoA dehydrogenase	1p31	1.3.99.3	201450
MCKAD deficiency	Medium-chain ketoacyl-CoA thiolase			602199
SCAD deficiency	Short-chain acyl-CoA dehydrogenase	12q22-qter	1.3.99.2	201470
SCHAD deficiency	Short-chain hydroxyacyl-CoA dehydrogenase	4q22-q26	1.1.1.35	601609
Deficiency of	HMG-CoA synthetase	1p13-p12	4.1.3.5	600234
Disorders of carbohydrate metabolism and transport				
Disorders in the metabolism of glucose, galactose, fructose, and glycerol				
Deficiency of	Pyruvate carboxylase, oxaloacetic decarboxylase	11q13.4–q13.5	6.4.1.1	266150
Deficiency of	Phosphoenolpyruvate carboxykinase, cytosolic	20q13.31	4.1.1.32	261680
Deficiency of	Fructose-1,6-diphosphatase	9q22.2–q22.3	3.1.3.11	229700
Deficiency of	Triosephosphate isomerase	12p13	5.3.1.1	190450
Deficiency of	Fructose-1,6-diphosphate aldolase, aldolase A	16q22-q24	4.1.2.13	103850
Deficiency of	Phosphoglycerate kinase	Xq13	2.7.2.3	311800
Deficiency of	Glucose-6-phosphate dehydrogenase	Xq28	1.1.1.49	305900
Deficiency of	Pyruvate kinase (erythrocytes)	1q21	2.7.1.40	266200

Deficiency of	Galactokinase	17q24	2.7.1.6	230200
Galactosemia	Galactose-1-phosphate uridyltransferase	9p13	2.7.7.12	230400
Deficiency of	UDP-galactose-4-prime-epimerase	1p36-p35	5.1.3.2	230350
Fructosuria	Fructokinase, ketohexokinase	2p23.3-p23.2	2.7.1.3	229800
Hereditary fructose intolerance	Aldolase B	9q22.3	4.1.2.13	229600
Hyperglycerolemia/glycerol intolerance	Glycerol kinase	Xp21.3-p21.2	2.7.1.30	307030
D-Glyceric aciduria	D-glycerate kinase			220120
Glycogen storage disorders				
Glycogen storage disease (GSD) type 0	Glycogen synthase 2 (liver)	12p12.2	2.4.1.11	240600 138571
GSD type Ia	Glucose-6-phosphatase	17q21	3.1.3.9	232200
GSD type Ib/c	Glucose-6-phosphate translocase	11q23.3	G6PU	232220 232240 602671
GSD type Ic	Phosphate transport			232240
GSD type II	Lysosomal acid alpha-1,4-glucosidase	17q21.2-q23	3.2.1.20	232300, 232330
GSD type IIb				
GSD type III	Glycogen debranching enzyme (Amylo-1,6-glucosidase, oligo-1,4-1,4-glucanotransferase)	1p21	3.2.1.33 2.4.1.25	232400

(continued)

Table B.1. *Continued.*

Disease name	Enzyme/protein	Gene locus	EC number/protein	OMIM
GSD type IV	Glycogen branching enzyme (Amylo-1,4-1,6-transglucosylase)	3p12	2.4.1.18	232500
GSD type V	Glycogen phosphorylase (muscle)	11q13	2.4.1.1	232600 153460
GSD type VI	Glycogen phosphorylase (liver)	14q21–q22	2.4.1.1	232700
GSD type VII	Phosphofructokinase muscle type	12q13.3	2.7.1.11	232800 171850
X-linked muscle GSD (GSD VIII)	Phosphorylase kinase alpha subunit muscle type	Xq13	KPB1	311870
X-linked liver GSD (GSD VIII)	Phosphorylase kinase alpha subunit liver type	Xp22.2–p22.1	KPB2	306000
Autos.-rec. liver and muscle GSD	Phosphorylase kinase beta subunit	16q12–q13	KPBB 172490	261750
Deficiency of	Phosphorylase kinase gamma subunit muscle type	7p12–q21	KPBG	172470
Deficiency of	Phosphorylase kinase gamma subunit liver/testis type	16p12.1–p11.2	KPBH	172471
GSD of heart	Phosphorylase kinase (heart)			261740
GSD Ixc	Phosphorylase kinase (generalized)		2.7.1.38	694549

Carbohydrate transport defects

Disease	Protein	Location	Symbol	MIM
Hypoglycorrhachia	Glucose transporter 1	1p35–p31.3	GTR1	138140
Fanconi-Bickel syndrome	Glucose transporter 2	3q26.1–q26.3	GTR2	138160
				227810
[No disease known]	Glucose transporter 3	12p13.3	GTR3	138170
Deficiency of	Glucose transporter 4	17p13	GTR4	138190
Deficiency of	Glucose transporter 5		GTR5	
Glucose/galactose malabsorption	Sodium-glucose cotransporter 1	22q13.1	SL51	182380
Renal glucosuria	Sodium-glucose cotransporter 2	16p11.2	SL52	182381
				233100
Pentosuria	L-Xylulose reductase			260800
Congenital lactose intolerance				150220
Disaccharide intolerance I	Sucrase-isomaltase	3q25–q26	3.2.1.48	222900
Disaccharide intolerance II	Lactase [processing defect]	2q21	3.2.1.62	223000
				603202
Disaccharide intolerance III	Lactase [hereditary (non-)persistence]	2q21	3.2.1.62	223100
Trehalose intolerance	Trehalase		3.2.1.28	275360
Mitochondrial disorders				
Pyruvate dehydrogenase (PDH) deficiency	Pyruvate decarboxylase (dehydrogenase) (lipoamide) E1 component alpha chain, E1A	Xp22.2-p22.13	1.2.4.1 ODPA	312170 208800
PDH deficiency	Pyruvate decarboxylase (dehydrogenase) (lipoamide) E1 component beta chain, E1B	3p13–q23	1.2.4.1 ODPB	179060

(continued)

Table B.1. *Continued.*

Disease name	Enzyme/protein	Gene locus	EC number/protein	OMIM
PDH deficiency	Dihydrolipoyl transacetylase (PDHC-E2 component)	7p14–p13	2.3.1.12 ODP2	245348
2-Ketoacid dehydrogenase deficiency	Dihydrolipoyl dehydrogenase (E3 component)	7q31–q32	1.8.4.1	246900
Deficiency of	PDH complex protein X	11p13	ODPX	245349
2-Ketoglutaric aciduria	2-Ketoglutarate dehydrogenase (lipoamide) E1 component	7p14–p13	1.2.4.2 ODO1	203740
KGDH deficiency	Dihydrolipoyl succinyltransferase (KGDH-E2 component)	14q24.3	2.3.1.61 ODO2	126063
Fumaric aciduria	Fumarase	1q42.1	4.2.1.2	136850
Malonic aciduria		16q24	4.1.1.9	248360
Complex-I deficiency	NADH-ubiquinone reductase (~43 proteins)		1.6.5.3	252010
Complex-II deficiency	Succinate-ubiquinone reductase (~5 proteins)		1.3.5.1	252011
Complex III deficiency	Ubiquinone dehydrogenase (~11 proteins)		1.10.2.2	124000
Cytochrome C deficiency	Cytochrome C oxidase (~13 proteins)		1.9.3.1	220110
Complex V deficiency	ATP-synthase		3.6.1.34	604273
MELAS syndrome				540000

Disease	Protein	Gene	Location	OMIM
MERRF syndrome				545000
NARP syndrome				551500
Pearson syndrome				557000
Kearns-Sayre syndrome				530000
Leber optic atrophy				535000
Leigh syndrome				256000
mt DNA breakage				550000
mt DNA depletion	DNA-polymerase gamma			251880
Disorders of cobalamin and folate metabolism				
Pernicious anemia	Intrinsic factor	IF	11q13	261000
Pernicious anemia	R protein			193090
Imerslund-Gräsbeck syndrome	Cubilin (intrinsic factor-vitamin B_{12} receptor)		10p12.1	261100
				602997
Pernicious anemia	Transcobalamin II	TCO2	22q11.2-qter	275350
Cobalamin F defect				277380
Cobalamin C defect				277400
Cobalamin D defect	Cob(III)alamin reductase			277410
Cobalamin A defect				251100
Cobalamin B defect				251110
Cobalamin E defect	Methionine synthase reductase		5p15.3-p15.2	236270
				602568

(continued)

Table B.1. *Continued.*

Disease name	Enzyme/protein	Gene locus	EC number/protein	OMIM
Cobalamin G defect	Methyltetrahydrofolate-homocysteine methyltransferase; methionine synthase	1q43	2.1.1.13	250940 156570
Hereditary folate malabsorption	Folic acid transport			229050
Deficiency of	Dihydrofolate reductase	5q11.2–q13.2	1.5.1.3	126060
Deficiency of	5,10-Methylenetetrahydrofolatereductase	1p36.3	1.5.1.20	236250
Deficiency of	Glutamate forminimotransferase			229100
Disorders of the transport or utilization of copper, iron, and zinc				
Disorders of copper metabolism				
Menkes syndrome, occipital horn syndrome	Cu^{2+} transporting ATPase, α-polypeptide	Xq12–q13	3.6.1.36	309400 304150 300011
Wilson disease	Cu^{2+} transporting ATPase, β-polypeptide	13q14.3–q21.1	3.6.1.36	277900
Disorders of iron metabolism				
Hereditary hemochromatosis		6p21.3	HFE	235200
Juvenile hemochromatosis		1q		602390
Neonatal hemochromatosis	Various enzymes of bile acid synthesis			231100

Disorders of zinc metabolism

Disorder	Enzyme/protein	Location	EC/gene	OMIM
Acrodermatitis enteropathica				201100
Hyperzincemia with functional zinc depletion				601979

DISORDERS OF THE BIOSYNTHESIS AND BREAKDOWN OF COMPLEX MOLECULES
Disorders of nucleotide metabolism
Disorders of purine metabolism

Disorder	Enzyme/protein	Location	EC/gene	OMIM
PRPP synthetase superactivity	Phosphoribosylpyrophosphate synthetase	Xq22–q24	2.7.6.1	311850
Deficiency of	Adenylosuccinate lyase	22q13.1	4.3.2.2	103050
Deficiency of	Adenosine monophosphate deaminase 1	1p21-p13	3.5.4.6	102770
Deficiency of	Adenosine deaminase	20q13.11	3.5.4.4	102700
Xanthinuria type I	Xanthine oxidase	2p23-p22	1.1.1.204 1.1.3.22	278300
Xanthinuria type II	Activation of xanthine + aldehyde oxidases			603692
Molybdenum cofactor deficiency type 1	Molybdenum cofactor synthesis step 1	6p21.3	*MOCS1* gene	252150 603707
Molybdenum cofactor deficiency type 2	Molybdopterin synthase	5q11	*MOCS2* gene	252150 603708
Familial juvenile hyperuricemic nephropathy				162000
Lesch–Nyhan syndrome	Hypoxanthine-guanine phosphoribosyltransferase	Xq26-q27.2	2.4.2.8	308000
Deficiency of	Purine-nucleoside phosphorylase	14q13.1	2.4.2.1	164050

(continued)

Table B.1. *Continued.*

Disease name	Enzyme/protein	Gene locus	EC number/protein	OMIM
Deficiency of	Adenine phosphoribosyltransferase	16q24.3	2.4.2.7	102600
Deficiency of	Inosine triphosphatase	20p		147520
Mercaptopurine sensitivity	Thiopurine S-methyltransferase	6p22.3	2.1.1.67	187680
Disorders of pyrimidine metabolism				
Orotic aciduria type I	Uridinemonophosphate (UMP) synthetase	3q13	2.4.2.10	258900
Orotic aciduria type II	UMP synthetase (orotidine-5′-decarboxylase)	3q13	4.1.1.23	258920
Deficiency of	Pyrimidine-5′ nucleotidase I		3.1.3.5	266120
Deficiency of	Dihydropyrimidine dehydrogenase	1p22	1.3.1.2	274270
Deficiency of	Dihydropyrimidinase	8q22	3.5.22	222748
Deficiency of	β-Ureidopropionase		3.5.1.6	
Hyperbetaalaninemia	β-Alanine-2-ketoglutarate transaminase			237400
Deficiency of	β-Aminoisobutyrate-pyruvate transaminase		2.6.1.40	210100
Other disorders of nucleotide metabolism				
(Gout)				138900
Nucleotide depletion	Nucleotidase			

Lysosomal disorders
Mucopolysaccharidoses (MPS)

MPS type I	α-L-Iduronidase	4p16.3	3.2.1.76	252800
MPS type II	Iduronate-2-sulfatase	Xq28	3.1.6.13	309900
MPS type IIIA	Heparan sulfate sulfatase	17q25.3	3.10.1.1	252900
MPS type IIIB	N-Acetyl-α-glucosaminidase	17q21	3.2.1.50	252920
MPS type IIIC	Acetyl-CoA:α-glucosaminide N-acetyltransferase	Chromos. 14		252930
MPS type IIID	N-Acetylglucosamine-6-sulfatase	12q14	3.1.6.14	252940
MPS type IVA	N-Acetylgalactosamine-6-sulfatase	16q24.3	3.1.6.4	253000
MPS type IVB (G$_{M1}$ gangliosidosis)	β-Galactosidase	3p21.33	3.2.1.23	252300 253010 230500
MPS type VI	N-Acetylgalactosamine 4-sulfatase (arysulfatase B)	5q11–q13	3.1.6.12	253200
MPS type VII	β-Glucuronidase	7q21.11	3.2.1.31	253220

Oligosaccharidoses

Aspartylglucosaminuria	Aspartylglucosaminidase	4q23–q33	3.5.1.26	208400
Fucosidosis	α-L-Fucosidase	1p34	3.2.1.51	230000
α-Mannosidosis	α-Mannosidase	19cen–q12	3.2.1.24	248500
β-Mannosidosis	β-Mannosidase	4q22–q25	3.2.1.25	248510
Schindler disease	N-Acetyl-α-D-galactosaminidase	22q11	3.2.1.49	104170

(continued)

Table B.1. *Continued.*

Disease name	Enzyme/protein	Gene locus	EC number/protein	OMIM
Sialidosis	Sialidase (α-neuraminidase)	6q21.3	3.2.1.18	256550
Nephrosialidosis				256150
Mucolipidoses				
I-cell-disease, Pseudo-Hurler dystrophy	N-Acetylglucosamine-1-phosphotransferase	4q21–q23		252500, 252600
Mucolipidosis type IV		19p13.3-13.2		252650
Sphingolipidoses				
Niemann–Pick type A/B	Sphingomyelin phosphodiesterase	11p15.4-15.1	3.1.4.12	257200 257050
Gaucher (type I, II, III)	Acid glucosidase, glucosylceramidase	1q21	3.2.1.45	230800, 230900 231000
Fabry	α-Galactosidase A	Xq22	3.2.1.22	301500
Farber	Ceramidase	8p22-p21.3	3.5.1.23	228000
G$_{M1}$ gangliosidosis (MPS IVB)	β-Galactosidase	3p21.33	3.2.1.23	230500 230600 230650

Disease	Protein/Enzyme	Location	EC/Gene	OMIM
G_{M2} gangliosidosis type 1/Tay–Sachs	β–Hexosaminidase α-chain (Hexosaminidase A)	15q23-q24	3.2.1.52	272800
G_{M2} gangliosidosis type AB/Tay–Sachs AB	G_{M2} activator protein	5q31.3–q33.1	SAP3	272750
G_{M2} gangliosidosis type 2/Sandhoff	β–Hexosaminidase β-chain (Hexosaminidase A+B)	5q13	3.2.1.52	268800
Galactosialidosis	Lysosomal protective protein	20q13.1	PRTP	256540
Krabbe	Galactocerebrosidase	14q31	3.2.1.46	245200
Metachromatic leukodystrophy	Arylsulphatase A	22q13.31-qter	3.1.6.8	250100, 156310
Metachromatic leukodystrophy	Prosaposin, saposin B, sphingolipid activator protein 1	10q22.1	SAP	249900
Multiple sulfatase deficiency				176801
				272200
Lipid storage disorders				
Niemann–Pick types C1, D		18q11–q12	NPC1	257220 257250 601015
Niemann–Pick type C2				278000
Wolman, cholesteryl ester storage disease	Acid lipase, acid cholesteryl ester hydrolase	10q24–q25	3.1.1.13	
CLN1—Santavuori–Haltia	Palmitoyl-protein thioesterase	1p32	3.1.2.22	256730 600722 600680
CLN2—Jansky–Bielschowsky		11p15.5		204500

(continued)

Table B.1. *Continued.*

Disease name	Enzyme/protein	Gene locus	EC number/protein	OMIM
CLN3—Batten, Spielmeyer–Vogt	Battenin	16p12.1	CLN3	204200
CLN4—Kufs				204300
CLN dominant/Parry				162350
CLN5—Finnish variant	CLN5 protein	13q21.1–q32	CLN5	256731
CLN6		15q21–23		601780
CLN8		8pter-p22		600143
Lysosomal transport defects				
Cystinosis	Cystinosin	17p13		219800
				219900
				219750
Salla disease, infantile sialic acid storage disorder	Solute carrier family 17 (anion/sugar transporter), member 5	6q14–q15		604369
				269920
				604322
Sialuria	UDP-N-acetylglucosamine-2-epimerase/ N-acetylmannosamine kinase	9p12-p11	5.1.3.14 2.7.1.60	269921 603824

Other (predominantly) lysosomal disorders

Disease	Protein	Chromosome	Gene	OMIM
Hermansky-Pudlak I	Hermansky-Pudlak syndrome protein	10q23.1–23.3	HPS	203300
Hermansky-Pudlak II	β-3a-Adaptin	Chromos. 5		603401

Peroxisomal disorders
Disorders of peroxisome biogenesis

Disease	Protein	Chromosome	Gene	OMIM
Zellweger syndrome				601539
Neonatal adrenoleukodystrophy				214100
Infantile Refsum disease				202370
	PEX1	7q21–q22	PEX1	266510
	PEX2, peroxisomal membrane protein 3	8q21.1	PEX2	602136
	PEX3		PEX3	170993
	PEX5, peroxisomal targeting signal 1 receptor	12p13.3	PEX5	603164
	PEX6, peroxisome assembly factor-2	6p21.1	PEX6	600414
	PEX10	Chromos. 1	PEXA	601498
	PEX11A, peroxisomal membrane protein 28			602859
	PEX11B	Chromos. 1		603866
	PEX12			603867
	PEX13	2p15	PEXC	601758
	PEX14		PEXD	601789
	PEX16		PEXE	601791
	PEX19, peroxisomal farnesylated protein PxF	1q22		603360
	Peroxisomal membrane protein 1, ABCD3	1p22–p21	ABD3	600279
				170995

(continued)

Table B.1. *Continued.*

Disease name	Enzyme/protein	Gene locus	EC number/protein	OMIM
Disorders of the activation and beta-oxidation of very-long-chain fatty acids				
X-chromosomal adrenoleukodystrophy	ATP-binding transporter	Xq28	ALD	300100
Pseudoneonatal adrenoleukodystrophy	Peroxisomal acyl-CoA oxidase	17q25	1.3.3.6	264470
Deficiency of	Peroxisomal branched-chain acyl-CoA oxidase	3p14.3		601641
Pseudo-Zellweger	Peroxisomal L-bifunctional enzyme	3q27	ECHP	261515
Pseudo-Zellweger	Peroxisomal d-bifunctional enzyme	5q2	DHB4	601860
	Enoyl-CoA hydratase	19q13.1	ECH1	600696
Pseudo-Zellweger	Peroxisomal 3-ketoacyl-CoA thiolase	3p23-p22	2.3.1.16	261510
				604054
Disorders of phytanic acid metabolism				
Refsum disease	Phytanoyl-CoA hydroxylase	10pter-p11.2	PAHX	266500
		10pter-p11.2		602026
Refsum disease with pipecolic acidemia				600964
Deficiency of	α-Methylacyl-CoA racemase	5p13.2–q11.1		604489

Disorders of ether-phospholipid biosynthesis

Rhizomelic chondrodysplasia punctata I	PEX7, peroxisomal targeting signal 2 receptor	6q22–24	PEX7	215100 601757
Rhizomelic chondrodysplasia punctata I	Dihydroxyacetonephosphate acyltransferase	Chromos. 1	2.3.1.42	222765 602744
Rhizomelic chondrodysplasia punctata I	Alkyl-dihydroxyacetonephosphate synthase	2q31	2.5.1.26	600121 603051

Disorders of the detoxification of oxygen radicals

Acatalasemia	Catalase	11p13	1.11.1.6	115500

Disorders of glyoxylate metabolism

Hyperoxaluria type I	Alanine:glyoxylate aminotransferase, serine:pyruvate aminotransferase	2q36–q37	2.6.1.44 2.6.1.51	259900 604285
Hyperoxaluria type II	D-Glycerate dehydrogenase, glyoxylate reductase/hydroxypyruvate reductase	9cen	1.1.1.79	260000 604296

Other peroxisomal disorders

Glutaric aciduria type III glutaryl CoA-oxidase				231690

Disorders of the metabolism of isoprenoids and sterols
Disorders of isoprenoid biosynthesis

Mevalonic aciduria, Hyper IgD syndrome	Mevalonate kinase	12q24	2.7.1.36	251170

(continued)

Table B.1. *Continued.*

Disease name	Enzyme/protein	Gene locus	EC number/ protein	OMIM
Disorders of sterol biosynthesis				
X-linked dominant chondrodysplasia punctata	3-β-Hydroxysteroid-Δ^8,Δ^7-isomerase	Xp11.23–p11.22		302960
Desmosterolemia	3β-Hydroxysterol-Δ^{24}-reductase	Chromos. 20		602398 125650
Smith–Lemli–Opitz syndrome	Sterol Δ^7-reductase	11q12–q13		270400 268670 602858
Disorders of bile acids and bilirubin metabolism, inherited cholestasis, and porphyrias				
Disorders of bile acid biosynthesis				
Neonatal hemochromatosis	Various enzymes of bile acid synthesis			231100
Deficiency of	Δ^4-3-Oxysterol 5-β-reductase	7q32–q33		235555 604741
Deficiency of	Oxysterol 7-α-hydroxylase	8q21.3	CP7B	603711
Deficiency of	Cholesterol 7-α-hydroxylase	8q11–q12	CP7A	118455
Cerebrotendinous xanthomatosis	Sterol 27-hydroxylase	2q33-qter		213700
Disorders of bilirubin metabolism and inherited cholestasis				
Crigler-Najjar type I	UDP-glucuronosyltransferase 1	Chromos. 2	2.4.1.17	218800

Disease	Description	Location	Gene/EC	OMIM
Crigler-Najjar type II				143500
Gilbert				197040
Dubin-Johnson	Canalicular multispecific organic anion transporter 1	10q24	MRP2	237500, 601107
Rotor				237450
Familial intrahepatic cholestasis 1, (progressive = PFIC1, Byler) (benign recurrent = BRIC)	Potential phospholipid-transporting ATPase IC	18q21	AT1C	211600, 243300, 602397
Familial intrahepatic cholestasis 2 (PFIC2)	Liver-specific ATP-binding cassette transporter (bile salt export pump)	2q24		601847, 603201
Familial intrahepatic cholestasis 3 (PFIC3)	Class III multidrug resistance P-glycoprotein	7q21.1	MDR3	602347, 171060
Recurrent intrahepatic cholestasis of pregnancy	Heterozygosity for mutations in one of the PFIC genes			147480
Arthrogryposis multiplex congenita with jaundice and renal dysfunction				208085
Porphyrias				
Erythropoietic protoporphyria	Ferrochelatase	18q21.3	4.99.1.1	177000
Porphyria variegata	Protoporphyrinogen oxidase	1q22	1.3.3.4	176200, 600923
Hereditary sideroblastic anemia	δ-Aminolevulinate synthase 2	Xp11.21	2.3.1.37	301300

(continued)

Table B.1. *Continued.*

Disease name	Enzyme/protein	Gene locus	EC number/protein	OMIM
Congenital erythropoietic porphyria (Günther)	Uroporphyrinogen III cosynthetase	10q25.2–q26.3	4.2.1.75	263700
Acute intermittent porphyria	Porphobilinogen deaminase	11q23.3	4.3.1.8	176000
Acute porphyria Chester type	Coproporphyrinogen oxidase	11q23.1	1.3.3.3	176010
Coproporphyria		3q12		121300
Porphyria cutanea tarda I				176090
Porphyria cutanea tarda II	Uroporphyrinogen decarboxylase	1p34	4.1.1.37	176100
Acute hepatic porphyria	Porphobilinogen synthase	9q34	4.2.1.24	125270
Congenital disorders of glycosylation (CDG)				
CDG Ia (CDGS1a)	Phosphomannomutase-2	16p13.3–p13.2	5.4.2.8	212065
				601785
CDG Ib (CDGS1b)	Mannosephosphate isomerase	15q22-qter	5.3.1.8	602579
				154550
CDG Ic (CDGS5)	Glucosyltransferase			603147
				604566
CDG Id (CDGS4)	Mannosyltransferase			601110
CDG Ie	Dolichol-phosphate mannose synthase		2.4.1.83	603503
CDG Ix				603585

Disease	Protein	Gene symbol	Location	EC number	MIM
CDG II (CDGS2)	N-Acetylglucosaminyltransferase II		14q21	2.4.1.143	212066 602616
CDG I/IIx (CDGS3)					212067
Disorders of lipoprotein metabolism					
Hypercholesterolemias and mixed hyperlipidemias					
Type II hyperlipoproteinemia					144400
Familial hypercholesterolemia	Lipoprotein (a)	APOA	6q27		152200
	LDL receptor	LDLR	19p13.2–p13.1		143890
Familial hypercholesterolemia	Ligand-defective apolipoprotein B	APB	2q24		107730
Sitosterolemia, phytosterolemia			2p21		210250
Mixed hyperlipidemias					
Familial combined hyperlipidemia	HYPLIP 1		1q21–q23		144250
	HYPLIP 2		11p		602491 604499
Dysbetalipoproteinemia	Apolipoprotein E	APE	19q13.2		107741
Deficiency of	Hepatic lipase		15q21–q23	3.1.1.3	151670
Hypertriglyceridemias					
Familial hypertriglyceridemia					145750
Hyperlipoproteinemia IV					144600

(continued)

Table B.1. *Continued.*

Disease name	Enzyme/protein	Gene locus	EC number/protein	OMIM
Familial chylomicronemia	Lipoprotein lipase	8p22	3.1.1.34	238600
Familial chylomicronemia	Apolipoprotein C-II	19q13.2	APC2	207750
Deficiency of	Apolipoprotein C-III	11q23	APC3	107720
Disorders of HDL metabolism				
Familial high-density lipoprotein deficiency, Tangier disease	ATP-binding cassette-1	9q22–q31	ABC1	205400 604091 600046
Hypoalphalipoproteinemia	Apolipoprotein A-I	11q23	APA1	107680
Norum disease, fish-eye disease	Lecithin:cholesterol acyltransferase	16q22.1	2.3.1.43	245900 136120
Hyperalphalipoproteinemia				143470
Deficiency of	Cholesteryl ester transfer protein	16q21	CETP	118470
Disorders with low LDL cholesterol and triglycerides				
Abetalipoproteinemia	Microsomal triglyceride transfer protein	4q22–q24	MTP	200100 157147
Hypobetalipoproteinemia	Apolipoprotein B	2q24	APB	107730
Anderson disease				246700

NEUROTRANSMITTER DEFICIENCIES AND RELATED DISORDERS

Disorders of glycine and serine metabolism

Nonketotic hyperglycinemia type I	Glycine cleavage system P-protein, glycine dehydrogenase (decarboxylating)	9p22	1.4.4.2	238300
Nonketotic hyperglycinemia type II	Glycine cleavage system T-protein, aminomethyltransferase	3p21.2–21.1	2.1.2.10	238310
Nonketotic hyperglycinemia type III	Glycine cleavage system, H-protein		GCSH	238330
Deficiency of	3-Phosphoglycerate dehydrogenase		1.1.1.95	601815
Deficiency of	3-Phosphoserine phosphatase	7p15.2–p15.1	3.1.3.3	172480
Sarcosinemia	Sarcosine dehydrogenase	9q33–q34	1.5.99.1	268900 604455

Disorders of the metabolism of pterins and biogenic amines

BH$_4$ deficiency, dopa responsive dystonia	Guanosine-5-triphosphate cyclohydrolase	14q22.1–q22.2	3.5.4.16	128230 233910 600225
BH$_4$ deficiency	6-Pyruvoyltetrahydropterin synthase	11q22.3–q23.3	4.6.1.10	261640
Deficiency of	Sepiapterin reductase	2p14–p12	1.1.1.153	182125
Deficiency of	Dihydropteridinreductase	4p15.31	1.6.99.7	261630
Primapterinuria	Pterin-4-α-carbinolamine dehydratase	10q22	4.2.1.96	264070 126090
Deficiency of	Tyrosine hydroxylase	11p15.5	1.14.16.2	191290

(continued)

Table B.1. *Continued.*

Disease name	Enzyme/protein	Gene locus	EC number/protein	OMIM
Deficiency of	Aromatic amino acid decarboxylase	7p11	4.1.1.28	107930
Deficiency of	Dopamine beta hydroxylase	9q34	1.14.17.1	223360
Disorders of γ-aminobutyrate (GABA) metabolism				
4-Hydroxybutyric aciduria	Succinic semialdehyde dehydrogenase	6p22	1.2.1.16	271980
Deficiency of	GABA transaminase	16p13.3	2.6.1.19	137150
Pyridoxine-dependent convulsions	Glutamate decarboxylase	(2q31)	(4.1.1.15)	266100
Other neurometabolic disorders				
Deficiency of	Sulfite oxidase			272300
Creatine synthesis defect	Guanidinoacetate methyltransferase	19p13.3	2.1.1.2	601240
Canavan disease	Aspartoacylase, aminoacylase II	17pter-p13	3.5.1.15	271900
OTHER INBORN ERRORS OF METABOLISM				
Trimethylaminuria	Flavin containing monooxygenase type III	1q23–25	1.14.13.8	602079
Deficiency of	α-1-Antitrypsin	14q32.1	A1AT	107400

Sjögren–Larsson syndrome	Fatty aldehyde dehydrogenase	17p11.2	1.2.1.3 DAH4	270200
Deficiency of	Pancreatic lipase		3.1.1.3	246600
No disease known	Pancreatic colipase	6pter-p21.1	COL	120105
Deficiency of	Cytosolic acetoacetyl-CoA thiolase	6q25.3–q26		100678
X-linked recessive chondrodysplasia punctata	Arylsulfatase E	Xp22.3	3.1.6.- ARSE	302950 300180

The table provides a comprehensive list of inborn errors of metabolism, sorted according to disease groups under the same headings as those used in the introduction of this book. It contains the following information:

- The common name used for the disorder. The words "deficiency of" indicate that no special disease name exists and that *deficiency* after the enzyme or protein is commonly used for the disease (e.g., "biotinidase deficiency").
- The name of the deficient enzyme or protein.
- The chromosomal location of the gene involved in the disease.
- The EC number of the deficient enzyme and/or the abbreviation of the deficient protein.
- The *online mendelian inheritance in man* number of the disease and/or the respective protein or gene.

Additional information can be obtained either through the respective ExPASy or OMIM sites or through a search of GeneCards at the Weizmann Institute of Science, Israel (http://bioinfo.weizmann.ac.il/cards/) using the OMIM number, EC number, or protein abbreviation. For further information on enzyme nomenclature and a systematic collation of enzymes, see http://www.chem.qmw.ac.uk/iubmb/enzyme/.

Abbreviations; ATP, adenosine triphosphate; Autos.-rec., autosomal-recessive; BH, tetrahydrobiopterin; Chromos., chromosome; CLN, ceroid lipofuscinosis; HDL, high-density lipoprotein; IgD, immunoglobulin D; KGDH, 2-ketoglutate dehydrogenase; LCHAD, long-chain hydroxyacyl-CoA dehydrogenase; LDL, low-density lipoprotein; MELAS, mitochondrial encephalomyopathy, lactic acidemia, and strokelike episodes; MERRF, myoclonic epilepsy with ragged red fibers; NADH, nicotinamide adinine dinucleotide; NARP, neurodegeration, ataxia, and retinitis pigmentosa.

Appendix C ♣ General References

Blau N, Duran M, Gibson KM, Blaskovics ME, eds. *Physician's guide to the laboratory diagnosis of metabolic diseases,* 2nd ed. Heidelberg: Springer, 2002.

Detailed collation of clinical and laboratory findings in individual disorders. Helpful for the metabolic specialist and the clinician with experiences with metabolic disorders; less well-suited to clinicians who do not regularly see patients with inborn errors of metabolism.

Bremer HJ, Duran M, Kamerling JP, Przyrembel H, Wadman SK. *Disturbances of amino acid metabolism: clinical chemistry and diagnosis.* Munich: Urban & Schwarzenberg, 1981.

A unique, detailed source of information on amino acids and aminoacidopathies. Contains large tables of normal values in various body fluids. Somewhat outdated and unfortunately out-of-print but worth the effort to get second-hand.

Brock DJH. *Molecular genetics for the clinician.* Cambridge: Cambridge University Press, 1993.

A well-written, helpfully illustrated small text. It is aimed at the clinician rather than the molecular biologist.

Clarke JTR. *A clinical guide to inherited metabolic diseases.* Cambridge: Cambridge University Press, 1996.

Hands-on description of five symptom-based presentations of metabolic diseases (central nervous system, heart disease, liver disease, the acutely ill neonate, and storage disorders). Sketchy on practically relevant information for physicians.

Desnick RJ, ed. *Treatment of genetic diseases.* New York: Churchill Livingstone, 1991.

A multiauthor distillation of the Asilomar meeting. Has some things not found elsewhere.

Fernandes J, Saudubray JM, Van den Berghe G, eds. *Inborn metabolic diseases,* 3rd ed. Heidelberg: Springer, 2000.

Accessible textbook that covers all major groups of metabolic disorders and is particularly helpful for clinicians who seek basic information on diagnosis and treatment of individual defects. Individual chapters are written by various authors and are of variable quality.

McKusick VA. *Mendelian inheritance in man,* 12th ed. Baltimore: The John Hopkins University Press, 1998.

The standard compilation of genetic disorders in print form. The number allocated to entries in the MIM catalog is used in scientific publications worldwide for the exact identification of individual genetic disorders. The online version "OMIM" is more up-to-date and comprehensive. It is available free of charge on the Internet at http://www. ncbi.nlm.nih.gov/Omim.

Nyhan WL, Ozand PT. *Atlas of metabolic diseases.* London: Chapman & Hall, 1998.

Detailed monographs of a wide range of individual metabolic disorders with excellent photographs.

Rimoin DL, Connor JM, Pyeritz RE, eds. *Emery and Rimoin's principles and practice of medical genetics,* 3rd ed. New York: Churchill Livingstone, 1996.

An excellent, comprehensive, and up-to-date textbook of clinical genetics. Quite expensive. New edition in 2001.

Schinzel A, ed. *Catalogue of unbalanced chromosome aberrations in man.* Berlin: de Gruyter, 1984.

The metabolic specialist finds that having a source book on chromosomes is useful.

Scriver CR, Beaudet AL, Sly WS, Valle D, eds. *The metabolic and molecular bases of inherited diseases,* 7th ed. New York: McGraw-Hill, 1995.

The standard three-volume textbook on inherited disorders. Special emphasis on molecular and pathophysiological aspects of individual disorders. Limited use in the clinical setting as the little practical advice for the clinician can get lost in the wealth of information. A CD-ROM version is also available.

Seashore MR, Wappner RS. *Genetics in primary care & clinical medicine.* Stanford: Appleton & Lange, 1996.

A well-written, concise book that covers a wide range of genetic disorders, including a large number of inborn errors of metabolism. Excellent introduction to clinical genetics.

Zschocke J, Hoffmann GF. *Vademecum metabolicum: manual of metabolic puediatrics.* Stuttgart: Schattauer, 1999.

A concise pocket book containing the essentials of metabolic pediatrics, with short descriptions of most inborn errors of metabolism.

Appendix D ♣ Internet Resources

OMIM (*http://www.ncbi.nlm.nih.gov/omim*)

This is the online version of *Mendelian inheritance in man,* the oldest and most widely used collation of genetic disorders; it is edited by Victor A. McKusick. It is freely available from NCBI, the National Center for Biotechnology Information. The database contains monographs of individual disorders and genes with references and extensive links to other online resources. OMIM has an emphasis on molecular information, but plenty of clinical data that are useful in daily practice are also available. The number allocated to entries in the OMIM catalog is used in scientific publications worldwide for the exact identification of individual genetic disorders.

GENECLINICS (*http://www.geneclinics.org*)

This expert-written, peer-reviewed medical database contains short descriptions of genetic disorders, including information on diagnosis, treatment, and genetic testing for these conditions. The information is very useful, particularly for clinicians and genetic counselors; the number of disorders included is limited but increasing thus far.

THE RARE DISEASE DATABASE
(*http://www.rarediseases.org*)

This is one of the largest clinical databases, containing information on more than 1,000 rare disorders. It is maintained by the National Organization for Rare Disorders (NORD), a federation of voluntary health organizations; it is not free of charge.

RARE GENETIC DISEASES IN CHILDREN
(*http://mcrcr2.med.nyu.edu/murphp01*)

This internet site contains links to various sources of information on rare genetic diseases that affect children.

SOCIETY FOR THE STUDY OF INBORN ERRORS
OF METABOLISM (SSIEM)(*http://www.ssiem.org.uk/*)

The homepage of the SSIEM provides excellent links to various internet resources that deal with inborn errors of metabolism, including laboratory directories.

GENETESTS (*http://www.genetests.org*)

GeneTests is a predominantly North American list of laboratories that offer molecular tests for genetic disorders. It is funded by the National Library of Medicine of the National Institutes of Health and by the U.S. Maternal and Child Health Bureau of the Department of Health and Human Services. Access is free of charge, but it is password-protected. The listed laboratories are not independently verified. GeneTests, like most similar lists, is not fully comprehensive, and some diagnostic laboratories in the United States are not included.

EUROPEAN DIRECTORY OF DNA LABORATORIES
(http://www.eddnal.com)

This is the European equivalent to GeneTests; it provides data on genetic services and molecular genetic laboratories in Europe and links to national databases in Europe. It is funded by the EMQN initiative (European Molecular Genetics Quality Network). Access is free of charge; it is not password-protected.

ORPHANET *(http://orphanet.infobiogen.fr)*

This French database is aimed at both researchers and clinicians; it contains information on a large number of genetic and nongenetic conditions, as well as on diagnostic services in France. The information is available in both English and French.

GENOME DATABASE (GDB) *(http://www.gdb.org)*

The scientific database was established in 1990 as the official repository for genomic mapping data resulting from the Human Genome Initiative. It comprises descriptions of regions of the human genome, as well as genetic maps, and is linked to OMIM and other sequence databases. It is directed mainly at researchers.

GENECARDS *(http://bioinfo.weizmann.ac.il/cards)*

This is a concise, gene-oriented database that contains information on various functions of human genes, including the respective proteins and associated disorders. Copious links to other internet databases are included. GeneCards are particularly useful for geneticists and researchers in the areas of functional genomics and proteomics.

HUGO MUTATION DATABASE INITIATIVE
(http://ariel.ucs.unimelb.edu.au:80/~cotton/mdi.htm)

The mutation database initiative is part of the Human Genome Organization (HUGO) and is concerned with the registration of mutations in human genes. Its website provides links to various locus-specific databases that provide mutation data and other information on individual genes and disorders.

HUMAN GENE MUTATION DATABASE
(HGMD)*(http://www.uwcm.ac.uk/uwcm/mg/hgmd0.html)*

This database, based in Cardiff, Wales, on mutations that cause human disorders was originally established for the study of mutational mechanisms in human genes. The website also provides links to locus-specific databases and other sites that are relevant to mutation studies.

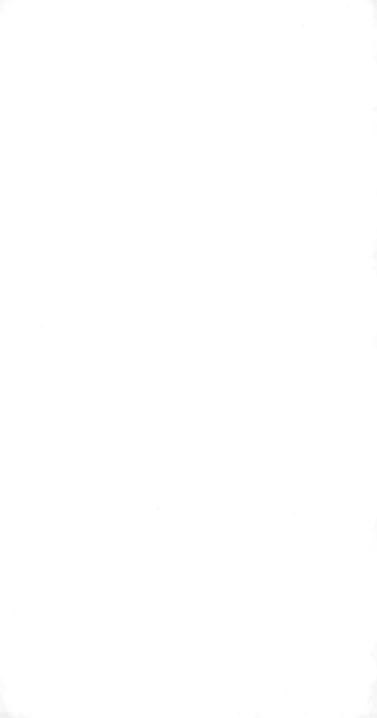

♣ Subject Index

Note: Page numbers followed by *f* indicate figures; those followed by *t* indicate tables.

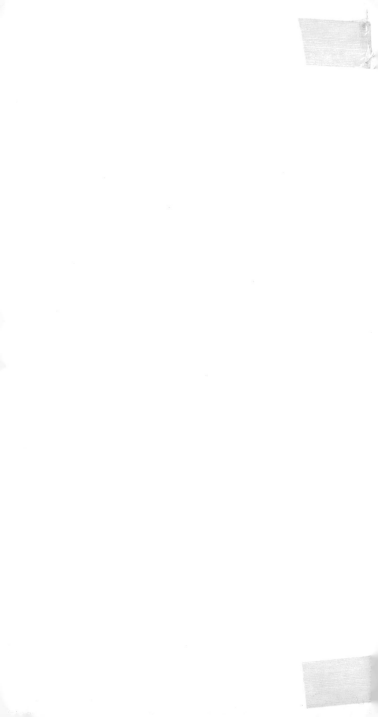